MW01156370

Human Parasitic Diseases
Sourcebook

Stephen A. Berger, MD

Director, Geographic Medicine
Tel Aviv Medical Center
Tel Aviv, Israel

John S. Marr, MD, MPH

Office of Epidemiology
Virginia Department of Health
Richmond, Virginia

Visiting Lecturer
Department of International and Public Health
School of Public Health
New York Medical College
Valhalla, New York

JONES AND BARTLETT PUBLISHERS
Sudbury, Massachusetts
BOSTON   TORONTO   LONDON   SINGAPORE

World Headquarters

Jones and Bartlett
Publishers
40 Tall Pine Drive
Sudbury, MA 01776
978-443-5000
info@jbpub.com
www.jbpub.com

Jones and Bartlett
Publishers Canada
6339 Ormindale Way
Mississauga, ON
L5V 1J2
Canada

Jones and Bartlett
Publishers International
Barb House, Barb Mews
London W6 7PA
United Kingdom

Jones and Bartlett's books and products are available through most bookstores and on-line booksellers. To contact Jones and Bartlett Publishers directly, call 800-832-0034, fax 978-443-8000, or visit our website www.jbpub.com.

Substantial discounts on bulk quantities of Jones and Bartlett's publications are available to corporations, professional associations, and other qualified organizations. For details and specific discount information, contact the special sales department at Jones and Bartlett via the above contact information or send an email to specialsales@jbpub.com.

Library of Congress Cataloging-in-Publication Data

Berger, Stephen A.
   Human parasitic diseases sourcebook / Stephen A. Berger, John S. Marr.
     p. ; cm.
   Includes bibliographical references and index.
   ISBN 0-7637-2962-0 (pbk. : alk. paper)
   1. Parasitic diseases—Handbooks, manuals, etc. 2. Medical parasitology—Handbooks, manuals, etc.   I. Marr, John S. II. Title.
   [DNLM: 1. Parasitic Diseases—diagnosis—Resource Guides.
2. Parasites—pathogenicity—Resource Guides. 3. Parasitic Diseases
—therapy—Resource Guides.   WC 39 B496h 2006]
RC119.B446 2006
616.9′6—dc22

2005019369

Production Credits
Publisher: Michael Brown
Production Director: Amy Rose
Associate Production Editor: Carolyn F. Rogers
Editorial Assistant: Kylah McNeill
Associate Marketing Manager: Marissa Hederson
Composition: Auburn Associates, Inc.
Cover Art: *Scolex*, Alexis Rockman
Cover Design: Kristin E. Ohlin
Text Design: Auburn Associates, Inc.
Printing and Binding: Malloy, Inc.
Cover Printing: Malloy, Inc.

Printed in the United States of America
09 08 07 06 05   10 9 8 7 6 5 4 3 2 1

CONTENTS

Parasites are listed from A-Z, with a letter to the right denoting the broad classification of each agent: (P = Protozoan, C = Cestode, T = Trematode, N = Nematode, A = Arthropod, O = Other). Annotated diagrams that outline the life cycles of all major parasites have been reproduced with permission from the Centers for Disease Control and Prevention web site: http://www.dpd.cdc.gov/dpdx/HTML/Frames/body_para_health.htm.

*TYPE: (P = Protozoan, C = Cestode, T = Trematode, N = Nematode, A = Arthropod, O = Other)

*TYPE: (P = Protozoan, C = Cestode, T = Trematode, N = Nematode, A = Arthropod, O = Other)

*TYPE: (P = Protozoan, C = Cestode, T = Trematode, N = Nematode, A = Arthropod, O = Other)

FOREWORD
Jay Keystone

As I write these words, 337 generic infectious diseases afflict humans worldwide. Ninety-three of these infections are due to parasites, and more than a third of these are caused by parasites that can be passed on to other humans. Current patterns of global travel and immigration virtually guarantee that physicians in industrialized countries will inevitably be confronted by patients presenting perplexing problems posed by parasites. During 2000, almost 700 million persons crossed at least one international border, many en route to a developing country where exotic parasites abound. In-migration from developing countries has increased dramatically over the past 20 years and increasingly brings people—and their parasites—in contact with healthcare professionals. With more outdoor recreational activities, other local, homegrown zoonoses might also present themselves to our healthcare systems. Beavers, the revered national symbols of Canada, are often responsible for the transmission of the well-known *Giardia lamblia*, one of the most common waterborne infections in North America. However, each year many North Americans acquire infection by lesser known parasites like *Toxocara canis, Diphyllobothrium latum,* and *Baylisascaris procyonis,* to name only a few emerging zoonoses. You will learn from this monograph that the term exotic is only a relative concept. Zoonotic parasitic infections are much more common than you might suspect, and likely to become even more common in the future.

Does the world need yet another textbook about parasites, and specifically, exotic parasites? No, the world needs a handbook, and this is it! Physicians, medical students, and residents, who often lack adequate knowledge of the subject, require an efficient way of formulating a useful, differential diagnosis for patients who have been exposed to a foreign environment, animals, foods, insects, etc. What better way to do this than to have all key information organized and summarized in a single handbook, virtually at one's fingertips?

Drs. Stephen Berger and John Marr have considerable expertise in the epidemiology, clinical presentation, diagnosis, and management of human parasitic infections. This book distills up-to-date epidemiological and parasitological information into a portable, inexpensive, and accurate compendium of the world's parasites that infect humans.

The authors have created an excellent, practical portrait of parasitology for the practitioner. This book offers easy access to relevant information and provides clinical "pearls," for students in training and health workers in the field. This useful handbook should easily find its way into the lab coats or study carousels of medical students and postgraduate trainees. I have been waiting for someone to write a useful and concise handbook on exotic human parasitic infections and I am pleased to see that Berger and Marr have taken up the challenge so successfully.

ACKNOWLEDGMENTS

The authors and the publisher would like to acknowledge the extraordinary contribution of Asim A. Jani, MD, MPH, FACP. This book could not have been written without his expert assistance. He brought fresh perspectives and keen insights in all aspects of the text and its preparation. His background in infectious diseases, clinical medicine, teaching, and public health practice enabled him to offer valuable advice and careful scrutiny to the project.

The authors would like to thank Chris Delcher for his masterful creation of parasite-specific mapping by country. All countries that have reported parasites in the recent past have been processed through GIS mapping and appear in clearly delineated regional maps created by Chris. Some might be surprised by seemingly odd disease distributions, but all country-specific reports have been verified in the literature. These lists are intended for the healthcare worker who suspects a parasite in a traveller or foreign visitor from a specific country. All maps will be updated as new reports are received.

The authors would also like to acknowledge the Centers for Disease Control and Prevention (CDC) for use of the pictorial and descriptive outlines of parasite life cycles. All life cycles have been obtained from the DPDx Laboratory Identification of Parasites of Public Health Concern website: http://www.dpd.cdc.gov/dpdx/HTML/Para_Health.htm.

Here, parasites of the intestinal tract, blood, and tissues are expertly and accurately displayed. It would have been a Herculean task to assemble and create new life cycles to essentially duplicate those already created by the CDC. Although we have removed the CDC signature logo from these figures in order to save some space and focus on the cycle itself, the readers should be aware that these were developed by the CDC. Though in the public domain, appreciation and proper acknowledgment should be given to their developers.

Chapter 1: Introduction

In biology, *parasite* is defined as an organism that obtains benefit from another, usually larger organism to which it usually causes injury. In medical practice a distinction is made between pathogenic viruses, bacteria and fungi (microbiology), and the protozoa, worms and arthropods that infect humans (parasitology). This book deals with all the common as well as lesser-known human protozoan, helminthic and arthropod infestations usually included within the rubric of parasitology.

Historically, humans acquired infectious diseases from their immediate environment. Millennia of nomadic slash and burn and hunter–gatherer existence exposed mankind to myriad parasites living in soil and on plant matter or within the tissues of land animals and fish. More intimate exposure to animal parasites occurred when animals were domesticated, farmed, and consumed without cooking. Peridomiciliary animals, such as rodents, were attracted to stored foods and inserted their own microbes and endo- and ectoparasites into human habitats. The rise of cities fostered the spread of microbes, including parasites, that could be transferred directly from human to human. Commerce (overland trade, shipping, and more recently, air travel), climate change, and war have also played a role in the dissemination of parasites. Today, globalization offers additional opportunities for once-exotic, niche parasites to appear and even establish themselves as cosmopolitan "strangers in a strange land" [Exodus 2: 21-22 (KJV)].

The field of parasitology largely fell out of medical favor as developed countries overcame their parasitic diseases, even as developing countries, mostly in tropical

1

climes, never escaped their parasitic burden. In recent years, air travel, commerce, destabilizing regional wars, and an appreciation of exotic cuisine have globalized virtually all human parasites.

The common, obvious, and well known parasites (viz. malaria, amebiasis, pinworm) are listed but not extensively addressed in this book since standard texts continue to give space to the major parasitic diseases. The *Human Parasitic Diseases Sourcebook* was created as a practical and portable book for healthcare workers and students who might encounter patients with parasitic disease. Every effort has been made to include lesser-known organisms which have been overlooked by standard texts—and some which are truly new, emerging parasites which have only recently been documented to infect humans.

The taxonomy used in this book has been coded to facilitate quick access and uniformity: Protozoa (P) are single-celled organisms; while most metazoan helminthic parasites are within the phylum *Annelida*, order *Helminthes*, families *Cestoda* (*C*—tapeworms), *Trematoda* (*T*—flukes), and *Nematoda* (*N*—round worms). Other groupings include *Arthropoda* (*A*—insects and arachnids) that invade tissue, as opposed to transient biters such as mosquitoes, flies, ticks, and bugs. A small number of other (O) parasites which are not subsumed under the preceding categories are also listed. An alphabetized index at the end of the text lists the names and conditions of all parasites included in the book, many of which have been subsumed under the simplified listing of major parasites.

Definitions

Vector: An arthropod or other living carrier that transports an infectious agent from an infected reservoir to a susceptible individual or immediate surroundings.

Vehicle: The mode of transmission for an infectious agent. This generally implies a passive and inanimate (ie, nonvector) mode.

Reservoir: Any animal, arthropod, plant, or substance in which an infectious agent normally lives and multiplies, on which it depends primarily for survival, and where it reproduces itself in such a manner that it can be transmitted to a susceptible host.

Diagnostic Clues
Modules have been created to assist in focusing on the differential diagnosis for defined clinical scenarios. These lists assume that a proper geographic distribution (especially considering those that can be worldwide), exposure history, physical examination, and laboratory data are available; and they arrange diseases in Chapter 2 according to parasites with **worldwide distribution** (page 5); **chief clinical complaint** (pages 6-15); presence of **hypereosinophilia** (pages 15-16); parasite **reservoirs** (pages 16-24); **vehicles** (pages 24-28); **vectors** (pages 28-29); and in Chapter 3 according to **clinical hints** (pages 31-49).

Treatment
Treatment is listed for each parasite. In addition, Chapter 6 examines the pharmacology and use of drugs. As of 2004, more than 55 generic drugs were marketed for the treatment of parasitic disease. These agents vary widely in therapeutic spectrum, dosage, toxicity, and effectiveness. The reader should note that many of the diseases in this text are self-limited, and few are directly contagious from one human to another. Thus, the need for treatment will often depend on the clinical features and severity of parasitism in the individual patient.

Chapter 2: Important Tables and Lists

Parasites with Worldwide Distribution (WWD)

Alariasis
Amoeba—free living
Anisakiasis
Ascariasis
Balantidiasis
Blastocystis hominis
   infection
Cercarial dermatitis
Cryptosporidiosis
Cutaneous larva migrans
Cyclospora infection
Cysticercosis
Demodex follicularum
Dientamoebal diarrhea
Diphyllobothriasis
Dipylidiasis
Dirofilariasis
Echinococcosis unilocular
Entamoebiasis—
   E. histolytica
Enterobiasis
Fascioliasis
Giardiasis
Gordian worms
Hirudinae infections

Hookworm (*A. duodenale*)
Hookworm
   (*N. americanus*)
Hymenolepis diminuta
   infection
Hymenolepis nana
   infection
Isosporiasis
Malaria
Microsporidiosis
Myiasis
Pediculosis
Pentastomiasis—
   Linguatula
Scabies
Schistosoma—avian species
Strongyloidiasis
Taeniasis (*T. saginata*)
Taeniasis (*T. solium*)
Toxocariasis
Toxoplasmosis
Trichinosis
Trichomoniasis
Trichuriasis

5

Parasites by Chief Clinical Complaint(s)

Hepatic Mass or Cyst

Amoebic abscess
Clonorchiasis
Fascioliasis
Echinococcosis—
    American polycystic

Echinococcosis—
    multilocular
Echinococcosis—
    unilocular
Opisthorchiasis

Biliary Disease

Amoebic abscess
Angiostrongyliasis—
    abdominal
Ascariasis
Clonorchiasis
Cryptosporidiosis
Cyclospora infection
Dicrocoeliasis
Diphyllobothriasis
Echinococcosis—
    American polycystic

Echinococcosis—
    multilocular
Echinococcosis—
    unilocular
Fascioliasis
Giardiasis
Isosporiasis
Microsporidiosis
Opisthorchiasis
Taeniasis
Trichostrongyliasis

Rectal or Anal Symptomatology

Amoebic colitis
Balantidiasis
Dipylidiasis
Enterobiasis
Schistosomiasis—
    intercalatum
Schistosomiasis—
    japonicum

Schistosomiasis—*mansoni*
Schistosomiasis—*mattheei*
Schistosomiasis—*mekongi*
Taeniasis
Trichuriasis

Meningitis or Meningismus

Amoeba—free living
Angiostrongyliasis
Baylisascariasis
Cysticercosis
Fascioliasis
Loiasis
Malaria
Paragonimiasis
Schistosomiasis—
    japonicum
Schistosomiasis—*mansoni*
Strongyloidiasis
Toxocariasis
Toxoplasmosis
Trichinosis
Trypanosomiasis—African
Trypanosomiasis—
    American

Lung Abscess, Mass, or Cyst

Amoebic abscess
Cysticercosis
Dirofilariasis
Echinococcosis—
    American polycystic
Echinococcosis—
    multilocular
Echinococcosis—
    unilocular
Fascioliasis
Gnathostomiasis
Paragonimiasis
Strongyloidiasis

Cerebral Mass or Cyst

Amoeba—free living
Amoebic abscess
Angiostrongyliasis
Coenurosis
Cysticercosis
Echinococcosis—
    unilocular
Fascioliasis
Gnathostomiasis
Paragonimiasis
Schistosomiasis—
    haematobium
Schistosomiasis—
    japonicum
Schistosomiasis—
    mansoni
Sparganosis
Toxoplasmosis

Uveitis or Retinitis

Alariasis
Amoeba—free living
Amoebic abscess
Angiostrongyliasis
Baylisascariasis
Coenurosis
Cysticercosis
Gnathostomiasis
Leishmaniasis—visceral

Loiasis
Onchocerciasis
Sparganosis
Thelaziasis
Toxocariasis
Toxoplasmosis
Trichinosis
Trypanosomiasis—African

Eye Worm or Ocular Mass

Alariasis
Amoeba—free living
Amoebic abscess
Angiostrongyliasis
Baylisascariasis
Coenurosis
Cysticercosis
Dirofilariasis
Echinococcosis—
    American polycystic
Fascioliasis

Gnathostomiasis
Loiasis
Mansonelliasis—
    M. perstans
Myiasis
Paragonimiasis
Pentastomiasis—
    Linguatula
Sparganosis
Thelaziasis
Toxocariasis

Splenomegaly or Splenic Lesion

Babesiosis
Capillariasis—
    extraintestinal
Fascioliasis
Leishmaniasis—visceral
Malaria

Schistosomiasis—
    haematobium
Schistosomiasis—
    intercalatum
Schistosomiasis—
    japonicum

Schistosomiasis—*mansoni*
Schistosomiasis—*mattheei*
Schistosomiasis—*mekongi*
Toxocariasis

Toxoplasmosis
Trypanosomiasis—African
Trypanosomiasis—
  American

Fever

Amoeba—free living
Amoebic abscess
Amoebic colitis
Angiostrongyliasis
Angiostrongyliasis—
  abdominal
Anisakiasis
Ascariasis
Babesiosis
Balantidiasis
Baylisascariasis
Capillariasis—
  extraintestinal
Capillariasis—intestinal
Clonorchiasis
Cryptosporidiosis
Cyclospora infection
Echinococcosis—
  unilocular
Fascioliasis
Filariasis—Bancroftian
Filariasis—*Brugia malayi*
Filariasis—*Brugia timori*
Giardiasis
Isosporiasis
Leishmaniasis—
  mucocutaneous
Leishmaniasis—visceral
Loiasis

Malaria
Mansonelliasis—
  M. ozzardi
Mansonelliasis—
  M. perstans
Mansonelliasis—
  M. streptocerca
Metorchiasis
Microsporidiosis
Oesophagostomiasis
Onchocerciasis
Opisthorchiasis
Paragonimiasis
Sarcocystosis
Schistosomiasis—
  haematobium
Schistosomiasis—
  intercalatum
Schistosomiasis—
  japonicum
Schistosomiasis—*mansoni*
Schistosomiasis—*mattheei*
Schistosomiasis—*mekongi*
Strongyloidiasis
Toxocariasis
Toxoplasmosis
Trichinosis
Trypanosomiasis—African
Trypanosomiasis—
  American

Jaundice

Amoebic abscess
Angiostrongyliasis—
  abdominal
Ascariasis
Babesiosis
Capillariasis—
  extraintestinal
Clonorchiasis
Dicrocoeliasis
Echinococcosis—
  American polycystic
Echinococcosis—
  multilocular
Echinococcosis—
  unilocular
Fascioliasis
Giardiasis
Leishmaniasis—visceral
Malaria
Microsporidiosis
Opisthorchiasis
Schistosomiasis—
  intercalatum
Schistosomiasis—
  japonicum
Schistosomiasis—*mansoni*
Schistosomiasis—*mattheei*
Schistosomiasis—*mekongi*
Toxoplasmosis
Trypanosomiasis—African

Diarrhea

Amoebic abscess
Amoebic colitis
Angiostrongyliasis—
  abdominal
Anisakiasis
Babesiosis
Balantidiasis
Bertielliasis
Blastocystis hominis
  infection
Capillariasis—intestinal
Clonorchiasis
Cryptosporidiosis
Cyclospora infection
Dientamoebal diarrhea
Dipylidiasis
Dracunculiasis
Echinostomiasis
Fascioliasis
Fasciolopsiasis
Gastrodiscoidiasis
Giardiasis
Heterophyid infections
Hymenolepis diminuta
  infection
Hymenolepis nana
  infection
Isosporiasis
Leishmaniasis—visceral
Malaria

Metagonimiasis
Metorchiasis
Microsporidiosis
Nanophyetiasis
Opisthorchiasis
Sarcocystosis
Schistosomiasis—*intercalatum*
Schistosomiasis—*japonicum*

Schistosomiasis—*mansoni*
Schistosomiasis—*mattheei*
Schistosomiasis—*mekongi*
Strongyloidiasis
Trichinosis
Trichostrongyliasis
Trichuriasis
Trypanosomiasis—American

Vomiting

Amoeba—free living
Amoebic abscess
Amoebic colitis
Angiostrongyliasis
Angiostrongyliasis—abdominal
Anisakiasis
Ascariasis
Babesiosis
Balantidiasis
Bertielliasis
Blastocystis hominis infection
Capillariasis—extraintestinal
Capillariasis—intestinal
Clonorchiasis
Coenurosis
Cryptosporidiosis
Cyclospora infection
Cysticercosis

Dicrocoeliasis
Dientamoebal diarrhea
Dracunculiasis
Echinococcosis—unilocular
Echinostomiasis
Fascioliasis
Fasciolopsiasis
Giardiasis
Gnathostomiasis
Heterophyid infections
Hymenolepis diminuta infection
Hymenolepis nana infection
Isosporiasis
Malaria
Metagonimiasis
Metorchiasis
Nanophyetiasis
Oesophagostomiasis

Opisthorchiasis
Pentastomiasis—*Armillifer*
Sarcocystosis
Schistosomiasis—
   intercalatum
Schistosomiasis—
   japonicum
Schistosomiasis—*mansoni*
Schistosomiasis—*mattheei*
Schistosomiasis—*mekongi*

Strongyloidiasis
Taeniasis
Toxoplasmosis
Trichinosis
Trichostrongyliasis
Trichuriasis
Trypanosomiasis—African
Trypanosomiasis—
   American

Hepatomegaly

Amoebic abscess
Angiostrongyliasis—
   abdominal
Ascariasis
Babesiosis
Baylisascariasis
Capillariasis—
   extraintestinal
Clonorchiasis
Echinococcosis—
   American polycystic
Echinococcosis—
   multilocular
Echinococcosis—
   unilocular
Fascioliasis
Leishmaniasis—visceral
Malaria

Mansonelliasis—
   M. ozzardi
Microsporidiosis
Opisthorchiasis
Schistosomiasis—
   intercalatum
Schistosomiasis—
   japonicum
Schistosomiasis—*mansoni*
Schistosomiasis—*mattheei*
Schistosomiasis—*mekongi*
Strongyloidiasis
Toxocariasis
Toxoplasmosis
Trypanosomiasis—African
Trypanosomiasis—
   American

Cough

Amoebic abscess
Anisakiasis
Ascariasis
Babesiosis
Balantidiasis
Capillariasis—
    extraintestinal
Cutaneous larva migrans
Dirofilariasis
Dracunculiasis
Echinococcosis—
    American polycystic
Echinococcosis—
    unilocular
Fascioliasis
Gnathostomiasis
Hookworm
Leishmaniasis visceral
Malaria
Mammomonogamiasis
Mansonelliasis—
    M. ozzardi

Metorchiasis
Microsporidiosis
Paragonimiasis
Pentastomiasis—
    Linguatula
Schistosomiasis—
    haematobium
Schistosomiasis—
    intercalatum
Schistosomiasis—
    japonicum
Schistosomiasis—*mansoni*
Schistosomiasis—*mekongi*
Strongyloidiasis
Taeniasis
Toxocariasis
Toxoplasmosis
Trichinosis
Trypanosomiasis—
    American

Skin or Subcutaneous Lesions

Alariasis
Amoeba—free living
Amoebic abscess
Baylisascariasis
Capillariasis—
    extraintestinal
Cercarial dermatitis
Cheyletiella

Cutaneous larva migrans
Dioctophyme renalis
    infection
Dracunculiasis
Fascioliasis
Gnathostomiasis
Hookworm
Leishmaniasis—cutaneous

Leishmaniasis—
   mucocutaneous
Leishmaniasis—visceral
Loiasis
Malaria
Mansonelliasis—
   M. ozzardi
Mansonelliasis—
   M. perstans
Mansonelliasis—
   M. streptocerca
Metorchiasis
Myiasis
Onchocerciasis
Pediculosis
Scabies
Schistosomiasis—
   haematobium

Schistosomiasis—
   intercalatum
Schistosomiasis—
   japonicum
Schistosomiasis—*mansoni*
Schistosomiasis—*mattheei*
Schistosomiasis—*mekongi*
Sparganosis
Strongyloidiasis
Taeniasis
Toxocariasis
Toxoplasmosis
Trichinosis
Trypanosomiasis—African
Trypanosomiasis—
   American
Tungiasis

Lymphadenopathy

Capillariasis—
   extraintestinal
Dracunculiasis
Fascioliasis
Filariasis—Bancroftian
Filariasis—*Brugia malayi*
Filariasis—*Brugia timori*
Leishmaniasis—cutaneous
Leishmaniasis—
   mucocutaneous
Leishmaniasis—visceral
Loiasis

Mansonelliasis—
   M. ozzardi
Mansonelliasis—
   M. streptocerca
Myiasis
Onchocerciasis
Opisthorchiasis
Scabies
Schistosomiasis—
   intercalatum
Schistosomiasis—
   japonicum

Schistosomiasis—*mansoni*
Schistosomiasis—*mattheei*
Schistosomiasis—*mekongi*
Toxoplasmosis
Trypanosomiasis—African
Trypanosomiasis—American

Headache

Amoeba—free living
Amoebic abscess
Angiostrongyliasis
Babesiosis
Balantidiasis
Baylisascariasis
Coenurosis
Cysticercosis
Echinococcosis—unilocular
Fascioliasis
Filariasis—Bancroftian
Filariasis—*Brugia malayi*
Gnathostomiasis
Hymenolepis nana infection
Isosporiasis
Loiasis
Malaria
Mansonelliasis—*M. ozzardi*
Mansonelliasis—*M. perstans*
Metorchiasis
Microsporidiosis
Paragonimiasis
Schistosomiasis—*japonicum*
Strongyloidiasis
Toxocariasis
Toxoplasmosis
Trichinosis
Trypanosomiasis—African
Trypanosomiasis—American

Parasites Inducing Hypereosinophilia*

Angiostrongyliasis—abdominal
Anisakiasis
Ascariasis
Baylisascariasis
Clonorchiasis
Fascioliasis
Filariasis—Bancroftian
Filariasis—*Brugia malayi*
Filariasis—*Brugia timori*
Gnathostomiasis
Hookworm

---

*≥3,000 eosinophiles per cu mm.

Loiasis
Metorchiasis
Onchocerciasis
Opisthorchiasis
Paragonimiasis
Schistosomiasis—
    haematobium
Schistosomiasis—
    intercalatum

Schistosomiasis—
    japonicum
Schistosomiasis—*mansoni*
Schistosomiasis—*mattheei*
Schistosomiasis—*mekongi*
Strongyloidiasis
Toxocariasis
Trichinosis

Reservoirs

Amphibian or Reptile

Alariasis
Angiostrongyliasis
Echinostomiasis

Gnathostomiasis
Pentastomiasis—*Armillifer*
Sparganosis

Ant

Dicrocoeliasis

Bird

Baylisascariasis
Cercarial dermatitis
Echinostomiasis

Microsporidiosis
Sparganosis
Toxoplasmosis

Cat

Baylisascariasis
Clonorchiasis
Cryptosporidiosis
Cutaneous larva migrans
Dipylidiasis
Dirofilariasis
Echinococcosis—
   multilocular
Echinococcosis—
   American polycystic
Echinostomiasis
Filariasis—*Brugia malayi*
Gnathostomiasis
Leishmaniasis—cutaneous
Metagonimiasis
Metorchiasis
Opisthorchiasis
Schistosomiasis—
   japonicum
Schistosomiasis—*mansoni*
Strongyloidiasis
Taenia crassiceps
Taenia taeniaebormis
Thelaziasis
Toxocariasis
Toxoplasmosis
Trichinosis
Trypanosomiasis—
   American

Carnivore—Wild

Alariasis
Ancylostoma caninum
Brugia—*zoonotic*
Coenurosis
Dioctophyme renalis
   infection
Diphyllobothriasis
Dirofilariasis
Echinococcosis—
   American polycystic
Echinococcosis—
   multilocular
Echinococcosis—
   unilocular
Filariasis—*Brugia malayi*
Gongylonemiasis
Leishmaniasis—cutaneous
Leishmaniasis—visceral
Metorchiasis
Microsporidiosis
Opisthorchiasis
Paragonimiasis
Taenia crassiceps
Trichinosis
Trypanosomiasis—African
Trypanosomiasis—
   American

Cattle

Babesiosis
Baylisascariasis
Cryptosporidiosis
Cutaneous larva migrans
Fascioliasis
Gongylonemiasis
Mammomonogamiasis
Pelodera strongyloides
Sarcocystosis

Schistosomiasis—*japonicum*
Schistosomiasis—*mansoni*
Schistosomiasis—*mattheei*
Taeniasis
Toxoplasmosis
Trichostrongyliasis
Trypanosomiasis—African

Copepod

Dracunculus medinensis

Deer

Babesiosis
Gongylonemiasis
Taeniasis
Thelaziasis

Dog

Ancylostoma caninum
Baylisascariasis
Clonorchiasis
Coenurosis
Cutaneous larva migrans
Diphyllobothriasis
Dipylidiasis
Dirofilariasis
Echinococcosis—American polycystic
Echinococcosis—multilocular

Echinococcosis—unilocular
Echinostomiasis
Fasciolopsiasis
Gnathostomiasis
Leishmaniasis—cutaneous
Leishmaniasis—visceral
Metagonimiasis
Metorchiasis
Microsporidiosis
Pelodera strongyloides

Opisthorchiasis
Paragonimiasis
Schistosomiasis—
    japonicum
Schistosomiasis—*mansoni*
Schistosomiasis—*mekongi*
Strongyloidiasis

Thelaziasis
Toxocariasis
Trichinosis
Trypanosomiasis—
    American
Tungiasis

Fish

Anisakiasis
Capillariasis—intestinal
Clonorchiasis
Gnathostomiasis
Heterophyid infections

Metagonimiasis
Metorchiasis
Microsporidiosis
Nanophyetiasis

Goat

Cryptosporidiosis
Echinococcosis—
    unilocular
Pentastomiasis—
    Linguatula

Schistosomiasis—*mattheei*
Toxoplasmosis
Trichostrongyliasis

Horse

Coenurosis
Echinococcosis—
    unilocular
Pelodera strongyloides

Schistosomiasis—
    japonicum
Schistosomiasis—*mattheei*

Human

Amebiasis
Ascariasis
Blastocystis hominis
  infection
Clonorchiasis
Cryptosporidiosis
Cyclospora infection
Cysticercosis
Dientamoebal diarrhea
Dioctophyme renalis
  infection
Diphyllobothriasis
Dracunculiasis
Echinostomiasis
Enterobiasis
Fasciolopsiasis
Filariasis—Bancroftian
Filariasis—*Brugia malayi*
Filariasis—*Brugia timori*
Giardiasis
Hookworm
Hymenolepis nana
  infection

Isosporiasis
Leishmaniasis—cutaneous
Leishmaniasis—
  mucocutaneous
Leishmaniasis—visceral
Loiasis
Malaria
Mansonelliasis—
  M. ozzardi
Mansonelliasis—
  M. perstans
Microsporidiosis
Onchocerciasis
Pediculosis
Scabies
Strongyloidiasis
Trichomoniasis
Trichuriasis
Trypanosomiasis—African
Trypanosomiasis—
  American

Mammal—Any

Alariasis
Angiostrongyliasis
Angiostrongyliasis—
  abdominal
Anisakiasis
Babesiosis
Balantidiasis

Baylisascariasis
Bertielliasis
Capillariasis—hepatic
Clonorchiasis
Coenurosis
Cryptosporidiosis
Cutaneous larva migrans
Cyclospora infection

Cysticercosis
Dicrocoeliasis
Dioctophyme renalis
  infection
Diphyllobothriasis
Dipylidiasis
Dirofilariasis
Echinococcosis—
  American polycystic
Echinococcosis—
  multilocular
Echinococcosis—
  unilocular
Echinostomiasis
Entamoeba polecki
  infection
Fascioliasis
Fasciolopsiasis
Filariasis—*Brugia malayi*
Gastrodiscoidiasis
Giardiasis
Gnathostomiasis
Gongylonemiasis
Hymenolepis diminuta
  infection
Hymenolepis nana
  infection
Leishmaniasis—cutaneous
Leishmaniasis—
  mucocutaneous
Leishmaniasis—visceral
Mammomonogamiasis
Mansonelliasis—
  M. streptocerca

Metagonimiasis
Metorchiasis
Microsporidiosis
Moniliformis moniliformis
Myiasis
Oesophagostomiasis
Opisthorchiasis
Paragonimiasis
Pentastomiasis—
  Armillifer
Pentastomiasis—
  Linguatula
Sarcocystosis
Schistosomiasis—
  haematobium
Schistosomiasis—
  japonicum
Schistosomiasis—*mansoni*
Schistosomiasis—*mattheei*
Schistosomiasis—*mekongi*
Strongyloidiasis
Taeniasis
Thelaziasis
Toxocariasis
Toxoplasmosis
Trichinosis
Trichostrongyliasis
Trypanosomiasis—
  African
Trypanosomiasis—
  American
Tungiasis

Marine Mammal

Anisakiasis
Trichinosis

Marsupial

Cryptosporidiosis
Leishmaniasis—cutaneous
Leishmaniasis—
   mucocutaneous

Toxoplasmosis
Trypanosomiasis—
   American

Pig

Balantidiasis
Clonorchiasis
Cysticercosis
Echinococcosis—
   unilocular
Entamoeba polecki
   infection
Fasciolopsiasis
Gastrodiscoidiasis
Gongylonemiasis
Paragonimiasis

Sarcocystosis
Schistosomiasis—
   japonicum
Schistosomiasis—*mansoni*
Taenia solium
Taenia asiatica
Toxoplasmosis
Trichinosis
Trypanosomiasis—
   American
Tungiasis

Primate—Nonhuman

Balantidiasis
Baylisascariasis
Bertielliasis
Cyclospora infection
Entamoeba polecki
   infection
Filariasis—*Brugia malayi*
Gongylonemiasis
Mansonelliasis—
   M. streptocerca

Microsporidiosis
Oesophagostomiasis
Ternidens diminutus
Schistosomiasis—
   haematobium
Schistosomiasis—*mansoni*
Strongyloidiasis

Rabbit or Hare

Babesiosis
Baylisascariasis
Microsporidiosis

Taenia serialis
Thelaziasis

Rodent

Angiostrongyliasis
Angiostrongyliasis—
    abdominal
Babesiosis
Balantidiasis
Baylisascariasis
Brugia—zoonotic
Capillariasis—hepatic
Cryptosporidiosis
Echinococcosis—
    American polycystic
Echinococcosis—
    multilocular
Echinostomiasis
Hymenolepis diminuta
    infection
Hymenolepis nana
    infection

Leishmaniasis—cutaneous
Leishmaniasis—
    mucocutaneous
Leishmaniasis—visceral
Microsporidiosis
Moniliformis moniliformis
Pelodera strongyloides
Pentastomiasis—*Armillifer*
Raillietina celebensis
Schistosomiasis—
    japonicum
Schistosomiasis—*mansoni*
Taenia serialis
Toxocariasis
Toxoplasmosis
Trichinosis
Trypanosomiasis—
    American

Sheep

Coenurosis
Dicrocoeliasis
Echinococcosis—
    unilocular
Fascioliasis
Pelodera strongyloides

Pentastomiasis—
    Linguatula
Schistosomiasis—*mattheei*
Toxoplasmosis
Trichostrongyliasis

Shellfish

Angiostrongyliasis
Anisakiasis
Paragonimiasis

Snail or Slug

Angiostrongyliasis—
  abdominal
Cercarial dermatitis
Clonorchiasis
Dicrocoeliasis
Echinostomiasis
Fascioliasis
Fasciolopsiasis
Gastrodiscoidiasis
Heterophyid infections
Metagonimiasis
Metorchiasis

Nanophyetiasis
Opisthorchiasis
Paragonimiasis
Schistosomiasis—
  haematobium
Schistosomiasis—
  intercalatum
Schistosomiasis—
  japonicum
Schistosomiasis—*mansoni*
Schistosomiasis—*mattheei*
Schistosomiasis—*mekongi*

Tick

Babesiosis

Vehicles

Ingested Reptile or Amphibian

Alariasis
Echinostomiasis
Gnathostomiasis

Mesocestoides
Pentastomiasis—*Armillifer*
Sparganosis

Ingested Insect, Mite, or Copepod

Acanthocephalaiasis
Bertielliasis
Dicrocoeliasis
Dipylidiasis
Dracunculiasis

Gongylonemiasis
Gordian worms
Hymenolepis diminuta
 infection

Fecal Matter

Amebiasis
Balantidiasis
Baylisascariasis
Blastocystis hominis
 infection
Cryptosporidiosis
Cysticercosis
Dientamoebal diarrhea

Entamoeba polecki
 infection
Enterobiasis
Giardiasis
Hymenolepis nana
 infection
Isosporiasis
Microsporidiosis

Fish

Anisakiasis
Capillariasis—intestinal
Clonorchiasis
Dioctophyme renalis
 infection
Diphyllobothriasis

Echinostomiasis
Gnathostomiasis
Heterophyid infections
Metorchiasis
Nanophyetiasis
Opisthorchiasis

Food—Any

Amebiasis
Angiostrongyliasis
Angiostrongyliasis—
 abdominal
Anisakiasis
Ascariasis

Balantidiasis
Bertielliasis
Blastocystis hominis
 infection
Capillariasis—hepatic
Capillariasis—intestinal

Clonorchiasis
Coenurosis
Dioctophyme renalis
  infection
Diphyllobothriasis
Echinostomiasis
Entamoeba polecki
  infection
Fascioliasis
Fasciolopsiasis
Gastrodiscoidiasis
Giardiasis
Gnathostomiasis
Heterophyid infections
Hymenolepis nana
  infection
Isosporiasis
Mammomonogamiasis

Mesocestoides
Metorchiasis
Microsporidiosis
Nanophyetiasis
Oesophagostomiasis
Opisthorchiasis
Paragonimiasis
Pentastomiasis—*Armillifer*
Pentastomiasis—
  Linguatula
Sarcocystosis
Sparganosis
Taeniasis
Toxocariasis
Toxoplasmosis
Trichinosis
Trichostrongyliasis
Trichuriasis

Meat

Gnathostomiasis
Mesocestoides
Pentastomiasis—
  Linguatula
Sarcocystosis

Sparganosis
Taeniasis
Taenia asiatica
Toxoplasmosis
Trichinosis

Shellfish

Angiostrongyliasis
Anisakiasis
Clonorchiasis

Cryptosporidiosis
Echinostomiasis
Paragonimiasis

Snail or Slug

Angiostrongyliasis
Angiostrongyliasis—abdominal
Echinostomiasis

Soil or Plant Matter

Baylisascariasis
Capillariasis—hepatic
Coenurosis
Cutaneous larva migrans
Cysticercosis
Echinococcosis—
    American polycystic
Echinococcosis—
    multilocular
Echinococcosis—
    unilocular

Hookworm
Micronemiasis
Oesophagostomiasis
Strongyloidiasis
Toxocariasis
Toxoplasmosis
Trichostrongyliasis
Trichuriasis
Tungiasis

Vegetables

Amebiasis
Angiostrongyliasis
Ascariasis
Cyclospora infection
Echinostomiasis
Fascioliasis
Fasciolopsiasis

Gastrodiscoidiasis
Giardiasis
Mammomonogamiasis
Pentastomiasis—*Armillifer*
Toxocariasis
Trichostrongyliasis
Trichuriasis

Water

Amoeba—free living
Amebiasis
Balantidiasis
Capillariasis—hepatic

Cercarial dermatitis
Coenurosis
Cryptosporidiosis
Cyclospora infection

Dracunculiasis
Echinostomiasis
Fascioliasis
Giardiasis
Hirudinae infections
Hymenolepis nana
   infection
Mammomonogamiasis
Oesophagostomiasis
Pentastomiasis—*Armillifer*
Sarcocystosis
Schistosomiasis—
   haematobium
Schistosomiasis—
   intercalatum
Schistosomiasis—
   japonicum
Schistosomiasis—*mansoni*
Schistosomiasis—*mattheei*
Schistosomiasis—*mekongi*
Sparganosis
Toxoplasmosis
Trichostrongyliasis

Vectors

Arthropods (insects and ticks) may mechanically transmit parasites to humans by their bites without being infected themselves. Mechanical transmission (M) implies transfer of the organism from one place to another. Biological transmission (B) implies that the organism has multiplied within the arthropod, and might or might not have caused illness in the vector. See Table 2-1.

Table 2-1   Vector Transmission

FLY

Amebiasis	M	*Musca domestica*
Leishmaniasis	B	*Phlebotomus/Lutzomyia* sp.
Loiasis	B	*Chrysops* spp.
Mansonelliasis	B	*Simulium* spp.
Onchocerciasis	B	*Simulim* spp.
Thelaziasis	B	*Musca/Fannia* sp.
Trypanosomiasis	B	*Glossina* sp.

GNAT/MIDGE

Mansonelliasis	B	Various genera

MOSQUITO

Dirofilariasis	B	Various genera
Filariasis	B	Various genera
Malaria	B	*Anopheles* sp.

TICK

Babesiosis	B	*Ixodes* spp.

BUG

American trypanosomiasis	B	Reduviid genera

Chapter 3: Clinical Hints*

PARASITE	CLINICAL HINT
Alariasis	Unilateral decreased vision due to neuroretinitis with pigmentary tracks. History of frog leg ingestion.
Amebiasis—free living	Severe, rapidly progressing meningoencephalitis (*Naegleria, Acanthamoeba* or *Balamuthia*) following swimming or diving in fresh water; or keratitis (*Acanthamoeba*), often following use of contaminated solutions to clean contact lenses.
Angiostrongy-liasis—*A. cantonensis*	Eosinophilic meningitis or encephalitis—generally self-limited; absent or low-grade fever; cranial nerve involvement (II, VI, V, and VII). Follows ingestion of slugs, snails, prawns or frogs.
Angiostrongyliasis—*A. costaricensis*	Mimics acute appendicitis, including presence of a right lower quadrant mass. Eosinophilia (uncommon in appendicitis) is prominent. Patient might recall recent ingestion of slugs or vegetation contaminated by slugs.

(continues)

*Modified from GIDEON—www.GideonOnline.com.

31

PARASITE	CLINICAL HINT
Anisakiasis	Allergic reactions or acute and chronic abdominal pain, often with peritoneal signs or hematemesis. Follows ingestion of undercooked fish (eg, sushi), squid, or octopus.
***Armillifer* infection**	Intestinal obstruction, pneumonia, and jaundice—related to mechanical obstruction by parasite; crescentic intraabdominal or intrathoracic calcifications on x-ray of chest or abdomen.
Ascariasis	An acute illness characterized by cough, wheezing, and eosinophilia; adult worms are associated with abdominal pain (occasionally obstruction) and pancreatic or biliary disease. Highest rates among children and in areas of crowding and poor sanitation.
Babesiosis	Fever, rigors, myalgia, hepatomegaly, and hemolysis. Might relapse repeatedly. Mimics malaria. Severe disease among asplenic patients—jaundice, renal failure, and death. European (*Babesia divergens*) invariably in splenectomized patients and usually fatal.
Balamuthia mandrillaris	Fulminant meningoencephalitis; rarely skin abscesses. Most patients have been immune competent.

Balantidiasis
Dysentery, often with vomiting. Mimics intestinal amebiasis. The disease is most common in pig-raising areas. Symptoms last for 1 to 4 weeks and might recur.

Baylisascariasis
Ocular, visceral, or neural larva migrans; eosinophilic meningitis; ocular disease characterized as diffuse unilateral subacute neuroretinitis (DUSN). Asymptomatic infection reported.

Bertiellosis
Abdominal pain, vomiting, diarrhea, or constipation following contact with primates.

Blastocystosis—*B. hominis*
Diarrhea and flatulence; usually no fever; illness similar to giardiasis. Increased risk among immune-suppressed patients. The exact role of this organism in disease is controversial.

Capillariasis—extraintestinal
Three infecting species produce bronchitis or pneumonia; acral pruritic rash; or tender hepatomegaly, abdominal distention, eosinophilia, and fever.

Capillariasis—hepatic
Tender hepatomegaly with hepatic dysfunction, abdominal distention, and eosinophilia. Splenomegaly and pneumonia have been reported.

(continues)

PARASITE	CLINICAL HINT
Capillariasis— intestinal	Diarrhea, weight loss, vomiting, and eosinophilia after ingestion of raw fresh-water fish. Malabsorption and wasting illness might follow. Case-fatality rates of 10 to 20% have been described.
Cercarial dermatitis	Pruritus, papules, vesicles (most commonly on legs) appearing one or more hours after swimming in fresh or salt water; lesions evolve and persist for 1 to 10 days.
Cheylettiella	Common mite of dogs, cats, and rabbits. Humans can acquire infection through close contact. Intensely pruritis macular, vesicular or bullous eruptions, but unlike scabies, dermal burrows not seen.
Clonorchiasis	Biliary symptomatology (obstruction or cholangitis) and eosinophilia beginning weeks to months after ingestion of raw fish. High association with cholangiocarcinoma.
Coenurosis	Mass in brain, eye, muscle, or subcutaneous tissue. Might present months to years after exposure in sheep-raising areas. Basilar arachnoiditis with internal hydrocephalus is common.

Cryptosporidiosis	Watery diarrhea, vomiting, abdominal pain. Although self-limited in healthy subjects, this is a chronic and wasting illness and can be associated with pulmonary disease among immunosuppressed (eg, AIDS) patients.
Cutaneous larva migrans	Erythematous, serpiginous, pruritic advancing lesion(s) or bullae—usually on the feet. Follows contact with moist sand or beachfront. Might recur or persist for months.
Cyclosporosis— *C. cayetanis*	Watery diarrhea (average six stools daily), abdominal pain, nausea, anorexia, and fatigue lasting up to 6 weeks (longer in AIDS patients). Most cases follow ingestion of contaminated water in underdeveloped countries.
Cysticercosis	Cerebral, ocular, or subcutaneous mass; usually no eosinophilia; calcifications noted on x-ray examination. Patient lives in area where pork is eaten. Concurrent *Taenia* infestation in 25 to 50% of patients.
Demodicosis	Unexplained onset of rosacea-like lesions on the face; eyelash loss; blepharitis; acne in older age groups. Facial lesions in dog owners, trainers.
Dicrocoeliasis	Abdominal pain, often accompanied by eosinophilia. Follows inadvertent ingestion of ants (with raw vegetables or fruit) in sheep-raising areas.

(continues)

35

PARASITE	CLINICAL HINT
Dientamoebiasis	Abdominal pain with watery or mucous diarrhea; eosinophilia might be present. Infestation can persist for more than 1 year.
Dioctophymiasis— D. renalis	Flank pain and hematuria beginning 3 to 6 months after eating raw fish or frog flesh. Subcutaneous infection has also been described.
Diplogonoriasis	As for *D latum*.
Dipylidiasis	Diarrhea, abdominal distention, and restlessness (in children); eosinophilia might be observed; proglottids might migrate out of anus.
Dirofilariasis	Most patients are asymptomatic; occasional instances of cough and chest pain, with solitary pulmonary coin lesion or multiple tender subcutaneous nodules; eosinophilia usually not present.
Drancontiasis— D. medinesis	Nausea and urticaria followed by the appearance of a papule or bulla (usually on the lower leg) which ruptures; calcified worm on x-ray; occasional eosinophilia. Worm can survive for 18 months in humans.
Dyphyllobothriasis— D. latum	Abdominal pain, diarrhea, and flatulence; vitamin B_{12} deficiency is noted in 0.02% of patients. Rare instances of intestinal obstruction have been described. Worm can survive for decades in human intestine.

Echinococcosis— *E. granulosis*	Calcified hepatic cyst or mass lesions in lungs and other organs; brain and lung involvement are common in pediatric cases.
Echinococcosis— *E. multilocularis*	Right upper quadrant pain and hepatic mass appearing years after acquisition in endemic area; jaundice might be present.
Echinostomiasis	Diarrhea and abdominal pain beginning approximately one month after eating raw mollusks or fish; eosinophilia might be present.
Encephalitozoon cuniculi	Should be included in the differential diagnosis for multisystem infection occurring in an immunosuppressed patient (eg, AIDS).
Entamoebiasis— *E. histolytica*	Abscess: Fever, local pain, weight loss. Liver abscess can be bacterial or amoebic—latter most often single and in right hepatic lobe. Colitis: Dysentery, abdominal pain, tenesmus—without hyperemia of rectal mucosa or fecal pus (ie, unlike shigellosis); liver abscess and dysentery rarely coexist in a given patient.
Entamoebiasis— *E. polecki*	Mucoid diarrhea and abdominal pain. Severe disease is unusual and should suggest another etiology.
Enterobiasis— *E. vermicularis*	Nocturnal anal pruritus; occasionally vaginitis or abdominal pain; eosinophilia is rarely, if ever, encountered.

(continues)

37

38

PARASITE	CLINICAL HINT
Fascioliasis	Fever, hepatomegaly, cholangitis, jaundice, and eosinophilia; urticaria occasionally observed during the acute illness. Parasite can survive more than 10 years in the biliary tract.
Fasciolopsiasis	Epigastric pain, diarrhea, nausea, and eosinophilia. Associated with ingestion of water chestnuts or other fresh water plants. Parasite can survive for 1 year in the human host.
Filariasis— *B. malayi*	Lymphangitis, lymphadenitis, eosinophilia, fever, and progressive lower extremity edema—usually spares the knee and elbow.
Filariasis— *Brugia* other	Painful regional lymphadenopathy of the neck, groin, or axilla, occasionally with eosinophilia.
Filariasis— *B. timori*	Recurrent lymphangitis, fever, and eosinophilia, late elephantiasis. The lymphangitis might follow a characteristic descending pattern.
Filariasis— *W. bancrofti*	Lymphangitis, lymphadenitis, eosinophilia, epididymitis, orchitis, and progressive edema. Episodes of fever and lymphangitis can recur over several years. Chyluria occasionally encountered.

Gastrodis-coidiasis	Diarrhea. Might be a history of ingesting raw water plants.
Giardiasis— *G. lamblia*	Foul-smelling, bulky diarrhea, nausea, and flatulence. Might wax and wane. Weight loss and low-grade fever are common.
Gnathostomiasis	Migratory nodules of skin, soft tissues, brain or eye; eosinophilia. Follows ingestion of raw meat, poultry, fish, or frog. Parasite can survive for more than 10 years in human tissue.
Gongylonemiasis	Protracted discomfort or sensation of movement in the buccal, oral, or gingival areas associated with a sensation of a foreign body.
Gordian worms	Passage of a 10- to 50-cm worm several days following inadvertent ingestion of insect or contaminated water.
Heterophyidiasis	Abdominal pain and mucous diarrhea with eosinophilia beginning 1 to 2 weeks after ingesting undercooked fish. Infestation resolves spontaneously within two months.
***Hirudinae* infections**	Overt, painless infestation by leeches following contact with fresh water. Secondary infection is rare.

(continues)

PARASITE	CLINICAL HINT
Hookworm— *N. americanus*	Pruritic papules (usually of feet); later cough and wheezing; abdominal pain and progressive iron-deficiency anemia; eosinophilia common; dyspnea and peripheral edema in heavy infections; *Ancylostoma caninum* implicated in eosinophilic enteritis.
Hookworm— *A. duodenale*	Pruritic papules (usually of feet); later cough and wheezing; abdominal pain and progressive iron-deficiency anemia; eosinophilia common; dyspnea and peripheral edema in heavy infections; *Ancylostoma caninum* implicated in eosinophilic enteritis.
Hymenolepisiasis— *H. diminuta*	Nausea, abdominal pain, and diarrhea; eosinophilia might be present. Primarily a pediatric disease in rodent-infested areas. Infestation resolves spontaneously within 2 months.
Hymenolepisiasis— *H. nana*	Nausea, abdominal pain, diarrhea, irritability, and weight loss; eosinophilia might be present. Infection is maintained by autoinfection (worm reproduces within the intestinal lumen).
Isosporiasis— *I. belli*	Myalgia, watery diarrhea, nausea, and leukocytosis; eosinophilia might be present. Prolonged and severe in AIDS patients.

Lagochilascariasis	Tender subcutaneous mass (usually limited to scalp and neck, occasionally pharynx or paranasal sinuses) with suppuration and fistulae; eosinophilia might be present.
Leishmaniasis— cutaneous (*Leishmania tropica*, et al); mucocutaneous (*Leishmania braziliensis*, et al)	Cutaneous: Chronic, ulcerating skin nodule, painless (*Leishmania tropica*) or painful (*L. major*); diffuse infection or regional lymphadenopathy occasionally encountered. Mucocutaneous: Skin ulceration or nasopharyngitis associated with purulent, mucoid exudates. The process could extend to underlying soft tissues. Metastatic lesions often involve the palate and pharynx.
Leishmaniasis— visceral	Chronic fever, weight loss, diaphoresis, hepatosplenomegaly, lymphadenopathy, and pancytopenia; grey pigmentation (kala-azar = black disease) might appear late in severe illness. Case-fatality rate = 5 (treated) to 90% (untreated).
Linguatulosis	Pharyngeal or otic itching, cough, rhinitis, or nasopharyngitis, which follows ingestion of undercooked liver.

(continues)

41

PARASITE	CLINICAL HINT
Loa loa	Migrating pruritic or painful subcutaneous nodules (Calabar swellings), fever, and eosinophilia; adult worms might exit to subconjunctival space.
Malaria— *Plasmodium spp.*	Fever, headache, rigors, vomiting, myalgia, diaphoresis, and hemolytic anemia; fever pattern (every other or every third day) and splenomegaly might be present. Clinical disease might relapse after 7 (*ovale* and *vivax*) to 40 (*malariae*) years.
Mammomono-gamiasis	Cough and hemoptysis associated with a laryngeal foreign body. Might persist for months.
Mansonelliasis— *M. ozzardi*	Arthralgia, pruritus, urticaria, rash, bronchospasm, headache, lymphadenopathy, and eosinophilia.
Mansonelliasis— *M. perstans*	Recurrent pruritic subcutaneous lesions, arthralgia, and eosinophilia; headache, fever, or abdominal pain might also be present.
Mansonelliasis— *M. streptocerca*	Pruritic dermatitis (usually over chest wall and shoulder area), hypopigmented macules, urticaria, and eosinophilia.
Mansonelliasis— other	Rare infection of the conjunctivae, ocular adnexae, brain or other organs—occasionally associated with microfilaremia.

Mesocestoidiasis	Abdominal pain and passage of motile proglottids—similar to taeniasis. Most infections reported from Japan and the United States.
Metagonimiasis	Mucous diarrhea and eosinophilia after eating raw fish. Infestation can persist for more than 1 year.
Metorchiasis	Abdominal pain, fever, headache, and eosinophilia beginning 1 to 15 days after ingestion of raw fish (sashimi). Symptoms can persist for more than 4 weeks.
Micronemiasis	Severe or fatal infection of the brain, meninges, heart, and liver. Most cases reported in the United States. Can be acquired through direct contact with decubitus ulcers or other wounds.
Microsporidiosis	In AIDS patients, infection is characterized by chronic diarrhea, wasting, and bilateral keratoconjunctivitis; hepatitis and myositis might be present.
Moniliformiasis— *M. moniliformis*	Most cases characterized by asymptomatic passage of a worm. Vague complaints such as periumbilical discomfort and giddiness have been described.
Myiasis	Pruritic or painful draining nodule; fever and eosinophilia might be present. Instances of brain, eye, middle ear, and other deep infestations are described.

(continues)

43

Parasite	Clinical Hint
Nanophyetiasis	Diarrhea, flatulence, and eosinophilia following ingestion of undercooked fish; recurrent diarrhea and weight loss can continue for more than 4 months.
Nosema spp.	Keratitis or conjunctivitis, often in the setting of immune compromise (eg, AIDS).
Oesophagostomiasis	Right lower quadrant abdominal pain and tenderness, often with intra-abdominal mass or peritoneal signs.
Onchocerca volvulus	Macular, papular, or dyschromic skin lesions; pruritus; lymphadenopathy; keratitis or uveitis; eosinophilia; firm nodules over bony prominences. Adult worms can survive for 15 years in the human host.
Opisthorchiasis	Right upper quadrant abdominal pain, hepatomegaly, cholangitis, and eosinophilia. Initial symptoms appear 3 to 4 weeks after ingestion of under-cooked freshwater fish. High association with cholangiocarcinoma.
Paragonimiasis	Pulmonary infection with bloody or rusty-looking sputum, central nervous system disease (eg, meningitis or seizures), and eosinophilia; subcutaneous nodules occasionally observed. Parasite can survive for decades in the human host.

Pediculosis

Pruritus in the setting of poor personal hygiene; adults or nits might be visible. Note that the body louse (*Pediculus humanus* var. *corporis*—not the head louse) transmits diseases such as epidemic typhus, trench fever, and relapsing fever.

Pleistophora spp.

Disseminated, multisystem disease in the setting of immune suppression (eg, AIDS).

Pseudoterranova decipiens

Allergic reactions or acute and chronic abdominal pain, often with peritoneal signs or hematemesis. Follows ingestion of undercooked fish (eg, sushi), squid, or octopus.

Raillietinaiasis

Passage of a tapeworm—usually in children.

Sarcocystosis

Diarrhea and abdominal pain of varying severity; muscle pain and eosinophilia occasionally encountered.

Scabies

Intensely pruritic papules, vesicles, and burrows—interdigital webs, wrists, elbows, axillae, perineal region, buttocks, penis. Pruritus most intense at night. Severe psoriaform infestation (Norwegian scabies) noted in debilitated patients.

(continues)

45

PARASITE	CLINICAL HINT
Schistosomiasis— *S. haematobium*	Early urticaria, fever, and eosinophilia; later, dysuria, hematuria, and obstructive nephropathy. Often complicated by bladder cancer in advanced cases. Parasite can survive for decades in the human host.
Schistosomiasis— *S. intercalatum*	Diarrhea (often bloody), abdominal pain, eosinophilia, and hepatosplenomegaly. Significant disease of liver, lung, or central nervous system is rare.
Schistosomiasis— *S. japonicum*	Early urticaria, fever, and eosinophilia; later, hepatosplenomegaly and portal hypertension. Parasite can survive for decades in the human host.
Schistosomiasis— *S. mansoni*	Early urticaria, fever, and eosinophilia; later, hepatosplenomegaly and portal hypertension. Parasite can survive for decades in the human host.
Schistosomiasis— *S. mattheei*	Diarrhea (often bloody), abdominal pain, eosinophilia, and hepatosplenomegaly. Significant disease of liver, lung, or central nervous system is rare.
Schistosomiasis— *S. mekongi*	Early urticaria, fever, and eosinophilia; later, hepatosplenomegaly and portal hypertension. Parasite can survive for decades in the human host.
Sparganosis	Painful or pruritic nodules and eosinophilia; worm present in skin, eye, brain, or other foci. Worm can survive for more than 5 years.

Strongyloidiasis— *S. stercoralis*	Diarrhea, gluteal, or perineal pruritus and rash; eosinophilia often present. Widespread dissemination encountered among immunosuppressed patients because of uncontrolled autoinfection (case-fatality rate for this complication = 80%).
Taeniasis—other	Passage of proglottids or ova; clinically similar to *Taenia saginata* infection.
Taeniasis— *T. solium*	Vomiting and weight loss. Often symptomatic or first appreciated due to passage of proglottids or tape segments. Parasite can survive for more than 25 years in the human intestine.
Taeniasis— *T. saginata*	Vomiting and weight loss. Often symptomatic or first appreciated due to passage of proglottids or tape segments. Parasite can survive for more than 25 years in the human intestine.
Ternidensiasis	Human disease is usually asymptomatic or characterized by colonic nodules and ulcers.
Thelaziasis	Conjunctivitis and lacrimation associated with the sensation of an ocular foreign body.
Toxocariasis	Cough, myalgia, seizures, urticaria, hepatomegaly, pulmonary infiltrates, or retrobulbar lesion; marked eosinophilia often present. Symptoms resolve after several weeks, but eosinophilia can persist for years.

(continues)

Parasite	Clinical Hint
Toxoplasmosis	Fever, lymphadenopathy, and hepatic dysfunction; chorioretinitis; cerebral cysts (patients with AIDS); congenital hydrocephalus, mental retardation, or blindness.
Trichinelliasis	Early diarrhea and vomiting; subsequent myalgia, facial edema, and eosinophilia. Onset 1 to 4 weeks following ingestion of undercooked meat (usually pork). Symptoms can persist for 2 months. Case-fatality rate for symptomatic infection = 2%.
Trichomoniasis	Vaginal pruritus, erythema, and thin or frothy discharge; mild urethritis can be present in male or female.
Trichuriasis	Abdominal pain, bloody diarrhea, rectal prolapse, or intestinal obstruction are occasionally encountered. The parasite can survive for as long as 5 years in the human host.
Trichostrongyliasis	Diarrhea, abdominal pain, and weight loss; eosinophilia is often present. Infestation can persist for years. Fatality and sequelae are not reported.
Trypanosomiasis— African	Chancre, myalgia, arthralgia, lymphadenopathy, and recurrent fever; later mental changes, sensory disorders, and heart failure. Disease due to

Trypanosoma brucei rhodesiense is more rapid and virulent than that due to *T.b. gambiense.*

Trypanosomiasis— American — Unilateral periorbital swelling (Romana's sign) with lymphadenopathy, hepatosplenomegaly, and encephalitis; later cardiomyopathy, megaesophagus, and megacolon. Progression to chronic stage in 20% of patients. Overall case-fatality rate = 10%.

Tungiasis — Painful papule or nodule, usually on the feet—can be multiple. Begins 1 to 2 weeks after walking on dry soil. Secondary infections and tetanus are described.

Vittaforma corneae — Keratitis or conjunctivitis, often in the setting of immune compromise (eg, AIDS).

Chapter 4: Parasites

Alariasis

Alaria americana, Alaria Infection

Agent
Trematode. *Alaria* species, alariasis infection, *Strigea* spp.

Reservoir
Mammalian carnivores (dogs, cats, foxes), rats and rabbits

Vector
None

Vehicle
Undercooked frogs' legs

Geographic Distribution
The precise distribution of these agents is not known. First reported cases from Canada and the United States. It is likely that this parasite has a worldwide distribution.

Incubation Period
Unknown. Acute manifestations can occur after a brief period. Chronic presentations or pathological findings occur after months or years.

Diagnostic Tests
Surgical removal and examination of shape, size (500 × 150 microns) of *mesocercariae*
Lung biopsy

Typical Therapy
There is no known therapy for alariasis.

Background

First human case report in 1976—fatal disseminated infection of thoracic, abdominal, peritoneal, and retroperitoneal tissues, and central nervous system. Associated with ingestion of undercooked frogs' legs. The adult trematode is found in paratenic mammalian carnivores. A recent case incriminated ingestion of undercooked wild goose. Humans act as a paratenic host. Adult flukes are normally found in the intestine of cats, dogs, foxes and mink in Europe, Africa, the Americas, Australia and Japan. Humans are infected by eating undercooked frogs (second intermediate hosts) that contain *mesocercariae.* These *mesocercariae* accumulate in various tissues of the paratenic hosts. Third paratenic intermediate hosts include reptiles, amphibians, birds, and mammals.

A related trematode, *Fibricola seoulensis,* is prevalent among rats in Korea, and is commonly acquired by local humans through ingestion of tadpoles infested with the second intermediate host. Clinical findings can include abdominal pain, diarrhea, fever, and eosinophilia.

Clinical Presentation

Although some cases have involved the eyes (retina and vitreous), systemic infections have produced bronchospasm, subcutaneous nodules, and infiltration of the cardiopulmonary, gastrointestinal, hepatobiliary, and central nervous systems. Complications have included hypersensitivity vasculitis, disseminated intravascular coagulation, and death.

Further Reading

Fernandes BJ, Cooper JD, Cullen JB, et al. Systemic infection with Alaria americana (Trematoda). *Can Med Assoc J.* 1976;115:1111-1114.

Freeman RS, Stuart PF, Cullen SJ, et al. Fatal human infection with mesocercariae of the trematode Alaria americana. *Am J Trop Med Hyg.* 1976;25:803-807.

Hong ST, Chai JY, Lee SH. Ten human cases of Fibricola seoulensis infection and mixed one with Stellantchasmus and Metagonimus. *Kisaengchunghak Chapchi.* 1986;24:95-97.

Hong ST, Cho TK, Hong SJ, Chai JY, Lee SH, Seo BS. Fifteen human cases of Fibricola seoulensis infection in Korea. *Kisaengchunghak Chapchi.* 1984;22:61-65.

Kramer MH, Eberhard ML, Blankenberg TA. Respiratory symptoms and subcutaneous granuloma caused by mesocercariae: a case report. *Am J Trop Med Hyg.* 1996;55:447-448.

McDonald HR, Kazacos KR, Schatz H, Johnson RN. Two cases of intraocular infection with Alaria mesocercaria (Trematoda). *Am J Ophthalmol.* 1994;117:447-55.

Amoebae—Free Living

Acanthamoeba, Acanthamoeba Infection, Balamuthia Infection, Hartmanella Infection, Leptomyxid Amoeba Infection, Naegleria Infection, Vahlkampfia Infection

Agent
Protozoa. *Centramoebida, Acanthamoebidae: Acanthamoeba* and *Balamuthia. Schizopyrenida, Vahkampfidae: Naegleria. A. palestinensis.*

Reservoir
Water and soil

Vector
None

Vehicle
Water (diving, swimming)

Geographic Distribution

The precise distribution of these agents is not known. Primary meningoencephalitis has been reported from the United States, Europe, Australia, Africa, New Zealand, and Central America.

Incubation Period

5–6d (range 2d–14d)

Diagnostic Tests

Wet preparation
Specialized cultures
Serology available in reference centers

Typical Therapy

Naegleria meningitis is treated with intravenous amphotericin B at a dosage of 1 mg/kg daily (maximum 50 mg/day) i.v.; supplemented with intrathecal amphotericin B, 0.1 mg given every other day. *Acanthamoeba* infections have been treated with pentamidine and topical preparations of chlorhexidine, ketoconazole, or itraconazole.

Background

- *Acanthamoeba* spp. are found worldwide, and have been identified in soil, dust, air, seawater, swimming pools, sewage, air conditioners, tap water, bottled water, dialysis units, vegetation, fish, amphibia, reptiles, contact lens cases, and the normal nose and throat of humans. Organisms feed on bacteria, algae, and yeasts. *Acanthamoeba* encephalitis occurs predominantly in debilitated or immunosuppressed individuals (AIDS, liver disease, diabetes, renal or bone marrow transplantation, steroid, or chemotherapy).

Acanthamoeba keratitis occurs in healthy people, with contact lens use accounting for more than 80% of cases. The annual incidence during 1985 through 1987 was estimated at 1.65 to 2.01 cases per million contact lens wearers. Species causing keratitis include *A. castellanii, A. polyphaga, A. hatchetti, A. culbertsoni, A. rhysodes, A. lungdunensis, A. quina,* and *A. griffini.*

- Corneal infection has been ascribed to *Acanthamoeba, Hartmanella,* and *Vahlkampfia* species.
- *Balamuthia mandrillaris* (leptomyxid amoeba) is primarily associated with central nervous system infection (rarely skin abscesses); however, unlike *Acanthamoeba,* most of the 13 cases reported to 1997 were in immunocompetent hosts. Seventy cases were reported up to 2000, from the United States, Mexico, Venezuela, and Peru. A single case of autochthonous *Balamuthia* encephalitis was reported in Europe (Czech Republic).
- *Naegleria fowleri* is found worldwide in soil, sewage, heating and ventilation units, swimming pools, power plant discharges, river, coastal and lake water, and thermally polluted water. *N. fowleri* grows at temperatures as high as 45°C, while *Acanthamoeba* are inhibited by temperatures above 35° to 39°C. *Naegleria* cysts are stable up to 8 months at 4°C. Serological surveys suggest that asymptomatic infection by both *Acanthamoeba* and *Naegleria* is common in the southern United States. As of 1997, approximately 179 cases of primary amoebic meningoencephalitis had been reported worldwide, with 81 cases in the United States.
- Bacterial species (*Legionella anisa* and *Bosea massiliensis*) associated with free-living amoeba can play a role in ventilator-associated pneumonia.

Causal Agents

Naegleria fowleri and *Acanthamoeba* spp., commonly found in lakes, swimming pools, tap water, and heating and air conditioning units. While only one species of *Naegleria* is known to infect humans, several species of *Acanthamoeba* are implicated, including *A. culbertsoni, A. polyphaga, A. castellanii, A. astronyxis, A. hatchetti,* and *A. rhysodes.* An additional agent of human disease, *Balamuthia mandrillaris,* is a related leptomyxid ameba that is morphologically similar in light microscopy to *Acanthamoeba* (CDC).

Life Cycle

Free-living amebae belonging to the genera *Acanthamoeba, Balamuthia,* and *Naegleria* are important causes of disease in humans and animals. *Naegleria fowleri* produces an acute, and usually lethal, central nervous system (CNS) disease called primary amebic meningoencephalitis (PAM). *N. fowleri* has three stages, cysts ❶ [Figure 4-1, left], ❷ trophozoites [left], and flagellated forms ❸ [left], in its life cycle. The trophozoites replicate by promitosis (the nuclear membrane remains intact) [left]. ❹ *Naegleria fowleri* is found in fresh water, soil, thermal discharges of power plants, heated swimming pools, hydrotherapy and medicinal pools, aquariums, and sewage. Trophozoites can turn into temporary flagellated forms which usually revert back to the trophozoite stage. Trophozoites infect humans or animals by entering the olfactory neuroepithelium ❺ and reaching the brain. *N. fowleri* trophozoites are found in cerebrospinal fluid (CSF) and tissue, while flagellated forms are found in CSF.

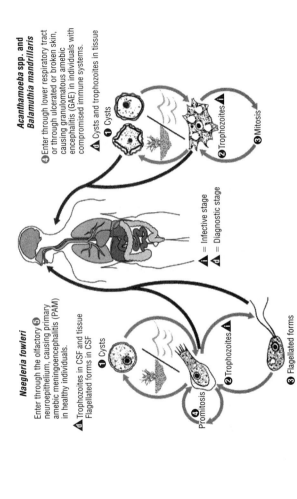

Acanthamoeba spp. and Balamuthia mandrillaris

④ Enter through lower respiratory tract or through ulcerated or broken skin, causing granulomatous amebic encephalitis (GAE) in individuals with compromised immune systems.

● Cysts and trophozoites in tissue

🔺d = Cysts and trophozoites in tissue

① Cysts 🔺

② Trophozoites 🔺

③ Mitosis

🔺 = Infective stage

🔺d = Diagnostic stage

Naegleria fowleri

Enter through the olfactory neuroepithelium, causing primary amebic meningoencephalitis (PAM) in healthy individuals. ❺

🔺d Trophozoites in CSF and tissue Flagellated forms in CSF

① Cysts 🔺

② Trophozoites 🔺

③ Flagellated forms

④ Promitosis

Figure 4-1   Life cycle of free-living amoeba.

57

Acanthamoeba spp. and *Balamuthia mandrillaris* are opportunistic free-living amebae capable of causing granulomatous amebic encephalitis (GAE) in individuals with compromised immune systems. *Acanthamoeba* spp. have been found in soil; fresh, brackish, and sea water; sewage; swimming pools; contact lens equipment; medicinal pools; dental treatment units; dialysis machines; heating, ventilating, and air conditioning systems; mammalian cell cultures; vegetables; human nostrils and throats; and human and animal brain, skin, and lung tissues. *B. mandrillaris* however, has not been identified in the environment but has been isolated from autopsy specimens of infected humans and animals. Unlike *N. fowleri*, *Acanthamoeba* and *Balamuthia* have only two stages, cysts ❶ [right] and trophozoites ❷ [right], in their life cycle. No flagellated stage exists as part of the life cycle. The trophozoites replicate by mitosis (nuclear membrane does not remain intact) ❸ [right]. The trophozoites are the infective forms and are believed to gain entry into the body through the lower respiratory tract, ulcerated or broken skin and invade the central nervous system by hematogenous dissemination ❹ [right]. *Acanthamoeba* spp. and *Balamuthia mandrillaris* cysts and trophozoites are found in tissue (CDC).

Clinical Presentation

Primary amoebic meningoencephalitis usually occurs in children and young adults who have been swimming in warm, fresh water. Infection is heralded by abnormal sensations of taste or smell followed by abrupt onset of fever, nausea, and vomiting. The majority of patients have headache, meningitis, and disorders of mental status changes. Coma and death can ensue within one week.

Granulomatous amoebic encephalitis due to *Acanthamoeba* occurs in immunocompromised and debilitated patients, and has a gradual onset characterized by focal neurologic deficits, mental status abnormalities, seizures, fever, headache, hemiparesis, and meningismus. Visual disturbances and ataxia are often encountered. Death can ensue within 7 to 120 days. *Acanthamoeba* infection has also been associated with skin ulcers, pneumonia, adrenalitis, vasculitis, osteomyelitis, and sinusitis.

Acanthamoeba keratitis is clinically similar to herpetic infection, and presents with a foreign-body sensation, eye pain, photophobia, tearing, blepharospasm, conjunctivitis, iritis, anterior uveitis, dendriform keratitis, and blurred vision.

Reference
Free-living amebic infections. Centers for Disease Control Web site. Available at: http://www.dpd.cdc.gov/dpdx/HTML/FreeLivingAmebic.htm. Accessed April 15, 2005.

Further Reading
Acanthamoeba infection. Centers for Disease Control Web site. Available at: http://www.cdc.gov/ncidod/dpd/parasites/acanthomoeba/factsht_acanthamoeba.htm. Accessed April 15, 2005.

Denney CF, Iragui VJ, Uber-Zak LD, et al. Amebic meningoencephalitis caused by Balamuthia mandrillaris: case report and review. *Clin Infect Dis.* 1997; 25:1354-1358.

Faude F, Sunnemann S, Retzlaff C, Meier T, Wiedemann P. Therapy refractory keratitis. Contact lens-induced keratitis caused by Acanthamoeba palestinensis. *Ophthalmologie.* 1997;94:448-449.

Ma P, Visvesvara GS, Martinez AJ, Theodore FH, Daggett PM, Sawyer TK. Naegleria and Acanthamoeba infections: review. *Rev Infect Dis.* 1990;12:490-513.

Marshall MM, Naumovitz D, Ortega Y, Sterling CR. Waterborne protozoan pathogens. *Clin Microbiol Rev.* 1997;10:67-85.

Naegleria infection fact sheet. Centers for Disease Control Web site. Available at: http://www.cdc.gov/ncidod/dpd/parasites/naegleria/default.htm. Accessed April 15, 2005.

Sharma S, Garg P, Rao GN. Patient characteristics, diagnosis, and treatment of non-contact lens related Acanthamoeba keratitis. *Br J Ophthalmol.* 2000;84:1103-1108.

Angiostrongylus (Panstrongylus) cantonensis

Angiostrongylose, Eosinophilic Meningitis, Panstrongyliasis, Parastrongyliasis

Agent
Nematoda. Phasmidea: *Angiostrongylus (Parastrongylus) cantonensis*

Reservoir
Rats, prawns, frogs

Vector
None

Vehicle
Snails, slugs, prawns, lettuce

Geographic Distribution

REGION I—NAm	USA
REGION IV—Carib	DOM, CUB, HTI, JAM, PRI
REGION V—NAfr	EGY
REGION VI—CAfr	CIV, COM, MDG, MUS, REU
REGION X—IndSub	IND, LKA

REGION XI—Asia	CHN, HKG, JPN, TWN
REGION XII—SEA	IDN, KHM, MYS, PHL, THA, VNM
REGION XIII—Poly	ASM, AUS, COK, FJI, GUM, NCL, PNG, PYF, VUT, WSM

Incubation Period
2w (range 5–35d)

Diagnostic Tests
Identification of parasite.
Serological tests have limited reliability.

Typical Therapy
Corticosteroids if severe CNS disease
Mebendazole 100 mg b.i.d. × 5d (age > 2 years)

Background

- *Parastrongylus (Angiostrongylus) cantonensis* was first identified in rats in Canton, China in 1933, and in humans in Taiwan in 1944. More than 2,500 cases had been reported in approximately 30 countries as of 1990.
- Epidemics occurred in Ponape (East Caroline Islands) during 1944 to 1948, and the parasite was widely disseminated by the African land snail (*Achatina fulica*).
- Infection of rats is now found throughout the Indo-Pacific basin, Madagascar, Cuba, Egypt, Puerto Rico, New Orleans, and Cuba. Following World War II, the parasite was identified in Southeast Asia and the Pacific, through Micronesia, Australia, and Polynesia. Cases were first identified in the Philippines, Saipan,

New Caledonia, Rarotonga, and Tahiti during the 1950s. During the 1960s, the disease was reported from Vietnam, Thailand, Cambodia, Java, Sarawak, Guam, and Hawaii.

- The parasite is common on a number of Caribbean islands. In 2000, 12 American tourists acquired angiostrongyliasis from contaminated Caesar salad in Jamaica.

- Adult worms reside in rat lungs, from which ova enter the pulmonary arteries. Larvae migrate via the trachea to the gastrointestinal tract, and are consumed by snails and slugs which feed on rat feces. Rats and humans are infected through ingestion of infective third-stage larvae in snails, or contaminated uncooked food. Only rodents or bandicoots can serve as the definitive hosts. Prawns and frogs are paratenic hosts, carrying only third-stage larvae. Lettuce (presumably contaminated with slug mucus), raw shrimp paste (notably Polynesian), land crabs, and coconut crabs can serve as vehicles.

- Rare instances of infection by an unrelated nematode, *Ascaris suum,* have also been characterized by eosinophilic meningitis.

Clinical Presentation

Disease is usually characterized by severe headache, neck and back stiffness, and paresthesias. Bell's palsy occurs in 5% of patients, and disturbances of vision or eye movement occur in 15%. Low-grade fever might be present. The worm has been found in the CSF and the eye. Cerebrospinal fluid usually has a pleocytosis with 25 to 100% eosinophiles; blood eosinophilia is not always present. The illness might last a few days to several months.

Note: Eosinophiles are not discernable in cerebrospinal fluid examination using routine methods. The clinician must request specific stains when cerebrospinal fluid eosinophilia is suspected.

Further Reading

Lowichik A, Siegel JD. Parasitic infections of the central nervous system in children. Part I: Congenital infections and meningoencephalitis. *J Child Neurol.* 1995;10:4-17.

Re VL III, Gluckman SJ. Eosinophilic meningitis. *Am J Med.* 2003;114:217-223.

Slom TJ, Cortese MM, Gerber SI, et al. An outbreak of eosinophilic meningitis caused by Angiostrongylus cantonensis in travelers returning from the Caribbean. *N Engl J Med.* 2002; 346:668-675.

Angiostrongylus (Panstrongylus, Morerastrongylus) costaricensis

Abdominal Angiostrongyliasis

Agent
Nematoda. Phasmidea: *Parastrongylus (Angiostrongylus, Morerastrongylus) costaricensis*

Reservoir
Cotton rats (*Sigmodon*), slugs

Vector
None

Vehicle
Slugs and slug excretions

Geographic Distribution
REGION II—CAm   BLZ, CRI, GTM, HND,
                       MEX, NIC, PAN, SLV

REGION III—SAm	BOL, BRA, CHL, COL, ECU, GUF, GUY, PER, PRY, SUR, URY, VEN
REGION IV—Carib	CUB, DMA, GLP, MTQ

Incubation Period
10–14d

Diagnostic Tests
Identification of ova or adults in surgical material
Serologic tests used in some endemic areas

Typical Therapy
Mebendazole 200 to 400 mg PO t.i.d. × 10d
Or thiabendazole 25 mg/kg t.i.d. (max 3 g/d) × 3d
Surgery for complications

Background

- Abdominal angiostrongyliais is found in Central America and South America, with most reported cases in Costa Rica. The disease occurs in both urban and rural areas, with highest incidence among male children and during the wet season.
- Larvae of *Parastrongylus costaricensis* develop in abdominal lymphatics, and then migrate to ileocecal arterioles where their ova degenerate and elicit inflammation and luminal narrowing.

Causal Agents

The nematode (roundworm) *Angiostrongylus cantonensis*, the rat lungworm, is the most common cause of human eosinophilic meningitis; whereas *Angiostrongylus*

(*Parastrongylus*) *costaricensis* is the causal agent of abdominal, or intestinal, angiostrongyliasis (CDC).

Life Cycle

Adult worms of *A. cantonensis* live in the pulmonary arteries of rats. The females lay eggs that release first-stage larvae in the terminal branches of the pulmonary arteries. The first-stage larvae migrate to the pharynx, are swallowed, and passed in the feces [Figure 4-2]. They penetrate or are ingested by an intermediate host (snail or slug). After two moults, third-stage larvae are produced, which are infective to mammalian hosts. When the mollusk is ingested by the definitive host, the third-stage larvae migrate to the brain where they develop into young adults. The young adults return to the venous system and then the pulmonary arteries where they become sexually mature. Of note, various animals act as paratenic (transport) hosts: after ingesting the infected snails, they carry the third-stage larvae which can resume their development when the paratenic host is ingested by a definitive host. Humans can acquire infection by eating raw or undercooked snails or slugs infected with the parasite; or by eating raw produce that contains a small snail or slug, or part of one. There is some question whether or not larvae can exit the infected mollusks in slime (infective to humans if ingested, for example, on raw produce). The disease can also be acquired by ingestion of contaminated or infected paratenic animals (crabs, freshwater shrimps). In humans, juvenile worms migrate to the brain, or rarely in the lungs, where they ultimately die. The life cycle of *Angiostrongylus* (*Parastrongylus*) *costaricensis* is similar, except that adult worms reside in the arterioles of the ileocecal area of the definitive host. In humans, *A. costaricensis* often reaches sexual maturity and releases eggs into the intestine. Eggs and larvae degenerate and cause intense local inflammatory reactions and do not appear to be shed in the stool (CDC).

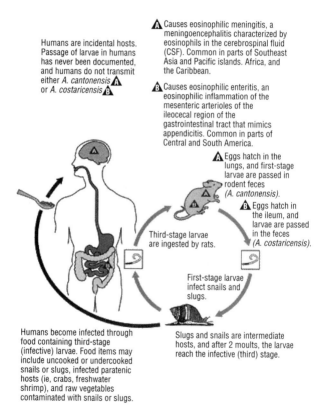

Figure 4-2   Life cycle of *Angiostrongylus (Panstrongylus, Morerastrongylus) costaricensis.*

Clinical Presentation

Clinical manifestations consist of abdominal pain, vomiting, fever, and a right lower quadrant mass (50% of cases). Most patients have been children. The syndrome suggests appendicitis or heavy infection by *Ascaris*; however, the former might be discounted by the presence of eosinophilia. Radiographic findings are nonspecific and show filling defects and spasticity of the ileum, cecum, or colon. Complications include intestinal perforation or obstruction. Ova and parasites are not found in feces, and diagnosis is made using serological tests or identification of parasites in surgical specimens.

Reference

Angiostrongyliasis. Centers for Disease Control Web site. Available at: http://www.dpd.cdc.gov/dpdx/HTML/angiostrongyliasis.htm. Accessed April 15, 2005.

Further Reading

Hulbert TV, Larsen RA, Chandrasoma PT. Abdominal angiostrongyliasis mimicking acute appendicitis and Meckel's diverticulum: report of a case in the United States and review. *Clin Infect Dis.* 1992;14:836-840.

Kramer MH, Greer GJ, Quinonez JF, et al. First reported outbreak of abdominal angiostrongyliasis. *Clin Infect Dis.* 1998;26:365-372.

Loria-Cortes R, Lobo-Sanahuja JF. Clinical abdominal angiostrongylosis. A study of 116 children with intestinal eosinophilic granuloma caused by Angiostrongylus costaricensis. *Am J Trop Med Hyg.* 1980;29:538-544.

Neafie RC, Marty AM. Unusual infections in humans. *Clin Microbiol Rev.* 1993;6:34-56.

Vazquez JJ, Boils PL, Sola JJ, et al. Angiostrongyliasis in a European patient: a rare cause of gangrenous ischemic enterocolitis. *Gastroenterology.* 1993;105:1544-1549.

Anisakiasis

Cod Worm Disease, Herring Worm Disease
Agent
Nematoda. Phasmidea: *Anisakis simplex, Pseudoterranova decipiens, Contracaecum* spp. and *Bolbosoma* spp.

Reservoir
Marine mammals

Vector
None

Vehicle
Undercooked saltwater fish, octopus, squid

Geographic Distribution
Worldwide. Although the disease is most common in countries where undercooked seafood is eaten, infection can also follow ingestion of marine fish imported from other countries.

Incubation Period
Hours–14d

Clinical Overview
Anisakiasis can present as an allergic reaction or as acute and chronic abdominal pain, often associated with peritoneal signs or hematemesis. The patient should be questioned regarding recent ingestion of undercooked or raw saltwater fish, octopus or squid (eg, sushi), or marinated saltwater fish (eg, ceviche).

Diagnostic Tests
Endoscopic identification of larvae

Typical Therapy
Endoscopic removal of larvae; surgery for complications

Background

- Anisakiasis was first recognized as a human disease in the Netherlands during the 1960s. Highest numbers are registered in Japan, the Netherlands, Germany, France, Spain, and the United States (notably California).
- Approximately 14,000 cases had been reported as of 2000—95% from Japan and 3.5% from Europe. More than 1,000 cases are registered each year in Tokyo—most from spotted chub mackerel (*Scomber japonicus*) and Japanese flying squid (*Todarodes pacificus*).
- Infection is usually caused by a single larva, which infects the gastrointestinal tract (rarely the lungs or peritoneal cavity).
- Gastric anisakiasis is the predominant form in Japan; intestinal anisakiasis is predominant in Europe (this could be an artifact of reporting and detection techniques).
- The two common species are *Anisakis* (acquired from cod, squid, herring, mackerel and salmon); and *P. (Phocanema, Terranova)* (acquired from cod, halibut, greenling, red snapper and flat fish).
- High risk dishes include sushi, sashimi, Dutch salt or smoked herring, Nordic gravlax (cured salmon), Hawaiian lomi-lomi (raw salmon), ceviche and *boquerones en vinagre* (pickled anchovies). Herring (*Clupea harengus*) is the principal vehicle in western Europe.

- Sensitization to the parasites has been identified in some cases of seafood allergy.
- *Anasakis simplex* and *A. physeteris* are parasites of whales, seals, walruses, sea lions and related mammals. *P. decipiens* is found exclusively in pinnipeds. Ova reach seawater in the feces of these animals, and develop into larvae, which are ingested by squid and other invertebrates—in turn ingested by fish, which can be eaten raw by humans.
- Nematodes of the genus *Eustrongylides* are parasitic as adults in the gastrointestinal tract of fish-eating birds and as larvae in the connective tissue or body cavity of *freshwater* fish. Amphibians, reptiles, and mammals (rarely) can become infected with larval *Eustrongylides* spp. and can play an ecological role as paratenic or transport hosts. Rare instances of intestinal disease in humans have followed ingestion of minnows, and were characterized by intense abdominal pain.

Causal Agents

Anisakiasis is caused by the accidental ingestion of larvae of the nematodes (roundworms) *Anisakis simplex* and *Pseudoterranova decipiens* (CDC).

Life Cycle

Adult stages of *Anisakis simplex* or *Pseudoterranova decipiens* reside in the stomach of marine mammals, where they are embedded in the mucosa, in clusters. Unembryonated eggs produced by adult females are passed in the feces of marine mammals ❶ [Figure 4-3]. The eggs become embryonated in water, and form first-stage larvae.

These molt, becoming second-stage larvae **2a**, and after hatching, become free-swimming forms **2b**. Larvae are ingested by crustaceans **3**, in which they develop into third-stage larvae that are infective to fish and squid **4**. The larvae migrate from the intestine to the peritoneal

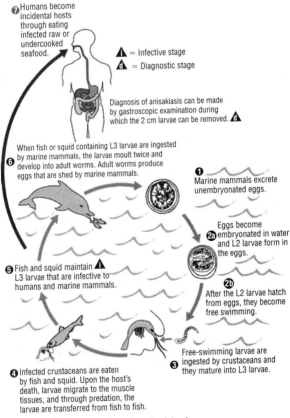

7 Humans become incidental hosts through eating infected raw or undercooked seafood.

⚠ = Infective stage
⚠d = Diagnostic stage

Diagnosis of anisakiasis can be made by gastroscopic examination during which the 2 cm larvae can be removed. ⚠d

6 When fish or squid containing L3 larvae are ingested by marine mammals, the larvae moult twice and develop into adult worms. Adult worms produce eggs that are shed by marine mammals.

1 Marine mammals excrete unembryonated eggs.

2a Eggs become embryonated in water and L2 larvae form in the eggs.

5 Fish and squid maintain ⚠ L3 larvae that are infective to humans and marine mammals.

2b After the L2 larvae hatch from eggs, they become free swimming.

3 Free-swimming larvae are ingested by crustaceans and they mature into L3 larvae.

4 Infected crustaceans are eaten by fish and squid. Upon the host's death, larvae migrate to the muscle tissues, and through predation, the larvae are transferred from fish to fish.

Figure 4-3   Life cycle of anisakiasis.

cavity, where they grow up to 3 cm in length. Upon the host's death, larvae migrate to the muscles, and through predation, are transferred from fish to fish. Fish and squid maintain third-stage larvae that are infective to humans and marine mammals ❺. When fish or squid containing larvae are ingested by marine mammals, the larvae moult twice and develop into adult worms. The adult females produce eggs, which are shed by marine mammals ❻. Humans become infected by eating raw or undercooked marine fish ❼. After ingestion, the anisakid larvae penetrate the gastric and intestinal mucosa, causing the symptoms of anisakiasis (CDC).

Clinical Presentation

The location of the worms and symptoms depend somewhat on the genus, with *Phocanema* more commonly associated with infection of the stomach, and *Anisakis* of the intestine. Symptoms occur within 48 hours after ingestion. Gastric anisakiasis is characterized by intense abdominal pain, nausea, and vomiting. Small intestinal involvement results in lower abdominal pain and signs of obstruction and might mimic appendicitis. Symptoms could last for months, rarely for years. The disease might also suggest tumor, regional enteritis or diverticulitis. Ingestion of *Anisakis* larvae with seafood is often responsible for acute allergic manifestations such as urticaria and anaphylaxis, with or without accompanying gastrointestinal symptomatology. Eosinophilia is usually not present in either gastric or intestinal anisakiasis; however, leukocytosis is noted in 67% of patients with intestinal involvement.

Reference

Anisakiasis. Centers for Disease Control Web site. Available at: http://www.dpd.cdc.gov/dpdx/HTML/Anisakiasis.htm. Accessed April 15, 2005.

Further Reading

Audicana MT, Ansotegui IJ, de Corres LF, Kennedy MW. Anisakis simplex: dangerous—dead and alive? *Trends Parasitol.* 2002;18:20-25.

Beaver PC, Otsuji T, Otsuji A, Yoshimura H, Uchikawa R, Sato A. Acanthocephalan, probably Bolbosoma, from the peritoneal cavity of man in Japan. *Am J Trop Med Hyg.* 1983;32:1016-1018.

Daschner A, Alonso-Gomez A, Cabanas R, Suarez-de-Parga JM, Lopez-Serrano MC. Gastroallergic anisakiasis: borderline between food allergy and parasitic disease—clinical and allergologic evaluation of 20 patients with confirmed acute parasitism by Anisakis simplex. *J Allergy Clin Immunol.* 2000;105(pt 1):176-181.

Lopez-Serrano MC, Gomez AA, Daschner A, et al. Gastroallergic anisakiasis: findings in 22 patients. *J Gastroenterol Hepatol.* 2000;15: 503-506.

Muraoka A, Suehiro I, Fujii M, et al. Acute gastric anisakiasis: 28 cases during the last 10 years. *Dig Dis Sci.* 1996;41:2362-2365.

Oldfield EC III. Emerging foodborne pathogens: keeping your patients and your families safe. *Rev Gastroenterol Disord.* 2001;1:177-186.

Tada I, Otsuji Y, Kamiya H, Mimori T, Sakaguchi Y, Makizumi S. The first case of a human infected with an acanthocephalan parasite, Bolbosoma sp. *J Parasitol.* 1983;69:205-208.

Takabe K, Ohki S, Kunihiro O, et al. Anisakidosis: a cause of intestinal obstruction from eating sushi. *Am J Gastroenterol.* 1998;93:1172-1173.

Armillifer Infection

Agent
Pentastomid worm. *Armillifer moniliformis* in Asia, *A. armillatus* and *A. grandis* in Africa.

Reservoir
Amphibians, reptiles, rodents

Vector
None

Vehicle
Snake meat, water, vegetation

Geographic Distribution

REGION III—SAm	GUY
REGION V—NAfr	EGY
REGION VI—CAfr	CMR, COD, COG, GMB, NGA, SEN, ZWE
REGION X—IndSub	IND
REGION XI—Asia	CHN, JPN
REGION XII—SEA	IDN, MYS, PHL

Incubation Period
Unknown

Diagnostic Tests
Identification of larvae in tissue

Typical Therapy
Excision as indicated

Background

- Pentastomids, arthropod-like worms which rarely infect humans, are divided into two genera: *Linguatula* (discussed later in this chapter) and *Armillifer*. The latter infects snakes and mammals as intermediate hosts.
- Human infection by *A. armillatus* has been reported from tropical Africa; *A. moniliformis* from Java, Sumatra, China, the Philippines and Malaysia; *A. grandis* from central Africa.

- Humans acquire infection through ingestion of uncooked snake meat or water contaminated by snake feces.

Clinical Presentation

Symptoms are related to mechanical pressure and might include intestinal obstruction or acute abdomen. Pneumonia, jaundice, pericarditis, and pleurisy have also been reported. C-shaped or coiled calcifications might be visible on x-rays.

Further Reading

Coker AO, Isokpehi RD, Thomas BN, Fagbenro-Beyioku AF, Omilabu SA. Zoonotic infections in Nigeria: overview from a medical perspective. *Acta Trop.* 2000;76:59-63.

Drabick JJ. Pentastomiasis. *Rev Infect Dis.* 1987;9:1087-1094.

Ma KC, Qiu MH, Rong YL. Pathological differentiation of suspected cases of pentastomiasis in China. *Trop Med Int Health.* 2002;7:166-177.

Self JT, Hopps HC, Williams AO. Pentastomiasis in Africans. *Trop Geogr Med.* 1975;27:1-13.

Ascaris lumbricoides

Agent

Nematoda. Phasmidea: *Ascaris lumbricoides.*

Reservoir

Humans

Vector

None

Vehicle

Vegetables, flies

Geographic Distribution
Worldwide

Diagnostic Tests
Stool microscopy

Typical Adult Therapy
Mebendazole 100 mg b.i.d. × 3d
Or albendazole 400 mg × 1 dose

Typical Pediatric Therapy
Mebendazole 100 mg b.i.d. × 3d (> age 2)
Or pyrantel pamoate 11 mg/kg (max 1 g) as single dose

Incubation Period
10–14d (range 7 ≥ 200d)

Background

- Symptomatic infection is most often associated with poor hygiene, ingestion of raw produce, and pediatric age group.
- *Ascaris* ova are resistant to cold and common disinfectants, but sensitive to sunlight and temperatures above 45°C.
- In 1947, it was estimated that 640 million humans were infested. In 1978, that number had grown to 800 million to 1 billion. By 1994, the estimated prevalence was 1.471 billion, with 12 million new cases per year. Rates are 45% in much of Latin America, and 95% in parts of Africa. The prevalence in sub-Saharan Africa is estimated at 26.7% (161 million cases).
- The case-fatality rate is estimated at 2/100,000—with 20,000 to 60,000 *Ascaris*-related deaths yearly (primarily females younger than 10 years) in 1985.

Fatal cases were estimated at 8,000 in 1998; and at 3,000 in 1999.

Causal Agent

Ascaris lumbricoides is the largest nematode (round-worm) which commonly parasitizes the human intestine. (Adult females: 20 to 35 cm; adult male: 15 to 30 cm.) (CDC)

Life Cycle

Adult worms ❶ [Figure 4-4] live in the lumen of the small intestine. A female may produce approximately 200,000 eggs per day, which are passed with the feces ❷. Fertile eggs embryonate and become infective after 18 days to several weeks ❸, depending on the environmental conditions (optimum: moist, warm, shaded soil). After infective eggs are swallowed ❹, larvae hatch ❺, invade the intestinal mucosa, and are carried via the portal, then systemic circulation to the lungs ❻. The larvae mature further in the lungs (10 to 14 days), penetrate the alveolar walls, ascend the bronchial tree to the throat, and are swallowed ❼. Upon reaching the small intestine, they develop into adult worms ❶. Between 2 and 3 months are required from ingestion of the infective eggs to oviposition by the adult female. Adult worms can live for 1 to 2 years (CDC).

Clinical Presentation

The pulmonary manifestations of ascariasis occur during the stage of larval migration through the lungs and resemble Loffler's syndrome: cough, wheezing, pulmonary

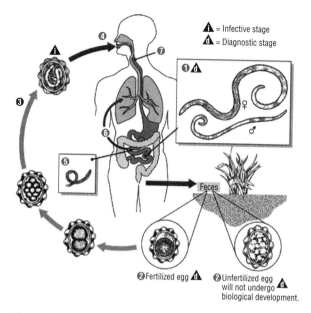

Figure 4-4   Life cycle of *Ascaris lumbricoides.*

infiltration, and eosinophilia. Children with heavy *Ascaris* infection experience impaired digestion and absorption of proteins, often with moderate steatorrhea. A mass of worms can block the lumen of the small bowel, resulting in acute intestinal obstruction, with vomiting, abdominal distention, and cramps. Worms can also invade and obstruct the biliary duct (pancreatic-biliary ascariasis), producing abdominal pain, which can be associated with ascending cholangitis, acute pancreatitis or, rarely, obstructive jaundice. Aberrant worms can appear at umbilical and hernial fistulas, the fallopian tubes, urinary bladder, lungs, nose, and other sites.

Reference

Ascariasis fact sheet. Centers for Disease Control Web site. Available at: http://www.dpd.cdc.gov/dpdx/HTML/ Ascariasis.htm. Accessed April 15, 2005.

Further Reading

Cox FE. History of human parasitology. *Clin Microbiol Rev.* 2002;15:595-612.

Crompton DW. Ascaris and ascariasis. *Adv Parasitol.* 2001;48:285-375.

Hall A, Holland C. Geographical variation in Ascaris lumbricoides fecundity and its implications for helminth control. *Parasitol Today.* 2000;16:540-544.

Partners for parasite control. World Health Organization Web site. Available at: http://www.who.int/ctd/intpara/. Accessed April 15, 2005.

Babesiosis

Agent

Protozoa. Sporozoa, Apicomplexa: *Babesia microti* or WA-1 (United States); or *B. divergens* and *B. bigemina* (Europe); or *Babesia* EU1.

Reservoir

Rodents (usually white-footed mouse = *Peromyscus leucopus*), rabbits, deer, cattle, ticks

Vector

Tick (*Ixodes scapularis* for *B. microti*; *Ixodes ricinus* for *B. divergens*)

Vehicle

Blood

Geographic Distribution

REGION I—NAm	CAN, USA
REGION II—CAm	MEX
REGION V—NAfr	EGY
REGION VII—SAfr	ZAF
REGION VIII—Eur	AUT, BEL, BIH, BLR, CHE, DEU, ESP, EST, FRA, GBR, GEO, HRV, HUN, IRL, ITA, LTU, LVA, MDA, MKD, POL, PRT, SVN, SWE, UKR, YUG
REGION IX—MidEast	ARM
REGION XI—Asia	AZE, CHN, JPN, KAZ, KGZ, RUS, TJK, TKM, TWN, UZB

Incubation Period

1–2w (range 1–9w)

Diagnostic Tests

Microscopy of stained blood smears
Animal inoculation
Serology
Nucleic acid amplification

Typical Adult Therapy

Atovaquone 750 mg b.i.d. + azithromycin 500 mg daily
    × 7–10d.
Or clindamycin 600 mg i.v. q8h × 7d + quinine 650 mg
    t.i.d. × 7d.
Exchange transfusion has been used in some cases.

Typical Pediatric Therapy

Clindamycin 10 mg/kg i.v. q8h × 7d + quinine 8 mg/kg
    t.i.d. × 7d

Background

- The first case of human babesiosis was reported in Yugoslavia in 1957 (fatal infection in a splenectomized patient).
- During 1975 to 1986, 214 cases were reported—200 in the United States and 14 in Europe (7 of these in France).
- As of 1997, more than 400 cases had been reported from the United States (*B. microti*). By 2001, 560 cases had been reported in New York State alone.
- As of 2003, 31 cases (9 fatal) of *B. divergens* infection had been reported in Europe (all in splenectomized patients—with most occurring during May to October, reflecting tick activity), in the countries of Belgium, France, Ireland, Poland, Scotland, Spain, Sweden, Switzerland, Russia, and Yugoslavia.
- Human infection by *B. microti* is rare in Europe because the principal enzootic vector (*Ixodes tranguliceps*) does not bite humans; however, *B. microti* is occasionally found in *I. ricinus* on the continent.
- Rates in Europe correspond to the cattle breeding season and periods of high tick activity.
- Most cases in Europe have involved splenectomized patients; 50% of European cases reported during 1957 to 1995 were fatal. No cases of transfusion-borne infection were reported as of 1999.
- Infections due to unnamed *Babesia* species have been reported in Washington state (*Babesia* WO1), California (*Babesia* CA1), and Missouri (*Babesia* MO1). Most infections due to these new species have occurred among splenectomized individuals; whereas 95% of *B. microti* infections are reported in persons with intact spleens. Infections in two asplenic men from Spain and Austria suggest a new strain (*Babesia* EU1) molecularly distinct from *B. microti* and *B. divergens*.

- To date, only ixodid tick species have been identified as vectors for *Babesia*: *I. dammini* (*I. scapularis*) for *B. microti*, and *I. ricinus* for *B. divergens*. Small terrrestrial mammals and subhuman primates can act as reservoirs for *B. microti*; cattle and rodents can act as reservoirs for *B. divergens*.

Causal Agents

Babesiosis is caused by hemoprotozoan parasites of the genus *Babesia*. While more than 100 species have been reported, only a few have been identified as causing human infections. *Babesia microti* and *Babesia divergens* have been identified in most human cases, but variants (considered different species) have been recently identified. Little is known about the occurrence of *Babesia* species in malaria-endemic areas where *Babesia* can easily be misdiagnosed as *Plasmodium* (CDC).

Life Cycle

The *Babesia microti* life cycle involves a tick and a rodent, usually the white-footed mouse, *Peromyscus leucopus*. During a blood meal, a *Babesia*-infected tick introduces sporozoites into the mouse host ❶ [Figure 4-5]. Sporozoites enter erythrocytes and undergo asexual reproduction (budding) ❷. Some parasites differentiate into male and female gametes, although these cannot be distinguished on routine microscopy ❸. The definitive host is the deer tick, *Ixodes dammini* (*I. scapularis*). Once ingested by a tick ❹, gametes unite and undergo a cycle which produces sporozoites ❺. Transovarial transmission (also known as "vertical," or hereditary, transmission) has been documented for "large" *Babesia* spp. but not for the "small" babesiae, such as *B. microti* **A**.

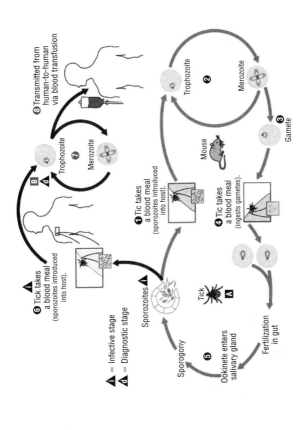

Figure 4-5 Life cycle of babesiosis.

83

Humans enter the cycle when bitten by infected ticks, which introduce sporozoites into the human host ❻. These enter erythrocytes ⒝ and undergo asexual replication (budding) ❼. Multiplication of the blood stage parasites is responsible for the clinical manifestations of the disease. Humans are, for all practical purposes, "dead-end hosts" and there is little, if any, subsequent transmission through ticks feeding on infected persons. In contrast, human to human transmission is well recognized to occur through blood transfusions ❽.

Note: Since deer are the natural hosts of these ticks, they are an integral part of the *Babesia* cycle, in that they influence the tick population. When deer populations increase, the tick population also increases, thus heightening the potential for transmission (CDC).

Clinical Presentation

Infection presents gradually, with malaise, fatigue, anorexia, shaking chills, fever, headache, myalgias, arthralgias, nausea, vomiting, abdominal pain, emotional lability, and dark urine. Photophobia, conjunctivitis, sore throat, and cough are also encountered. Adult respiratory distress syndrome, shock, petechiae, splinter hemorrhages, and ecchymoses have occasionally been noted. Splenomegaly and hepatomegaly are also described, but lymphadenopathy is not seen. Hemolytic anemia and elevated reticulocyte counts are noted. In most cases, 1 to 10% of erythrocytes are parasitized, but as many as 85% infection rates have been encountered in severe cases. The leukocyte count might be normal or decreased, and thrombocytopenia is common. Urinalysis reveals proteinuria and hemoglobinuria, and blood urea nitrogen and serum creatinine levels might be elevated. Mild hepatic dysfunction might also be seen.

Reference
Babesiosis. Centers for Disease Control Web site. Available at: http://www.dpd.cdc.gov/dpdx/HTML/Babesiosis.htm. Accessed April 15, 2005.

Further Reading

Babesia infection. Centers for Disease Control Web site. Available at: http://www.cdc.gov/ncidod/dpd/parasites/babesia/default.htm. Accessed April 15, 2005.

Gorenflot A, Moubri K, Precigout E, Carcy B, Schetters TP. Human babesiosis. *Ann Trop Med Parasitol.* 1998;92: 489-501.

Gray J, von Stedingk LV, Granstrom M. Zoonotic babesiosis. *Int J Med Microbiol.* 2002; 291(suppl)33:108-111.

Kjemtrup AM, Conrad PA. Human babesiosis: an emerging tick-borne disease. *Int J Parasitol.* 2000;30:1323-1337.

Pruthi RK, Marshall WF, Wiltsie JC, Persing DH. Human babesiosis. *Mayo Clin Proc.* 1995;70:853-862.

White DJ, Talarico J, Chang HG, Birkhead GS, Heimberger T, Morse DL. Human babesiosis in New York State: review of 139 hospitalized cases and analysis of prognostic factors. *Arch Intern Med.* 1998;158:2149-2154.

Balantidiasis

Ciliary Dysentery

Agent
Protozoa. Ciliate: *Balantidium coli.*

Reservoir
Pigs, nonhuman primates, rodents

Vector
None

Vehicle
Water, food

Geographic Distribution
Worldwide

Incubation Period
1–7d (range 1–60d)

Diagnostic Tests
Microscopy of stool or colonic aspirates

Typical Adult Therapy
Tetracycline 500 mg q.i.d. $\times$ 10d
Or metronidazole 750 mg t.i.d. $\times$ 5d
Or iodiquinol 650 mg t.i.d. $\times$ 20d

Typical Pediatric Therapy
Age $\geq$ 8 years: tetracycline 10 mg/kg q.i.d. (max 2g/d) $\times$
    10d
Age < 8 yrs, metronidazole 15 mg/kg t $\times$ 5d; or
    iodoquinol 13 mg/kg t.i.d. $\times$ 20d

Background

- Balantidiasis is found worldwide, but is most common
  in areas of poor sanitation, particularly in proximity to
  pigs. The pigs themselves do not manifest clinical
  illness. Other potential reservoirs include rodents and
  nonhuman primates.
- Carriage by pigs in some areas can range from 40 to
  90%; however, the organism is rarely present in more
  than 1% of humans in these areas. Trophozoites reside
  in the lumen of the large intestine of humans and

animals, where they replicate by binary fission with occasional conjugation.
- Cysts are formed and passed with feces. The cyst is the infectious stage and is acquired by the host through ingestion of contaminated food or water. Following ingestion, excystation occurs in the small intestine, and the trophozoites colonize the large intestine.
- Fewer than 1,000 cases had been reported prior to 1988. Worldwide prevalence is estimated at 0.02 to 0.12%.

Causal Agent

Balantidium coli, a large ciliated protozoan parasite (CDC).

Life Cycle

Cysts are the parasite stage responsible for transmission of balantidiasis ❶ [Figure 4-6]. The host most often acquires the cyst through ingestion of contaminated food or water ❷. Following ingestion, excystation occurs in the small intestine ❸. The trophozoites then reside in the lumen of the large intestine of humans and animals, where replication by binary fission, and conjugation occur ❹. Trophozoites undergo encystation to produce infective cysts ❺. Some trophozoites invade the colonic wall and multiply; while others return to the lumen and disintegrate. Mature cysts are passed with feces ❶ (CDC).

Clinical Presentation

Most cases are asymptomatic. Clinical manifestations, when present, include persistent diarrhea, occasionally

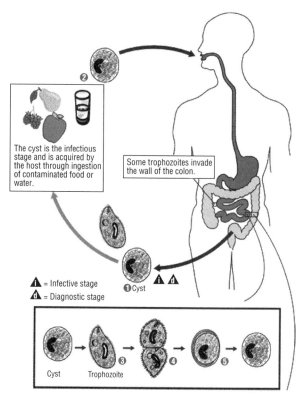

Figure 4-6   Life cycle of balantidiasis.

dysentery, abdominal pain, and weight loss. Symptoms can be severe in debilitated individuals. *Balantidium* pneumonia has been reported in immune-compromised patients.

Diagnosis is based on detection of trophozoites in stool specimens or in tissue collected during endoscopy. Cysts are less frequently encountered. *B. coli* is passed intermittently and once outside the colon is rapidly destroyed. Thus stool specimens should be collected repeatedly, and immediately examined or preserved.

Reference

Balantidiasis. Centers for Disease Control Web site. Available at: http://www.dpd.cdc.gov/dpdx/HTML/Balantidiasis.htm. Accessed April 15, 2005.

Further Reading

Balantidium infection. Centers for Disease Control Web site. Available at: http://www.cdc.gov/ncidod/dpd/parasites/balantidium/default.htm. Accessed April 15, 2005.

Garcia LS. Flagellates and ciliates. *Clin Lab Med.* 1999;19:621-638.

Kaur R, Rawat D, Kakkar M, Uppal B, Sharma VK. Intestinal parasites in children with diarrhea in Delhi, India. *Southeast Asian J Trop Med Public Health.* 2002;33:725-729.

Nakauchi K. The prevalence of Balantidium coli infection in fifty-six mammalian species. *J Vet Med Sci.* 1999;61:63-65.

Weiss LM, Keohane EM. The uncommon gastrointestinal protozoa: Microsporidia, Blastocystis, Isospora, Dientamoeba, and Balantidium. *Curr Clin Top Infect Dis.* 1997;17:147-187.

Baylisascaris procyonis

Agent
Nematoda. Phasmidea: *B. procyonis.*

Reservoir
Mammals (more than 40 species), birds

Vector
None

Vehicle
Animal feces (usually raccoon)

Geographic Distribution
To date, the parasite has been identified in Canada, Germany, the United States, and the Netherlands.

REGION I—NAm	CAN, USA
REGION VIII—Eur	DEU, NLD

Incubation Period
Unknown

Diagnostic Tests
Serology or identification of larvae in tissue

Typical Therapy
Although therapeutic guidelines have not been established, levamisole, albendazole, mebendazole, and thiabendazole are effective in animal models. Corticosteroids might be helpful. Laser ablation has been suggested for retinal larva.

Background

- A variety of *Baylisascaris* species are found in as many as 90 species of mammals, including raccoons (*B. procyonis*), skunks (*B. columnaris*), martens (*B. devosi*), and bears (*B. laevis*). *B. procyonis* is distributed throughout North America and Europe, with a predominance in northern areas. Human and animal infestation have been described in the United States, Germany, and the Netherlands. Infested animals have also been reported in Canada.
- As many as 50 to 60% of raccoons (*Procyon lotor*) in endemic areas are asymptomatically infected. In the

raccoon, the organism lives in the small intestine. The adult worm can grow to 14 to 18 cm long by 0.8 cm diameter. Eggs are ovoid, with a finely pitted outer shell, and measure 70 × 55 microns. Infected raccoons shed millions of eggs daily. After 3 to 4 weeks in the environment, the eggs are infective and are eaten by young raccoons. Older raccoons are frequently infected by eating an intermediate host such as mouse, squirrel, or bird that is infected with the larvae. Eggs can survive for years in soil.

• A single adult female worm produces 115,000 to 877,000 eggs daily; an infected raccoon can shed as many as 45,000,000 eggs daily. The infective dose for humans is estimated at fewer than 5,000 eggs. Humans acquire infection through ingestion of eggs in contaminated soil. In humans, dogs, and intermediate hosts, larvae invade other organs, the central nervous system, and the eye. Migrating larvae reach a length of 1.5 to 2.0 mm in size;. 5 to 7% of the larvae migrate to the brain.

Causal Agent

Human baylisascariasis is caused by larvae of *Baylisascaris procyonis*, an intestinal nematode of raccoons (CDC).

Life Cycle

Baylisascaris procyonis completes its life cycle in raccoons (*Procyon lotor*), with humans acquiring the infection as accidental hosts. Following ingestion by an animal (over 50 species of birds and mammals, especially rodents, have been identified as intermediate hosts) eggs hatch and larvae penetrate the gut wall [Figure 4-7] and migrate into various tissues, where they encyst. The life cycle is completed when raccoons eat infected tissues. Larvae develop into egg-laying adult worms in the small intestine and eggs are eliminated in raccoon feces. Humans are accidentally infected when they ingest infective eggs from the environment; typically in the setting of young children playing in the dirt. After ingestion, the eggs hatch and larvae penetrate the gut wall and migrate to a wide variety of tissues (liver, heart, lungs, brain, eyes), to produce visceral (VLM) and ocular (OLM) larva migrans syndromes, similar to that associated with toxocariasis. In contrast to *Toxocara* larvae, *Baylisascaris* larvae continue to grow during their time in the human host. Tissue damage and the signs and symptoms of baylisascariasis are relatively severe because of the size of *Baylisascaris* larvae, their tendency to wander widely, and the fact that they do not readily die (CDC).

Clinical Presentation

This diagnosis should be considered in patients with signs suggestive of visceral larva migrans who live in areas inhabited by raccoons. Clinical manifestations include eosinophilic encephalitis, ocular disease, and eosinophilic cardiac pseudotumor. Eosinophilic meningitis might be present. Eye involvement is referred to as diffuse unilateral subacute neuroretinitis (DUSN). Asymptomatic infection has been reported.

Reference

Baylisascariasis. Centers for Disease Control Web site. Available at: http://www.dpd.cdc.gov/dpdx/HTML/Baylisascariasis. htm. Accessed April 15, 2005.

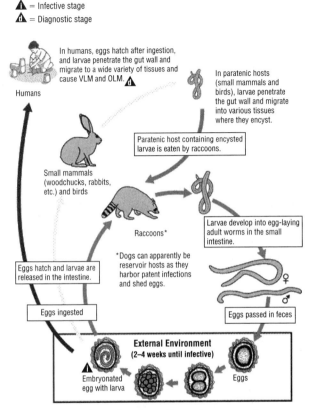

Figure 4-7   Life cycle of *Baylisacaris procyonis.*

Further Reading

Baylisascaris infection: raccoon roundworm infection. Centers
for Disease Control Web site. Available at: http://www.
cdc.gov/ncidod/dpd/parasites/baylisascaris/default.htm.
Accessed April 15, 2005.

Gavin PJ, Shulman ST. Raccoon roundworm (Baylisascaris procyonis). *Pediatr Infect Dis J*. 2003;22:651-652.

Park SY, Glaser C, Murray WJ, et al. Raccoon roundworm (Baylisascaris procyonis) encephalitis: case report and field investigation. *Pediatrics*. 2000;106:E56.

Sorvillo F, Ash LR, Berlin OG, Morse SA. Baylisascaris procyonis: an emerging helminthic zoonosis. *Emerg Infect Dis*. 2002;8:355-359.

Bertielliasis

Agent
Platyhelminthes, Cestoda. Cyclophyllidea, Anoplocephalidae: *Bertiella studeri* (rarely *B. mucronata*, from monkeys).

Reservoir
Nonhuman primates

Vector
None

Vehicle
Ingestion of mites

Geographic Distribution

REGION I—NAm	USA
REGION III—SAm	ARG, BRA, ECU, GUY, PRY
REGION IV—Carib	CUB, KNA
REGION VI—CAfr	COG, GAB, GNQ, KEN, MUS
REGION IX—MidEast	YEM
REGION X—IndSub	IND, LKA
REGION XI—Asia	SGP
REGION XII—SEA	IDN, MYS, PHL, THA

Incubation Period
Unknown

Diagnostic Tests
Identification of ova or proglottids in stool

Typical Therapy
Not established

Background

- *Bertiella* are tapeworm parasites of monkeys and other primates. Human infection is thought to result from inadvertant ingestion of infected orabitid (forest litter) mites. Ingested larvae then develop into adults measuring 20 to 30 cm.
- The first case of human bertielliasis was reported in 1913. As of 1997, 45 cases had been reported in the world's literature.
- Of 39 cases ascribed to *B. studeri*, four were reported from Mauritius, 11 in India, 9 in Sumatra, 2 in Java, 1 each in Borneo, Singapore, St. Kitts, the Philippines, Malaysia, Sri Lanka, Yemen, Equatorial Guinea, Thailand, and Gabon.
- Of five cases ascribed to *B. mucronata*, two were reported from Brazil, and one each from Argentina, Cuba, and Paraguay.
- A related cestode, *Inermicapsifer madagascariensis* (*Raillietina madacasariensis*), a parasite of rodents, is acquired through accidental ingestion of insects. Human infection has been reported in Africa, Central America, and South America. Most cases have been asymptomatic, with some complaining of anorexia and mild abdominal pain. *R. celebensis* infection has been reported in French Polynesia, and *R. demeriensis* infection in Ecuador.

Clinical Presentation

The few cases reported have ranged from asymptomatic infection to moderate abdominal pain, vomiting and diarrhea. Symptoms might be intermittent or continuous. Adult tapeworms are known to live for at least two years. Diagnosis is based on finding worms, worm segments, or ova in stool.

Further Reading

Bandyopadhyay AK, Manna B. The pathogenic and zoonotic potentiality of Bertiella studeri. *Ann Trop Med Parasitol.* 1987;81:465-456.

Galan-Puchades MT, Fuentes MV, Mas-Coma S. Human Bertiella studeri in Spain, probably of African origin. *Am J Trop Med Hyg.* 1997;56:610-612.

Panda DN, Panda MR. Record of Bertiella studeri (Blanchard, 1891), an anaplocephalid tapeworm, from a child. *Ann Trop Med Parasitol.* 1994;88:451-452.

Blastocystis hominis

Agent

Protozoa. Chromista, Bigyra, Blastocystea: *B. hominis* (taxonomic status remains uncertain).

Reservoir

Humans

Vector

None

Vehicle

Fecal–oral

Geographic Distribution

Worldwide

Incubation Period
Unknown

Diagnostic Tests
Stool microscopy

Typical Adult Therapy
Metronidazole 750 mg t.i.d. × 10d.
Cotrimoxazole has also been used.

Typical Pediatric Therapy
Metronidazole 15 mg/kg/d × 10d.
Cotrimoxazole has also been used.

Background

- *B. hominis* is found worldwide—its role in disease is controversial. As many as 1.5 to 10% of people in developed countries carry the parasite. A search for alternative etiologies (including other infectious agents) should always be made in such patients.
- Morphologically, *B. hominis* could be confused with *Dientamoeba fragilis*. The organism was once classified as a fungus, and its taxonomic status remains uncertain. Some authorities place *Blastocystis* in a separate kingdom (Chromista) distinct from the Protozoa.

Causal Agent

The taxonomic classification of *Blastocystis hominis* is mired in controversy. It has been previously considered as yeasts, fungi, or ameboid, flagellated, or sporozoan protozoa. Recently, however, based on molecular studies, especially dealing with the sequence information on the complete SSUrRNA gene, *B. hominis* has been placed within an informal group, the stramenopiles (Silberman et al. 1996). Stramenopiles are defined, based on molecular phylogenies, as a heterogeneous evolutionary assemblage of unicellular and multicellular protists including brown algae, diatoms, chrysophytes, water molds, slime nets, etc. (Patterson, 1994). Cavalier-Smith (1998) considers stramenopiles to be identical to his infrakingdom Heterokonta under the kingdom Chromista. Therefore, according to Cavalier-Smith, *B. hominis* is a heterokontid chromista (CDC).

Life Cycle

The following is the presumed life cycle of *B. hominis*. The classic form found in human stools is the cyst, which varies from 6 to 40 μm in diameter ❶ [Figure 4-8]. Presumably, cysts in stool ❶ are responsible for external transmission through ingestion of contaminated water or food ❷. Cysts infect epithelial cells of the digestive tract and multiply asexually (❸, ❹). Vacuolar forms of the parasite give origin to multi vacuolar ❺a and ameboid ❺b forms. The multi-vacuolar form develops into a pre-cyst ❻a which evolves to a thin-walled cyst ❼a, thought to be responsible for auto infection. The ameboid form evolves to a pre-cyst ❻b, which develops into thick-walled cyst through schizogony ❼b. The thick-walled cyst is excreted in feces ❶ (CDC).

Clinical Presentation
Some authorities in the field have ascribed symptoms such as leucocyte-negative diarrhea, nausea, flatulence, and abdominal distention to overgrowth of this protozoan. Symptoms usually last for 3 to 10 days, but might persist for weeks or months.

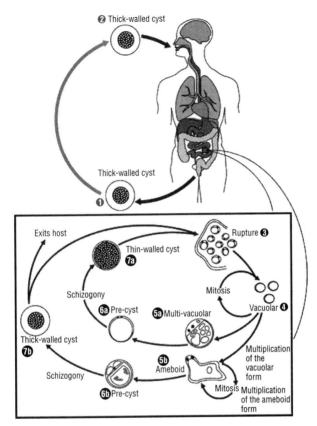

Figure 4-8   Life cycle of *Blastocystis hominus*.
Source: Blastocystis hominis stages were reproduced
from Singh M, Suresh K, Ho LC, Ng GC, Yap EH.
Elucidation of the life cycle of the intestinal protozoan Blastocystis hominis. *Parasitol Res.* 1995;81:449.
Copyright held by Springer-Verlag and reproduced
here by permission of Springer-Verlag and M. Singh.

References

Blastocystis hominis infection. Centers for Disease Control Web site. Available at: http://www.dpd.cdc.gov/dpdx/HTML/Blastocystis.htm. Accessed April 15, 2005.

Cavalier-Smith T. A revised six-kingdom system of life. *Biol Rev Camb Philos Soc.* 1998;73:203-266.

Patterson DJ. Protozoa, evolution and systematics. In: Housmann K, Hulsmann N, eds. *Progress in Protozoology.* Stuttgart, Germany: Fischer; 1994:1-14.

Silberman JD, Sogin ML, Leipe DD, Clark CG. Human parasite finds taxonomic home. *Nature.* 1996;380:398.

Capillaria hepatica

Calodiasis, Capillary Liver Worm, Hepatic Capillariasis

The Agent
Nematoda. Aphasmidia: *Capillaria (Calodium) hepatica*

Reservoir
Rats

Vector
None

Vehicle
Soil

Geographic Distribution
Capillariasis—hepatic

REGION I—NAm	USA
REGION II—CAm	MEX
REGION III—SAm	BRA
REGION VI—CAfr	NGA

REGION VII—SAfr	ZAF
REGION VIII—Eur	CHE, CZE, GRC, ITA, SVK
REGION IX—MidEast	TUR
REGION X—IndSub	IND
REGION XI—Asia	JPN, KOR, PRK

Incubation Period
21–28d

Diagnostic Tests
Visualization of ova or adults in liver tissue

Typical Therapy
None available

Background

- The first case of human infection was reported in 1924. Only 28 cases were reported worldwide as of 1999.
- Human infection is rare, and has been reported from Africa, Asia, Europe, and the Americas. Humans acquire the disease through ingestion of embryonated eggs in soil, food or water. Asymptomatic passage of eggs might follow ingestion of infected liver. Eggs can remain viable in soil for several months.
- *C. hepatica* is found in rodents worldwide, and is a common parasite of rats, and less commonly of squirrels, muskrats, hares, beavers, chimpanzees and monkeys. The infestation rate in rats (*Rattus norvegicus*) is 7 to 90%.
- *C. aerophila* is found in cats, dogs, foxes (notably domestic *Vulpes vulpes*) and other carnivores. Ova are passed with feces and ingested by earthworms. When mature ova are ingested by a dog (or accidentally by a human) larvae are released and migrate to the lungs.

- *Anatrichosoma cutaneum* produces subcutaneous tracts in the soles and palms of monkeys (notably macaques). Ova emerge from skin exudate to the soil, and appear to infect the host by ingestion. Only two cases of human infection had been reported to 2003.

Causal Agents

The nematode (roundworm) *Capillaria philippinensis* causes human intestinal capillariasis. Two other *Capillaria* species parasitize animals, with rare reported instances of human infections. They are *C. hepatica*, which causes in humans hepatic capillariasis, and *C. aerophila*, which causes in humans pulmonary capillariasis (CDC).

Life Cycle

Typically, unembryonated eggs are passed in the human stool ❶ [Figure 4-9] and become embryonated in the external environment ❷. After ingestion by freshwater fish, larvae hatch, penetrate the intestine, and migrate to the tissues ❸. Ingestion of raw or undercooked fish results in infection of the human host ❹. The adults of *Capillaria philippinensis* (males: 2.3 to 3.2 mm; females: 2.5 to 4.3 mm) reside in the human small intestine, where they burrow into the mucosa ❺. Females deposit unembryonated eggs, some of which become embryonated in the intestine, and release larvae that can cause autoinfection or hyperinfection (a massive number of adult worms) ❻. *Capillaria philippinesis* is currently considered a parasite of fish-eating birds, which seem to be the natural definitive host ❼.

Adults of *Capillaria hepatica* reside in the livers of various animals, especially rats. The females produce eggs that are

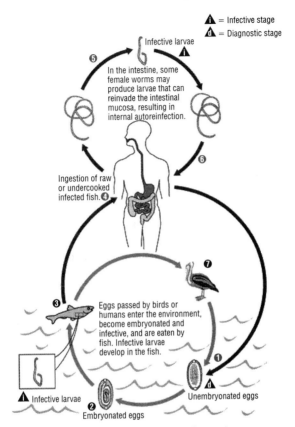

= Infective stage

= Diagnostic stage

Infective larvae

⑤ In the intestine, some female worms may produce larvae that can reinvade the intestinal mucosa, resulting in internal autoreinfection.

Ingestion of raw or undercooked infected fish. **④**

⑥

⑦

③

Eggs passed by birds or humans enter the environment, become embryonated and infective, and are eaten by fish. Infective larvae develop in the fish.

①

Unembryonated eggs

Infective larvae **②**

Embryonated eggs

Figure 4-9   Life cycle of *Capillaria hepatica*.

retained in the liver parenchyma. When the infected animal is eaten by another animal, the eggs are released by digestion, excreted in the feces of the second animal, and become embryonated in the soil. Alternatively, eggs can be released following the death and decomposition of the

first animal, and mature in the soil. Following ingestion
by a subsequent host, these infective eggs release larvae in
the intestine that migrate through the portal circulation
to the liver, where they develop into adults.

Adults of *C. aerophila* reside in the epithelium of the
tracheo-bronchial tree of various animals. Eggs are produced, coughed up, swallowed by the animal, and excreted
in its feces. The eggs become embryonated in the soil.
Ingestion of infective eggs completes the cycle. Transport
or paratenic hosts may also intervene in the cycle (CDC).

Clinical Presentation
The spectrum of infestation extends from asymptomatic
infestation to fatal disease. Symptoms include fever, tender hepatomegaly with hepatic dysfunction, abdominal
distention, and eosinophilia. Splenomegaly and pneumonia have been reported.

   C. aerophila infection is characterized by cough,
bronchitis, fever, and eosinophilia.

   A. cutaneum infection is characterized by dermal lesions and pruritis of the fingers or feet.

Reference
Capillariasis. Centers for Disease Control Web site. Available
   at: http://www.dpd.cdc.gov/dpdx/HTML/Capillariasis.htm.
   Accessed April 15, 2005.

Further Reading
Attah EB, Nagarajan S, Obineche EN, Gera SC. Hepatic capillariasis. *Am J Clin Pathol.* 1983;79:127-130.

Bhattacharya D, Patel AK, Das SC, Sikdar A. Capillaria hepatica, a parasite of zoonotic importance—a brief overview.
   J Commun Dis. 1999; 31:267-269.

Kokai GK, Perisic VN. How frequent is Capillaria hepatica infestation in Europe? *Eur J Pediatr.* 1990;150:72.

Capillaria philippinensis

Aonchotheciasis, Intestinal Capillariasis

Agent
Nematoda. Aphasmidia: *Capillaria (Aonchotheca) philippinensis.*

Reservoir
Not well established; possibly birds or fish

Vector
None

Vehicle
Food; possibly poorly cooked small fish

Geographic Distribution
REGION III—SAm	COL
REGION V—NAfr	EGY
REGION IX—MidEast	ARE, IRN
REGION X—IndSub	IND
REGION XI—Asia	JPN, KOR, PRK, TWN
REGION XII—SEA	IDN, PHL, THA

Incubation Period
Usually a few weeks

Diagnostic Tests
Identification of ova or adults in stool, tissue or duodenal aspirate

Typical Therapy
Mebendazole 200 mg b.i.d. × 20d
Or albendazole 200 mg b.i.d. × 10d
Or thiabendazole 12.5 mg/kg b.i.d. × 30d

Background

- Intestinal capillariasis was first described in the Philippines in 1964. The parasite is found in Thailand, the Philippines, Korea, Indonesia, and India, with rare reports from Japan, Egypt, and Iran (presumably related to ingestion of imported fish).
- *C. philippinensis* is a parasite of the human small intestine. Both males and females measure about 4 mm in length. Eggs and larvae are passed in the feces. Eggs embryonate when they reach water and are eaten by fish. The eggs hatch in the fish, and juveniles mature into infective forms in a few weeks. The definitive host is infected when it eats the fish containing infective larvae. Larvae can reinfect the host directly (autoinfection), resulting in massive infections reminiscent of strongyloidiasis.
- In the Philippines, the disease is endemic to north Luzon, Agusan del Norte (Mindanao) and St. Bernard (Leyte). Cases have also been reported in Compostela Valley Province. In Northern Luzon during 1967–1990, 1,884 cases (110 fatal) were registered. A male/female ratio of 2/1 is ascribed to ingestion of kinilaw (raw fish) while working.

Clinical Presentation

Asymptomatic infestation is reported. Heavy infections are manifest as watery diarrhea, abdominal cramps, malaise, eosinophilia, hypoalbuminemia, and malabsorption syndromes. Case-fatality rates of 10 to 20% have been registered.

Further Reading

Capillariasis. Centers for Disease Control Web site. Available at: http://www.dpd.cdc.gov/dpdx/HTML/Capillariasis.htm. Accessed April 15, 2005.

Cross JH. Intestinal capillariasis. *Clin Microbiol Rev.* 1992;5:120-129.

Dronda F, Chaves F, Sanz A, Lopez-Velez R. Human intestinal capillariasis in an area of nonendemicity: case report and review. *Clin Infect Dis.* 1993;17:909-912.

McCarthy J, Moore TA. Emerging helminth zoonoses. *Int J Parasitol.* 2000;30:1351-1360.

Cercarial Dermatitis

Clam Digger's Itch, Duck Itch, Schistosome Dermatitis, Swimmer's Itch

Agent
Platyhelminthes, Trematoda. Avian schistosomes: *Trichobilharzia, Heterobilharzia, Orientobilharzia, Diplostomum spathaceum, et al, Schistosoma spindale.*

Reservoir
Aquatic birds and snails (various)

Vector
None

Vehicle
Water—skin contact

Geographic Distribution
Although reports have been published by the following countries, cercarial dermatitis is felt to have a near worldwide distribution among countries having suitable bodies of water, water fowl, etc.: Argentina, Australia, Canada, China, Colombia, Denmark, France, Germany, Iceland, Japan, Malaysia, Netherlands, New Zealand, Poland, Russian Federation, Scotland, South Africa, Suriname, Switzerland, Taiwan, United Kingdom, United States, Venezuela

Incubation Period
A few hours (range 1h–5d)

Diagnostic Tests
No test available

Typical Therapy
Supportive

Background

- Cercarial dermatitis is acquired from saltwater and freshwater bodies worldwide.
- Indigenous peoples (ie, in Africa) are rarely affected.
- Although human schistosomiasis is also characterized by an initial stage of cercarial dermatitis, the local symptoms associated with avian schistosomes are more intense.
- The most common genus causing human infection is *Trichobilharzia*, which has a worldwide distribution. Other genera include *Heterobilharzia* (North America), *Orientobilharzia* (Asia), *Schistosomatium* (North America), *Austrobilharzia* (worldwide), *Bilharziella* (Northern Hemisphere), *Microbilharzia* (North America), and *Gigantobilharzia* (worldwide).

Clinical Presentation
Symptoms of pricking sensation and pruritis associated with rash might begin from within 1 hour to as long as 5 days following exposure. The rash can be macular, ur-ticarial, or manifest as diffuse erythema—with progres-sion to papules and vesicles. Lesions are most common on the legs and feet. Systemic symptoms are uncommon; however, fever and lymphadenopathy are seen following repeated exposure.

Further Reading

Anonymous. Cercarial dermatitis outbreak at a state park—Delaware, 1991. *MMWR Morb Mortal Wkly Rep.* 1992;41(14):225-228.

Baird JK, Wear DJ. Cercarial dermatitis: the swimmer's itch. *Clin Dermatol.* 1987;5:88-91.

Folster-Holst R, Disko R, Rowert J, Bockeler W, Kreiselmaier I, Christophers E. Cercarial dermatitis contracted via contact with an aquarium: case report and review. *Br J Dermatol.* 2001;145:638-640.

Gonzalez E. Schistosomiasis, cercarial dermatitis, and marine dermatitis. *Dermatol Clin.* 1989;7:291-300.

Levesque B, Giovenazzo P, Guerrier P, Laverdiere D, Prud'Homme H. Investigation of an outbreak of cercarial dermatitis. *Epidemiol Infect.* 2002;129:379-386.

Mulvihill CA, Burnett JW. Swimmer's itch: a cercarial dermatitis. *Cutis.* 1990;46:211-213.

Schistosomiasis. Centers for Disease Control Web site. Available at: http://www.cdc.gov/ncidod/dpd/parasites/schistosomiasis/default.htm. Accessed April 15, 2005.

Clonorchis sinensis

Chinese Liver Fluke

Agent
Platyhelminthes, Trematoda. Plagiorchiida, Opisthorchiidae: *C. (Opisthorchis) sinensis.*

Reservoir
Humans, cats, dogs, pigs, snails (*Bythnia, Alocinma, Semisulcospira*)

Vector
None

Vehicle
Freshwater fish; occasionally crayfish

Geographic Distribution

REGION IX—MidEast	IRN
REGION XI—Asia	CHN, HKG, JPN, KOR, MAC, PRK, RUS, SGP, TWN
REGION XII—SEA	IDN, KHM, LAO, MMR, MYS, PHL, THA, VNM

Incubation Period
21–28d (range 10–2y)

Diagnostic Tests
Identification of ova in stool or duodenal aspirate

Typical Adult Therapy
Praziquantel 25 mg/kg t.i.d. × 1d
Or albendazole 10 mg/kg × 7d

Typical Pediatric Therapy
Praziquantel 25 mg/kg t.i.d. × 1d

Background

- Human infection by *C. sinensis* was first discovered in 1875. Adult parasites live in the smaller intrahepatic bile ducts of the final hosts (humans, cats, dogs, other fish-eating mammals).
- Most susceptible fish belong to the family Cyprinidae (less commonly, Anabantidae), with prevalence rates dependent on season, fish species, and water quality. Ova are viable in water for 5 weeks, and miracidia for

20 minutes. Infective cysts can withstand heating to 70°C for 15 minutes.

- Although infection has been largely eliminated from Japan and Korea, clonorchiasis remains prevalent in parts of Taiwan, Hong Kong, Vietnam, and China. Infection is generally first noted among teenagers, and rates increase with age. An association with cholangiocarcinoma has been established.

- The principal intermediate (snail) hosts are *Parafossarulus manchouricus* and *Bulinus fuschsiana*. *Bythnia longicornis*, *Assiminea lutea*, and *Melanoides tuberculatus* can also be involved in transmission.

Causal Agent

The trematode *Clonorchis sinensis* (Chinese or oriental liver fluke) (CDC).

Life Cycle

Embryonated eggs are discharged via the biliary ducts to the stool ❶ [Figure 4-10]. Eggs are ingested by a suitable snail intermediate host ❷, of which there there are more than 100 species. Each egg releases a miracidium ❷ⓐ, which goes through several developmental stages (sporocysts ❷ⓑ, rediae ❷ⓒ, and cercariae ❷ⓓ). The cercariae are released from the snail, and after a short period of free-swimming in water, come in contact and penetrate the flesh of freshwater fish, where they encyst as metacercariae ❸. Infection of humans occurs by ingestion of undercooked, salted, pickled, or smoked freshwater fish ❹. After ingestion, the metacercariae excyst in the duodenum ❺ and ascend the biliary tract through the ampulla of Vater ❻. Maturation takes approximately 1 month. Adult flukes (measuring 10 to 25 mm by 3 to 5 mm) reside in

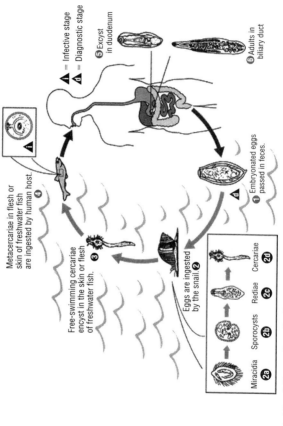

Metacercariae in flesh or skin of freshwater fish are ingested by human host.

❹

Free-swimming cercariae encyst in the skin or flesh of freshwater fish.

❸

▲ = Infective stage
◢ = Diagnostic stage

❺ Excyst in duodenum

❻ Adults in biliary duct

❼ Embryonated eggs passed in feces.

Eggs are ingested by the snail ❷

Miracidia ❷ⓐ Sporocysts ❷ⓑ Rediae ❷ⓒ Cercariae ❷ⓓ

Figure 4-10   Life cycle of *Clonorchis sinensis*.

112

small and medium sized biliary ducts. In addition to humans, carnivorous animals serve as reservoir hosts (CDC).

Clinical Presentation

Initial symptoms include fever, epigastric and right upper quadrant pain, eosinophilia and diarrhea. Chronic infection is often asymptomatic, but might be manifest as cholangitis, cholecystitis, pancreatitis and biliary obstruction. Adults are known to survive for as long as 25 years in the human host. Complications include secondary bacterial infection and cholangiocarcinoma.

Reference

Clonorchiasis. Centers for Disease Control Web site. Available at: http://www.dpd.cdc.gov/dpdx/HTML/Clonorchiasis.htm. Accessed April 15, 2005.

Further Reading

Clonorchis infection. Centers for Disease Control Web site. Available at: http://www.cdc.gov/ncidod/dpd/parasites/clonorchis/default.htm. Accessed April 15, 2005.

Keiser J, Utzinger J. Chemotherapy for major food-borne trematodes: a review. *Expert Opin Pharmacother.* 2004;5:1711-1726.

Wang KX, Zhang RB, Cui YB, Tian Y, Cai R, Li CP. Clinical and epidemiological features of patients with clonorchiasis. *World J Gastroenterol.* 2004;10:446-448.

Watanapa P, Watanapa WB. Liver fluke-associated cholangiocarcinoma. *Br J Surg.* 2002;89:962-970.

Coenurosis

Agent

Platyhelminthes, Cestoda. Cyclophyllidea, Taeniidae: *Multiceps* spp.

Reservoir
Sheep, wild carnivores, horses, dogs

Vector
None

Vehicle
Water, food, soil (contaminated by dogs)

Geographic Distribution

REGION I—NAm	USA
REGION II—CAm	MEX
REGION III—SAm	BRA, GUY
REGION VI—CAfr	AGO, BDI, COD, COG, GAB, KEN, NGA, RWA, UGA
REGION VII—SAfr	ZAF
REGION VIII—Eur	GBR, FRA

Incubation Period
Unknown

Diagnostic Tests
Identification of parasite in biopsy material

Typical Therapy
Excision

Background

- Human coenurosis has been reported from western Europe, the United States, and sub-Saharan Africa.
- *Taenia multiceps* is a parasite of dogs, which acquire the infection from sheep. The latter often have a cyst in the hindbrain which is clinically manifested as staggers.

- Extracranial disease is encountered in tropical Africa, but not elsewhere—suggesting that more than one species could be involved.
- Adult forms of *T. multiceps serialis* are found in canids in North America, with larval forms in hares, rabbits, and squirrels. Six cases of human infection were reported in North America to 1998.
- *T. crassiceps*, a tapeworm of canids in North America, rarely infects humans and presents as a cyst of the eye, brain, or subcutaneous tissues. Cases have been reported in Canada and France, including an AIDS patient with cysticerci in the soft tissues.

Clinical Presentation

Human infection has a predilection for the cysterna magna and presents as basal arachnoiditis and hydrocephalus. Subcutaneous tissue, muscle, and eye infections are also reported, characterized as cystic masses (often containing daughter cysts) which can attain the size of a hen's egg.

Further Reading

Francois A, Favennec L, Cambon-Michot C, et al. Taenia crassiceps invasive cysticercosis: a new human pathogen in acquired immunodeficiency syndrome? *Am J Surg Pathol.* 1998;22:488-492.

Hermos JA, Healy GR, Schultz MG, Barlow J, Church WG. Fatal human cerebral coenurosis. *JAMA.* 1970;213:1461-1464.

Ing MB, Schantz PM, Turner JA. Human coenurosis in North America: case reports and review. *Clin Infect Dis.* 1998;27:519-523.

Pau A, Turtas S, Brambilla M, Leoni A, Rosa M, Viale GL. Computed tomography and magnetic resonance imaging of cerebral coenurosis. *Surg Neurol.* 1987;27:548-552.

Cryptosporidiosis

Agent
Protozoa. Sporozoa, Apicomplexa: *Cryptosporidium parvum* (rarely *C. muris, C. felis, C. meleagridis, et al*).

Reservoir
Mammal (79 species identified as of 1997)

Vector
None

Vehicle
Water, feces, oysters, flies

Geographic Distribution
Worldwide

Incubation Period
5–10d (range 2–14d)

Diagnostic Tests
Stool/duodenal aspirate for acid-fast, direct fluorescence
  staining, or antigen assay
Nucleic acid amplification

Typical Adult Therapy
Nitazoxanide 500 mg PO b.i.d. $\times$ 3 days

Typical Pediatric Therapy
Nitazoxanide 100 mg PO b.i.d. $\times$ 3 days (for age $\geq$ 4 years)

Background

- *Cryptosporidium* was first recognized as a human
  pathogen in 1976. Only seven cases were reported
  during 1976 to 1982. Many thousands of cases of
  infection are now routinely reported, worldwide.

- *Cryptosporidium* oocysts are resistant to most disinfectants, including the usual levels of chlorine present in swimming pools. Oocysts can remain dormant for months in moist environments; but are susceptible to heat, cold, and drying (inactivated within 2 hours in dry atmosphere).
- Patients continue to excrete oocysts for weeks after symptoms resolve. The principal reservoirs are cattle and other domestic animals.
- Illness is acquired from food or water contaminated with fecal material. Transmission also can occur from person to person, animal to person, or contact with contaminated environmental surfaces. Infection is common among health-care workers, children and staff in nurseries, and tourists to developing countries.
- Infective *C. parvum* oocysts are found in mussels (*Mytilus galloprovincialis*) and cockles (*Cerastoderma edule*) from the shellfish-producing region (Galicia, northwest Spain, bounded by the Atlantic Ocean) that accounts for the majority of European shellfish production.
- Cryptosporidiosis accounts for 2 to 31.5% of pediatric diarrhea in Latin America. The organism is found in 1 to 3% of stool specimens in Europe and North America, and 5 to 10% in Asia and Africa; and is implicated in 14 to 24% of AIDS-associated diarrhea (6.6% in Europe). The highest rate of asymptomatic carriage (31.6%) has been documented in the Bolivian Altiplano.
- An outbreak of cryptosporidiosis in Wisconsin in 1993 consisted of 403,237 cases from contaminated water. This was the largest American waterborne outbreak ever described.
- Antibody is present in 32 to 58% of adults in developed countries. As of 1997, 79 species of mammals have been found to carry *C. parvum*.

- *C. parvum* is the usual species responsible for human infection. *C. parvum* genotype 1 is found only in humans, while genotypes 1 and 2 are found in both humans and animals.
- *C. muris* has recently been implicated (Indonesia, Thailand, France, Peru, and Kenya).
- Sporadic infections by *C. canis*, *C. felis* and *C. meleagridis* have been reported among immunocompromised patients, with rare cases in immunocompetent patients.

Causal Agent

Many species of *Cryptosporidium* exist that infect humans and a wide range of animals. Although *Cryptosporidium parvum* and *Cryptosporidium hominis* (formerly known as *C. parvum* anthroponotic genotype or genotype 1) are the most prevalent species causing disease in humans, infections by *C. felis*, *C. meleagridis*, *C. canis*, and *C. muris* have also been reported (CDC).

Life Cycle

Sporulated oocysts, containing 4 sporozoites, are excreted by the infected host through feces and possibly other routes such as respiratory secretions ❶ [Figure 4-11]. Transmission of *Cryptosporidium parvum* and *C. hominis* occurs mainly through water (eg, drinking or recreational water). Occasionally food sources, such as chicken salad, may serve as vehicles for transmission. Many outbreaks in the United States have occurred in water parks, community swimming pools, and day-care centers. Zoonotic and anthroponotic transmission of *C. parvum* and anthroponotic transmission of *C. hominis* occur through exposure to infected animals or exposure to water contaminated by animal feces ❷. Following ingestion (and possibly inhalation) by a suitable host ❸, excystation ❹ occurs. Sporozoites are released and parasitize epithelial cells (❺,❻) of the gastrointestinal tract or other tissues such as the respiratory tract. In these cells, the parasites undergo asexual multiplication (schizogony or merogony) (❻, ❼, ❽) and sexual multiplication (gametogony) producing microgamonts (male) ❾ and macrogamonts (female)❿. Upon fertilization of macrogamonts by the microgametes (⓫), oocysts (⓬,⓭) develop, which sporulate in the infected host. Two different forms of oocyst are produced: thick-walled, which is commonly excreted from the host ⓬, and thin-walled oocyst⓭, which is primarily involved in autoinfection. Oocysts are infective upon excretion, thus permitting direct and immediate fecal–oral transmission.

Note that oocysts of *Cyclospora cayetanensis*, another important coccidian parasite, are unsporulated at the time of excretion and do not become infective until sporulation is completed. Refer to the life cycle of *Cyclospora cayentanensis* for further details (CDC).

Clinical Presentation

Cryptosporidiosis affects the gastrointestinal tract and can be asymptomatic or associated with watery diarrhea and abdominal cramps. Fever and anorexia are uncommon, and fecal leukocytes are not seen. Although vomiting is not common among adults, it is often encountered in children. The disease persists for 1 to 20 days (mean 10) in immunocompetent individuals; however, protracted, severe diarrhea leading to malabsorption, dehydration, extraintestinal (ie, biliary or pulmonary) and fatal infection can develop in immunocompromised individuals.

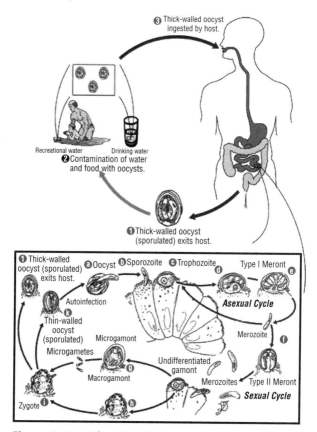

Figure 4-11   Life cycle of cryptosporidiosis. *Source:* Cryptosporidium stages were reproduced from Juranek DD. Cryptosporidiosis. In: Strickland GT, ed. *Hunter's Tropical Medicine and Emerging Infectious Diseases*, 8th ed. Philadelphia: WB Saunders; 2000. Originally adapted from the life cycle that appears in Current WL, Garcia LS. Cryptosporidiosis. *Clinc Microbiol Rev.* 1991;4:325-358.

Reference

Cryptosporidiosis. Centers for Disease Control Web site. Available at: http://www.dpd.cdc.gov/dpdx/HTML/ Cryptosporidiosis.htm. Accessed January 15, 2005.

Further Reading

Clark DP, Sears CL. The pathogenesis of cryptosporidiosis. *Parasitol Today.* 1996;12:221-225.

Cryptosporidiasis (Cryptosporidium infection). Centers for Disease Control Web site. Available at: http://www.cdc.gov/ ncidod/diseases/submenus/sub_crypto.htm. Accessed April 15, 2005.

Ramirez NE, Ward LA, Sreevatsan S. A review of the biology and epidemiology of cryptosporidiosis in humans and animals. *Microbes Infect.* 2004;6:773-785.

Xiao L, Fayer R, Ryan U, Upton SJ. Cryptosporidium taxonomy: recent advances and implications for public health. *Clin Microbiol Rev.* 2004;17:72-97.

Cutaneous Larva Migrans

Creeping Eruption, Plumber's Itch

Agent
Nematoda. Phasmidea: *Ancylostoma braziliense, A. caninum, Bunostomum phlebotomum, Strongyloides myopotami, et al.*

Reservoir
Cat, dog, cattle

Vector
None

Vehicle
Soil—contact

Incubation Period
2–3d (range 1–6d)

Diagnostic Tests
Biopsy is usually not helpful.

Typical Adult Therapy
Ivermectin 200 µg/kg as single dose
Or thiabendazole topical, and oral 25 mg/kg b.i.d. × 5d
   (max 3 g)
Or albendazole 200 mg b.i.d. × 3d

Typical Pediatric Therapy
Weight > 15 kg: ivermectin 200 µg/kg once
Or thiabendazole topical, and oral 25 mg/kg b.i.d. × 5d
   (max 3 g)
Or albendazole 2.5 mg/kg b.i.d. × 3d

Background

- Cutaneous larva migrans is most commonly acquired after skin (foot) contact with moist soil or beaches where dogs or cats are common. Most cases occur in warm, humid, tropical, and subtropical areas.
- The most common infecting species is *Ancylostotoma braziliense*. Other species which have been implicated include *A. caninum*, *Uncinaria stenocephala* (dogs), *A. ceylanicum* (dogs, cats, other carnivores), *Necator suillum* (pigs) and *B. phlebotomum* (cattle).

Life Cycle

Eggs are passed in the stool ❶ [Figure 4-12], and under favorable conditions (moisture, warmth, shade), larvae hatch in 1 to 2 days. The released rhabditiform larvae grow in the feces and/or the soil ❷, and after 5 to 10 days (and two molts) they become filariform (third-stage) larvae that are infective ❸. These infective larvae can survive 3 to 4 weeks in favorable environmental conditions. On contact with the human host, the larvae penetrate the skin and are carried through the veins to the heart and then to the lungs. They penetrate into the pulmonary alveoli, ascend the bronchial tree to the pharynx, and are swallowed ❹. The larvae reach the small intestine, where they reside and mature into adults. Adult worms live in the lumen of the small intestine, where they attach to the intestinal wall with resultant blood loss by the host ❺. Most adult worms are eliminated in 1 to 2 years, but longevity records can reach several years.

Some *A. duodenale* larvae, following penetration of the host skin, can become dormant (in the intestine or muscle). In addition, infection by *A. duodenale* may probably also occur by the oral and transmammary route. *N. americanus*, however, requires a transpulmonary migration phase (CDC).

Clinical Presentation
Erythematous, serpiginous, pruritic advancing lesion(s) or bullae—usually on feet; follows contact with moist sand or beachfront; can recur or persist for months. Lesions due to *A. braziliensis* and *A. caninum* are well defined and slow moving and can persist for months. Rare instances of retinitis and folliculitis caused by *A. caninum* have been reported.

Lesions of *Strongyloides* are less well defined, are rapidly moving, associated with a red flare, and persist for only a few hours (rare cases of *S. myopotami* and *S. procyornis* infection can be more persistent).

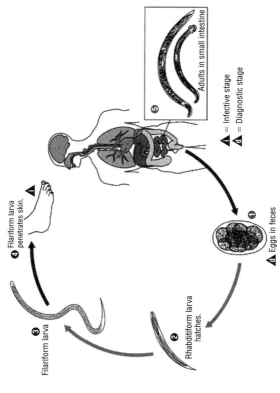

Figure 4-12   Life cycle of cutaneous larva migrans.

Adults in small intestine

▲ = Infective stage
△ = Diagnostic stage

⑤

① Eggs in feces

② Rhabditiform larva hatches.

③ Filariform larva

④ Filariform larva penetrates skin.

124

The initial lesions of human hookworm infestation (ground itch) are characterized by an irritating vesicular rash which can persist for a few days.

Gnathostomiasis might be associated with intermittent, pruritic or painful deep swellings which can persist for 1 to 4 weeks and then reappear elsewhere on the body after 1 week to several months. Occasionally, more superficial lesions might resemble those of *A. braziliensis* infection.

Occasionally, myiasis caused by *Gasterophilus* (acquired from horse contact) can mimic cutaneous larva migrans and persist for long periods. *Hypoderma ovis* and *H. lineatum* are occasionally associated with cattle contact and tend to produce deeper subcutaneous lesions.

Reference

Hookworm. Centers for Disease Control Web site. Available at: http://www.dpd.cdc.gov/dpdx/HTML/Hookworm.htm. Accessed April 15, 2005.

Further Reading

Heukelbach J, Wilcke T, Feldmeier H. Cutaneous larva migrans (creeping eruption) in an urban slum in Brazil. *Int J Dermatol*. 2004;43:511-515.

Hookworm. Centers for Disease Control Web site. Available at: http://www.dpd.cdc.gov/dpdx/HTML/Hookworm.htm. Accessed April 15, 2005.

Romano C, Albanese G, Gianni C. Emerging imported parasitoses in Italy. *Eur J Dermatol*. 2004;14:58-60.

Sherman SC, Radford N. Severe infestation of cutaneous larva migrans. *J Emerg Med*. 2004;26:347-349.

Cyclospora cayetanensis

Agent

Protozoa. Sporozoa, Apicomplexa: *Cyclospora cayetanensis*.

Reservoir
Humans, nonhuman primates

Vector
None

Vehicle
Water, vegetables

Incubation Period
1–11d

Geographic Distribution
The precise distribution is unknown; however, infection has been reported in most countries.

Diagnostic Tests
Identification of organism in stool smear.
Cold acid fast stains and ultraviolet microscopy could be helpful.

Typical Adult Therapy
Sulfamethoxazole/trimethoprim 800/160 mg b.i.d. × 7d

Typical Pediatric Therapy
Sulfamethoxazole/trimethoprim 10/2 mg/kg b.i.d. × 7d

Background

- Initially identified in Nepal as cyanobacterium-like bodies during the 1980s, *C. cayetanensis* is increasingly identified as an important cause of gastroenteritis worldwide. Various related species have been found in reptiles, moles, rodents, and chimpanzees, however it is unknown if any of these play a role in causing human disease. In retrospect, the first cases (three) were described in Papua New Guinea during 1977 to 1978.

- Water appears to be the principal vehicle for transmission; however, other routes for fecal–oral spread (eg, fruit) are also reported. Extensive outbreaks in the United States have been caused by raspberries imported from Guatemala.
- Cyclospora has been implicated in a number of sporadic cases and outbreaks of diarrhea in Nepal, Peru, Solomon Islands, Morocco, and other countries in North America, Central America, and South America, eastern Europe, and Asia, including India, Pakistan, and Cambodia.
- Initially, infections were associated with travel or residence in developing countries; however, more recent reports link the organism to ingestion of various fruits which were sprayed or washed with contaminated water.
- Cyclosporiasis displays a seasonal variability with more cases occurring in the warm and humid months of the year.

Causal Agent

The causal agent has been only recently identified as a unicellular coccidian parasite. The species designation *Cyclospora cayetanensis* was given in 1994 to Peruvian isolates of human-associated *Cyclospora*. It appears that all human cases are caused by this species (CDC).

Life Cycle

When passed in stools, the oocyst is not infective ❶ [Figure 4-13] (thus, direct fecal–oral transmission cannot occur; in contrast to another coccidian parasite, *Crypto-sporidium*). In the environment ❷, sporulation occurs after days or weeks at temperatures between 22°C to 32°C, resulting in division of the sporont into two sporo-cysts, each containing two elongate sporozoites ❸. Fresh produce and water can serve as vehicles for transmission ❹. Sporulated oocysts are ingested ❺ and excyst in the gastrointestinal tract, freeing sporozoites which invade epithelial cells of the small intestine ❻. Within these cells, parasites undergo asexual multiplication and develop-ment to mature oocysts, which will be shed in stools ❼. The potential mechanisms of contamination of food and water are still under investigation (CDC).

Clinical Presentation

The incubation period ranges from 1 to 7 days with the onset of symptoms occurring abruptly in 68% of cases. Patients usually present with intermittent watery diar-rhea, with eight or more stools per day. Other symptoms might include anorexia, nausea, abdominal cramps, bloating, flatulence, mild to moderate weight loss, fatigue, and myalgia. Fever is rare.

In the immunocompetent patient, the diarrhea might last from a few days to up to 3 months, with the or-ganism detectable in the stool for up to 2 months. Acalcu-lous *Cyclospora* cholecystitis has been demonstrated in a patient with AIDS. In immune-compromised individu-als, particularly AIDS patients, the disease can persist for weeks to several months.

Reference

Cyclosporiasis. Centers for Disease Control Web site. Available at: http://www.dpd.cdc.gov/dpdx/HTML/ Cyclosporiasis.htm. Accessed April 15, 2005.

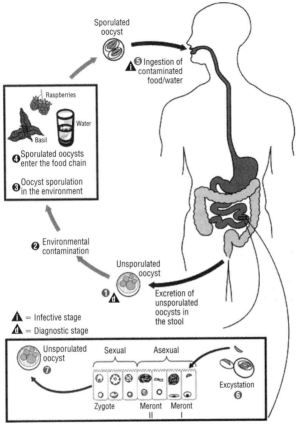

Figure 4-13 Life cycle of *Cyclospora cayetanensis*.
Source: Some of the elements in this figure are based
on an illustration by Ortega et al. Cyclospora cayeta-
nensis. In: Baker JR, Muller R, Rollinson D (eds.).
*Advances in Parasitology: Opportunistic Protozoa in
Humans.* San Diego: Academic Press; 1998:399-418.

Further Reading

Cyclospora infection or cyclosporiasis. Centers for Disease Control Web site. Available at: http://www.cdc.gov/ncidod/dpd/parasites/cyclospora/default.htm. Accessed April 15, 2005.

Ho AY, Lopez AS, Eberhart MG, et al. Outbreak of cyclosporiasis associated with imported raspberries, Philadelphia, Pennsylvania, 2000. *Emerg Infect Dis.* 2002;8:783-788.

Ribes JA, Seabolt JP, Overman SB. Point prevalence of Cryptosporidium, Cyclospora, and Isospora infections in patients being evaluated for diarrhea. *Am J Clin Pathol.* 2004;122:28-32.

Shields JM, Olson BH. Cyclospora cayetanensis: a review of an emerging parasitic coccidian. *Int J Parasitol.* 2003;33:371-391.

Cysticercosis

Agent
Platyhelminthes, Cestoda. Cyclophyllidea, Taeniidae: *Taenia solium.*

Reservoir
Pigs, humans

Vector
None

Vehicle
Soil (contaminated by pigs), fecal–oral contact, flies

Incubation Period
3m–3y

Geographic Distribution
Worldwide

Diagnostic Tests
Serology (blood or CSF) or biopsy

Typical Therapy
Albendazole 5 mg/kg t.i.d. × 30d
Or praziquantel 20 mg/kg t.i.d. × 14d (15–30d for
   neurocysticercosis)
Surgery as indicated

Background

- Cysticercosis is most often found in pig-raising areas
  with poor sanitation.
- The worldwide prevalence is estimated at 400,000. The
  age-adjusted prevalence in tropical countries is 10 to
  15 per 1,000.
- Seventy-five million persons live in endemic areas of
  Latin America. Neurocysticercosis is responsible for an
  estimated 50,000 deaths annually.
- This parasite is the principal cause of acquired seizure
  disorder (epilepsy) in several countries. Seizures occur
  in 50 to 70% of persons with neurocysticercosis.
- Each adult *T. solium* releases one to five proglottids
  daily—with 40,000 fertile ova per proglottid. Ova are
  highly resistant to environmental conditions and
  remain viable for up to 8 months in warm, humid
  climates. Humans and pigs acquire cysticercosis when
  they ingest ova present in human fecal material
  (including the patient's own feces) present on fingers
  or in food or water. Reverse peristalsis associated with
  vomiting in a patient with taeniasis might also allow
  ova to reach the upper gastrointestinal tract and initiate
  cysticercosis. Thus, 25 to 50% of patients with
  cysticercosis will be found to have concurrent taeniasis.

- *T. taeniaeformis* is a parasite of cats. Three cases of human cysticercosis due to this species have been reported from Argentina, Sri Lanka, and Czechoslovakia.

Causal Agent

The cestode (tapeworm) *Taenia solium* (pork tapeworm) is the main cause of human cysticercosis. In addition, the larval stage of other *Taenia* species (e.g., *multiceps*, *serialis*, *brauni*, *taeniaeformis*, *crassiceps*) can infect humans in various sites of localization including the brain, subcutaneous tissue, eye, or liver (CDC).

Life Cycle

Cysticercosis is an infection of both humans and pigs with the larval stages of the parasitic cestode, *Taenia solium*. This infection is caused by ingestion of eggs shed in the feces of a human tapeworm carrier ❶ [Figure 4-14]. Pigs and humans become infected by ingesting eggs or gravid proglottids ❷. Humans are infected either by ingestion of food contaminated with feces, or by autoinfection. In the latter case, a human infected with an adult *T. solium* may ingest eggs produced by that same tapeworm, either through fecal contamination or, possibly, via proglottids carried into the stomach by reverse peristalsis. Once eggs are ingested, oncospheres hatch in the intestine ❸, invade the intestinal wall, and migrate to striated muscles, brain, liver, and other tissues, where they develop into cysticerci. Brain cysts result in a condition known as neurocysticercosis. The parasite life cycle is completed, resulting in human tapeworm infection, when humans ingest undercooked pork containing cys-

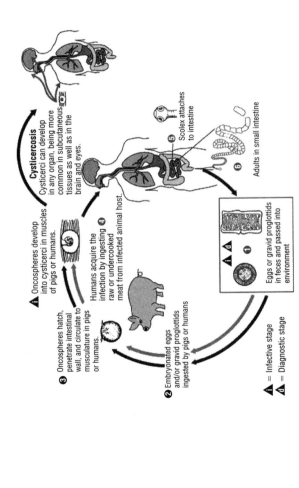

Figure 4-14 Life cycle of cysticercosis.

133

ticerci ❹. Cysts evaginate and attach to the small intestine
via their scolex ❺. Adult tapeworms develop (up to 2 to 7
m in length and produce less than 1000 proglottids, each
with approximately 50,000 eggs), and reside in the small
intestine for years ❻ (CDC).

Clinical Presentation
Cysticercosis is manifest as painless, rubbery (average 2
cm) nodules in skin and soft tissues or other body sites.
Central nervous system infection might present as
seizures, increased intracranial pressure, altered mental
status, eosinophilic meningitis, focal neurological defects,
spinal cord mass, or encephalitis. The eyes are infested in
15 to 45% of patients.

Reference
Cystercercosis. Centers for Disease Control Web site. Available
at: http://www.dpd.cdc.gov/dpdx/HTML/Cysticercosis.htm.
Accessed April 15, 2005.

Further Reading
Cysticercosis. Centers for Disease Control Web site. Available
at: http://www.cdc.gov/ncidod/dpd/parasites/
cysticercosis/default.htm. Accessed April 15, 2005.

Garcia HH, Gonzalez AE, Gilman RH, for the Cysticerosis
Working Group in Peru. Diagnosis, treatment and control of
Taenia solium cysticercosis. *Curr Opin Infect Dis.*
2003;16:411-419.

Raether W, Hanel H. Epidemiology, clinical manifestations and
diagnosis of zoonotic cestode infections: an update. *Parasitol
Res.* 2003;91:412-438.

White AC, Jr. Neurocysticercosis: updates on epidemiology,
pathogenesis, diagnosis, and management. *Annu Rev Med.*
2000;51:187-206.

Demodicosis

Demondicid, Demodectic Mange; Red Mange (Canines)

Agent
Arachnida. Acarina (mite), Demodex; *Demodex follicularum hominis; D. brevis. D. canis.*

Reservoir
Humans, dogs (*D. canis*)

Vector
None

Vehicle
Contact

Geographic Distribution
Worldwide

Incubation Period
Variable. Life cycle of the parasite is 15 days.

Diagnostic Tests
Skin scraping and microscopic slide to identify the organism

Typical Therapy
Gentamicin ointment; 0.5% selenium sulfide cream, metronidazole gel

Background
Humans harbor *D. follicularum* as an asymptomatic infection, ususally on the face. The microscopic mite (0.1–0.4 mm) lives in the secretory ducts of sebaceous glands (*D. follicularum*) and hair follicles (*D. brevis*). Controversy exists

as to the extent of disease this mite can cause, although cases of blepharitis, rosacea, and atypical acne, especially in older individuals, have been reported to be due to *Demodex* spp. Cases of skin eruptions on the face and neck in dog owners and handlers have been described due to *D. canis.*

The prevalence of *Demodex* in people with rosacea has been reported as significantly higher than people without rosacea (51%), eczema (28%), and lupus discoides (31%), but given the universality and prevalence of this mite, cause and effect are unclear.

Clinical Presentation

Maculopapular lesions on the face, nose, around eyelashes, and face. Unexplained eyelash loss. Onset of acne in dog handlers.

Further Reading

Demmler M, Mino de Kaspar H, Möhring C, Klaus V. Blepharitis. Demodex foliculorum, assoziiertes Erregerspektrum und spezifische Therapie. *Ophthalmologe.* 1997;94:191-196.

English FP. Demodex folliculorum and oedema of the eyelash. *Brit J Ophthalmol.* 1971;55:742-749.

English FP, Iwamoto T, Darrell RW, DeVoe AG. The vector potential of Demodex folliculorum. *Arch Ophthalmol.* 1970;84:83-85.

Norn MS. Incidence of demodex folliculorum on skin of lids and nose. *Acta Ophthalmlogica.* 1982;60:575-583.

Dicrocoeliasis

Lancet Liver Fluke

Agent

Platyhelminthes, Trematoda. Plagiorchiida, Dicrocoeliidae: *Dicrocoelium dendriticum* and *D. hospes.*

Reservoir
Sheep, snails, ants

Vector
None

Vehicle
Ingested ants

Geographic Distribution

REGION I—NAm	CAN, USA
REGION III—SAm	BRA
REGION V—NAfr	EGY
REGION VI—CAfr	CAF, GHA, KEN, SLE
REGION VIII—Eur	BLR, CZE, ESP, EST, FRA, GEO, LTU, LVA, LVA, MDA, SVK, UKR
REGION IX—MidEast	ARM, IRN, SAU
REGION XI—Asia	AZE, KAZ, KGZ, RUS, TJK, TKM, UZB
REGION XII—SEA	PHL

Incubation Period
Unknown

Diagnostic Tests
Identification of ova in stool, bile or duodenal aspirate

Typical Therapy
Praziquantel 25 mg/kg PO t.i.d. $\times$ 1d (investigational)

Background

- Dicrocoeliasis is caused by *D. dendriticum* and *D. hospes.*

- *D. dendriticum* is found in Europe, the former Soviet Union, China, Australia, Japan, Indonesia, Malaysia, North America, South America, and Cuba. The parasite has been identified in South American camelids (llamas and alpacas) in Switzerland and Germany.

- *D. hospes* is found in East Africa, Ghana, and Sierra Leone.

- *Dicrocoelium* species cause hepato-biliary damage (ending in cirrhosis) in sheep, goats, cattle, buffaloes, camels, hares, and other herbivorous animals (rarely in humans). Animal infection has been described in Africa, Asia, and Europe (in Italy, especially in Sardinia, the trematode affects sheep farms).

- A related parasite, *Eurytrema pancreaticum*, lives in the biliary and pancreatic ducts of cattle, sheep, water buffaloes, goats, and camels in Asia. Human infection has been reported in Japan and southern China.

- Adult worms (5 to 15 mm long and 1.5 to 2.5 mm wide) live in the bile ducts of herbivorous animals where they lay eggs that are eliminated with feces. The eggs are ingested by various species of land snails (genus *Helicella*) and hatch in the digestive tract of the first intermediate host releasing the miracidium. The latter transforms into a sporocyst, a daughter sporocyst, and finally into cercariae (0.7 mm). Land snails release the cercariae in slimeballs, which are eaten by ants. Cercariae develop into metacercariae within the abdominal cavity of the ant. Herbivorous animals (ie, the definitive hosts) ingest grass containing the infected ants; and after rupturing of the cyst wall of the metacercariae, young adults migrate to the biliary tree where they develop to adult flukes.

- The parasite favors areas of dry and calcareous or alkaline soils which favor the intermediate hosts. Eggs survive over winter and can remain viable for as long as 20 months. Peak fecal excretion by ruminants occurs during the winter in Mediterranean countries. More than 90 mollusc intermediates have been identified, including *Cochlicopa lubrica* (worldwide), *Helicella corderoi* (Spain), *Zebrina Hohenackeri* (Caucasus), *H. obvia* (Germany), and *Cernuella virgata* (Italy, Spain, and Turkey).

Clinical Presentation

Human infection occurs after accidental ingestion of infected ants. Spurious infections are more frequently observed and are the consequence of the ingestion of raw or undercooked animal liver. Symptoms and signs of hepatobiliary involvement are usually mild and limited to hepatomegaly, bloating, and abdominal discomfort. Eosinophilia is present during the early stages of infection.

Further Reading

Bada JL. Dicroceliasis: a fluke diagnosis or a false infection? *JAMA*. 1988;259:2998-2999.

Drabick JJ, Egan JE, Brown SL, Vick RG, Sandman BM, Neafie RC. Dicroceliasis (lancet fluke disease) in an HIV seropositive man. *JAMA*. 1988;259:567-568.

el-Shiekh-Mohamed AR, Mummery V. Human dicrocoeliasis: report on 208 cases from Saudi Arabia. *Trop Geogr Med*. 1990;42:1-7.

Manga-Gonzalez MY, Gonzalez-Lanza C, Cabanas E, Campo R. Contributions to and review of dicrocoeliosis, with special reference to the intermediate hosts of Dicrocoelium dendriticum. *Parasitology*. 2001;123(suppl):S91-S114.

Dientamoeba fragilis

Agent

Protozoa. Archezoa, Parabasalia, Trichomonadea, Flagellate: *D. fragilis*.

Reservoir
Humans

Vector
None

Vehicle
Fecal–oral contact—possibly attached to pinworm ova

Incubation Period
8–25d

Geographic Distribution
Dientamoebal diarrhea appears to have a worldwide distribution; however, identification of the parasite is relatively uncommon—perhaps reflecting its unfamiliarity to routine laboratory staff.

Diagnostic Tests
Identification of trophozoites in stool.
Alert laboratory when this diagnosis is suspected.

Typical Adult Therapy
Stool precautions
Iodoquinol 650 mg PO t.i.d. × 20d
Or tetracycline 500 mg q.i.d. × 10d
Or paromomycin 10 mg/kg t.i.d. × 7d

Typical Pediatric Therapy
Stool precautions
Iodoquinol 13 mg/kd PO t.i.d. × 20d
Or (age > 8) tetracycline 10 mg/kg q.i.d. × 10d
Or paromomycin 10 mg/kg t.i.d. × 7d

Background

- Although *D. fragilis* resembles an amoeba-like protozoan, it is currently classified as an aberrant trichomonad. Morphologically the organism might be confused with *Blastocystis hominis*.
- *D. fragilis* is probably transmitted by fecal–oral route, and transmission via helminth eggs (eg, *Ascaris lumbricoides, Enterobius vermicularis*) has been postulated. *D. fragilis* has been found to persist in the intestinal canal of pinworms for more than 84 days.
- The disease is found worldwide and is particularly common in closed institutions.

Causal Agent

Despite its name, *Dientamoeba fragilis* is not an ameba but a flagellate. This protozoan produces trophozoites, but cysts have not been identified. Infection is often asymptomatic (CDC).

Life Cycle

The complete life cycle of this parasite has not yet been determined, but assumptions are made based on clinical data. To date, the cyst stage has not been identified, and the trophozoite is the only stage found in stools of infected individuals ❶ [Figure 4-15]. *D. fragilis* is probably transmitted by the fecal–oral route ❷ and transmission via helminth eggs (eg, *Ascaris, Enterobius* spp.) is postulated ❸. Trophozoites of *D. fragilis* contain either one or two nuclei (❶,❹), and are found in children complaining of intestinal (eg, intermittent diarrhea, abdominal pain) and other symptoms (eg, nausea, anorexia, fatigue, malaise, poor weight gain) (CDC).

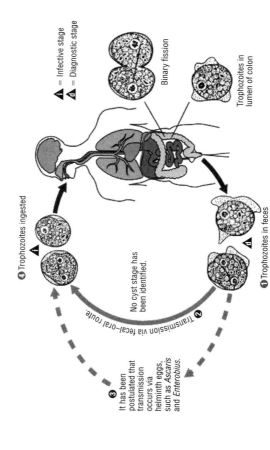

Figure 4-15 Life cycle of *Dientamoeba fragilis*.

▲ = Infective stage
△ = Diagnostic stage

Binary fission

Trophozoites in lumen of colon

❹ Trophozoites ingested

No cyst stage has been identified.

❷ Transmission via fecal–oral route.

❸ It has been postulated that transmission occurs via helminth eggs, such as *Ascaris* and *Enterobius*.

❶ Trophozoites in feces

Clinical Presentation

Most infections are asymptomatic; however, some might be characterized by diarrhea and abdominal pain. Eosinophilia might be present; infestation may persist for more than one year. The occurrence of diarrhea in patients with enterobiasis should suggest the possibility of *D. fragilis* gastroenteritis.

Reference

Dientamoeba. Centers for Disease Control Web site. Available at: http://www.dpd.cdc.gov/dpdx/HTML/Dientamoeba.htm. Accessed April 15, 2005.

Further Reading

Butler WP. Dientamoeba fragilis: an unusual intestinal pathogen. *Dig Dis Sci.* 1996;41:1811-1813.

Dickinson EC, Cohen MA, Schlenker MK. Dientamoeba fragilis: a significant pathogen. *Am J Emerg Med.* 2002;20:62-63.

Dientamoeba fragilis infection. Centers for Disease Control Web site. Available at: http://www.cdc.gov/ncidod/dpd/parasites/dientamoeba/default.htm. Accessed April 15, 2005.

Norberg A, Nord CE, Evengard B. Dientamoeba fragilis—a protozoal infection which may cause severe bowel distress. *Clin Microbiol Infect.* 2003;9:65-68.

Weiss LM, Keohane EM. The uncommon gastrointestinal Protozoa: Microsporidia, Blastocystis, Isospora, Dientamoeba, and Balantidium. *Curr Clin Top Infect Dis.* 1997;17:147-187.

Dioctophyme renalis

Giant Kidney Worm

Agent

Nematoda. Phasmidea: *D. renalis.*

Reservoir
Dogs, mink

Vector
None

Vehicle
Food (fish which have ingested aquatic worms)

Geographic Distribution

REGION I—NAm	CAN, USA
REGION III—SAm	ARG, BRA, URY
REGION VIII—Eur	DEU
REGION IX—MidEast	IRN
REGION XI—Asia	CHN, JPN, RUS

Incubation Period
3–6m

Diagnostic Tests
Identification of ova in urine or adults in tissue

Typical Therapy
Excision as required

Background

- Infective ova of *D. renalis*, the giant kidney worm (adults may grow to a length of 100 cm), are shed in the urine of a variety of small carnivores. Ova are then ingested by aquatic worms, which are, in turn, eaten by fish or frogs.
- Humans are infected through ingestion of the latter. Cases have been reported in Asia, Europe, and the Americas.

- In severe infections, the kidney is completely destroyed.
- At least four cases of subcutaneous infection have been reported.

Clinical Presentation

Flank pain and hematuria begin 3 to 6 months after eating raw fish or frog flesh. Subcutaneous infection has also been described.

Further Reading

Anonymous. The giant kidney worm. *Semin Dial.* 2002;15(2):120.

Fernando SS. The giant kidney worm (Dioctophyma renale) infection in man in Australia. *Am J Surg Pathol.* 1983;7:281-284.

Hanjani AA, Sadighian A, Nikakhtar B, Arfaa F. The first report of human infection with Dioctophyma renale in Iran. *Trans R Soc Trop Med Hyg.* 1968;62:647-648.

Ignjatovic I, Stojkovic I, Kutlesic C, Tasic S. Infestation of the human kidney with Dioctophyma renale. *Urol Int.* 2003;70:70-73.

Narvaez JA, Turell LP, Serra J, Hidalgo F. Hyperdense renal cystic lesions caused by Dioctophyma renale. *AJR Am J Roentgenol.* 1994;163:997-998.

Sun T, Turnbull A, Lieberman PH, Sternberg SS. Giant kidney worm (Dioctophyma renale) infection mimicking retroperitoneal neoplasm. *Am J Surg Pathol.* 1986;10:508-512.

Diphyllobothrium latum

Fish Tapeworm

Agent

Platyhelminthes, Cestoda. Pseudophyllidea, Diphyllobothriidae: *D. latum.*

Reservoir
Humans, dogs, bears, fish-eating mammals

Vector
None

Vehicle
Freshwater fish—notably perch, burbot and pike

Incubation Period
4–6w (range 2w–2y)

Geographic Distribution
Widespread, notably in countries where freshwater fish are found

Diagnostic Tests
Identification of ova or proglottids in feces

Typical Therapy
Praziquantel 10 mg/kg PO as single dose

Background

- Diphyllobothriasis is common where freshwater fish are consumed. Highest endemicity (prevalence > 2%) is found in Scandinavia, the Baltic countries, North America, Japan, Chile, and areas of Siberia.
- It is estimated that 9 million people are infested worldwide.
- *D. dendriticum* is acquired from salmon, char, and trout and is found in the subarctic region.
- *D. klebanovskii* is acquired from salmon and is found in eastern Siberia.

- *D. nihonkaiense* is acquired from salmon and is found in Japan.
- *D. ursi* is acquired from salmon and is found in Canada and Alaska.
- *D. cordatum* (intermediate host unknown) is found in Greenland and Alaska.
- *D. dalliae* is acquired from blackfish and is found in Alaska and eastern Siberia.
- *D. pacificum*, a large tapeworm of seals, is often found as an accidental parasite of humans. This is the principal agent of diphyllobothriasis in South America. Associated symptoms consist of abdominal pain, flatulence, and diarrhea.
- *D. ursi* is a natural parasite of bears. Human infection has been reported in Canada.

Causal Agents

The cestode *Diphyllobothrium latum* (the fish or broad tapeworm), the largest human tapeworm. Several other *Diphyllobothrium* species have been reported to infect humans, but less frequently; they include *D. pacificum, D. cordatum, D. ursi, D. dendriticum, D. lanceolatum, D. dalliae,* and *D. yonagoensis* (CDC).

Life Cycle

Immature eggs are passed in feces ❶ [Figure 4-16]. Under appropriate conditions, these mature (approximately 18 to 20 days) ❷ to yield oncospheres which develop into coracidia ❸. After ingestion by a suitable freshwater crustacean (the copepod first intermediate host) coracidia develop into procercoid larvae ❹. Following ingestion of the cope-

pod by a suitable second intermediate host, typically minnows and other small freshwater fish, procercoid larvae are
released from the crustacean and migrate into the fish flesh
where they develop into plerocercoid larvae (sparganum)
❺. Plerocercoid larvae are the infective stage for humans.
Because humans do not generally eat undercooked minnows and similar small freshwater fish, these do not represent an important source of infection. Nevertheless, these
small second intermediate hosts can be eaten by larger
predator species, eg, trout, perch, walleyed pike ❻. In this
case, the sparganum will migrate to the musculature of the
larger predator fish; and humans can acquire the disease
by eating these tissues in the form of raw or undercooked
fish ❼. After ingestion, the plerocercoids develop into mature adult tapeworms which reside in the small intestine.
Adults of *D. latum* attach to the intestinal mucosa by
means of the two bilateral groves (bothria) of their scolex
❽. Adults can reach more than 10 m in length, and contain
more than 3,000 proglottids. Immature eggs are discharged from the proglottids (up to 1,000,000 eggs per day
per worm) ❾ and passed in the feces ❶. Eggs begin to appear in the feces 5 to 6 weeks after infection. In addition to
humans, many other mammals may serve as definitive
hosts for *D. latum* (CDC).

Clinical Presentation
Most infestations are asymptomatic; however, some
patients may experience abdominal pain, diarrhea, and
flatulence. Vitamin B_{12} deficiency is noted in 0.02% of
patients. Rare instances of intestinal obstruction have
been described. The adult worm may survive for decades
in human intestine.

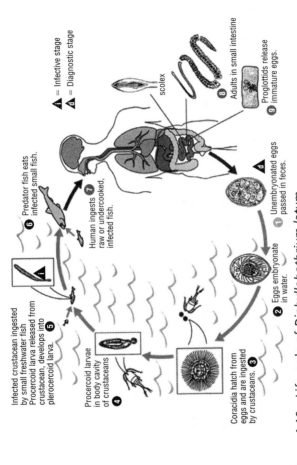

1 Unembryonated eggs passed in feces. **d**

2 Eggs embryonate in water.

3 Coracidia hatch from eggs and are ingested by crustaceans.

4 Procercoid larvae in body cavity of crustaceans.

5 Infected crustacean ingested by small freshwater fish. Procercoid larva released from crustacean, develops into plerocercoid larva. **A**

6 Predator fish eats infected small fish.

7 Human ingests raw or undercooked, infected fish.

8 Adults in small intestine

9 Proglottids release immature eggs.

scolex

A = Infective stage

d = Diagnostic stage

Figure 4-16   Life cycle of *Diphyllobothrium latum.*

Reference

Diphyllobothriasis. Centers for Disease Control Web site. Available at: http://www.dpd.cdc.gov/dpdx/HTML/ diphyllobothriasis.htm. Accessed April 15, 2005.

Further Reading

Bruckner DA. Helminthic food-borne infections. *Clin Lab Med*. 1999;19:639-660.

Raether W, Hanel H. Epidemiology, clinical manifestations and diagnosis of zoonotic cestode infections: an update. *Parasitol Res*. 2003;91:412-438.

Vuylsteke P, Bertrand C, Verhoef GE, Vandenberghe P. Case of megaloblastic anemia caused by intestinal taeniasis. *Ann Hematol*. 2004;83:487-488.

Diplogonoporiasis

Diplogonoporus

Diplogonoporus grandis shares clinical and epidemiological features with *Diphyllobothrium latum*. Human infection was first reported in humans in 1892, and as of 2002, approximately 180 cases were reported, all originating in Japan. Adults measure 3 to 10 meters in length. Suspected secondary intermediate hosts include sardines, mackerel, horse mackerel, bonito and yellowtail. Ova are indistinguishable from those of *D. latum*. Rare instances of human infection by *Diplogonoporus balaenopterae*, a pathogen of whales, have been reported.

Geographical Distribution

Japan

Further Reading

Clavel A, Bargues MD, Castillo FJ, Rubio MD, Mas-Coma S. Diplogonoporiasis presumably introduced into Spain: first confirmed case of human infection acquired outside the Far East. *Am J Trop Med Hyg.* 1997;57:317-320.

Kobayashi H, Nakamura N, Nagasawa K. A mass occurrence of human infection with Diplogonoporus grandis (Cestoda: Diphyllobothriidae) in Shizuoka Prefecture, central Japan. *Parasitol Int.* 2002;51:73-79.

Dipylidium caninum

Cucumber Tapeworm, Dog Tapeworm, Double-pored Dog Tapeworm

Agent
Platyhelminthes, Cestoda. Cyclophyllidea, Dipylidiidae: *D. caninum.*

Reservoir
Dogs, cats

Vector
None

Vehicle
Ingested fleas (*Ctenocephalides* spp.)

Geographic Distribution
D. caninum appears to have a worldwide distribution; however, human infection is relatively uncommon.

Incubation Period
21–28d

Diagnostic Tests
Identification of proglottids in feces

Typical Therapy
Praziquantel 10 mg/kg PO as single dose

Background

- Dipylidiasis is common in dogs, cats, foxes, and jackals. Human infection is most often described among European children, but also occurs in the Far East, Africa, North America, and South America.
- The mature worm is segmented and 20 to 50 cm long. Humans acquire infection through accidental ingestion of insects, which in turn are hosts to cysticerci of the parasite. Pets may exhibit behavior to relieve anal pruritis (such as scraping anal region across grass or carpeting).
- The dog is the principal definitive host for *D. caninum*. Other potential hosts include cats, foxes, and humans (mostly children). The adult tapeworms (measuring up to 60 cm in length and 3 mm in width) reside in the small intestine of the host. The proglottids mature, become gravid, detach from the tapeworm, and migrate to the anus or are passed in the stool. Subsequently, they release typical egg packets.
- Following ingestion of an egg by the intermediate host (larval stages of the dog louse = *Trichodectes canis*, dog flea = *Ctenocephalides canis*, cat flea = *C. felis*, or human flea = *Pulex irritans*), an oncosphere is released into the flea's intestine. The oncosphere penetrates the intestinal wall, invades the insect's hemocoel (body cavity), and develops into a cysticercoid larva. The vertebrate host becomes infected by ingesting the adult flea containing the cysticercoid. In the small intestine of the vertebrate host, the cysticercoid develops into the adult

tapeworm which reaches maturity about 1 month after infection.

Causal Agent

Dipylidium caninum (the double-pored dog tapeworm) mainly infects dogs and cats, but is occasionally found in humans (CDC).

Life Cycle

Gravid proglottids are passed intact in the feces or emerge from the anal verge of the host ❶ [Figure 4-17], and release characteristic egg packets ❷. Occasionally, proglottids rupture and egg packets are seen in stool samples. Following ingestion of an egg by the intermediate host (larval stages of the dog or cat flea *Ctenocephalides* spp.), an oncosphere is released into the flea's intestine. The oncosphere penetrates the intestinal wall, invades the insect's hemocoel (body cavity), and develops into a cysticercoid larva ❸. The larva then develops into an adult, and the adult flea harbours the infective cysticercoid ❹. Vertebrate hosts become infected by ingesting the adult flea containing the cysticercoid ❺. The dog is the principal definitive host for *Dipylidium caninum*. Other potential hosts include cats, foxes, and humans (usually children) ❻, ❼. Humans acquire infection by ingesting the infected flea, often during close contact between children and their infected pets. In the small intestine of the vertebrate host the cysticercoid develops into the adult tapeworm, which reaches maturity after 1 month ❽. Adult tapeworms (measuring up to 60 cm in length and 3 mm in width) reside in the small intestine of the host, each attached by a scolex. Proglottids (segments) have two genital pores (hence the name

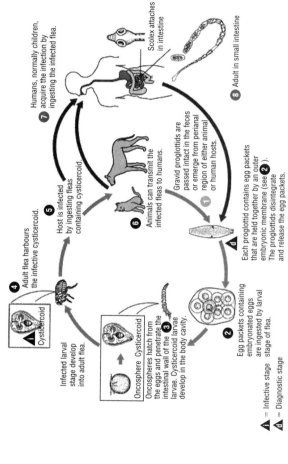

Figure 4-17   Life cycle of *Dipylidium caninum.*

Humans, normally children, acquire the infection by ingesting the infected flea. **7**

Scolex attaches in intestine

8 Adult in small intestine

Gravid proglottids are passed intact in the feces or emerge from perianal region of either animal or human hosts. **1**

Host is infected by ingesting fleas containing cysticercoid **5**

Animals can transmit the infected fleas to humans. **6**

Each proglottid contains egg packets that are held together by an outer embryonic membrane (see **2**). The proglottids disintegrate and release the egg packets. **d**

Adult flea harbours the infective cysticercoid. **4**

Infected larval stage develop into adult flea.

Cysticercoid **A**

Egg packets containing embryonated eggs are ingested by larval stage of flea. **2**

Oncosphere   Cysticercoid

Oncospheres hatch from the eggs and penetrate the intestinal wall of the larvae. Cysticercoid larvae develop in the body cavity. **3**

A = Infective stage
A = Diagnostic stage

154

"double-pored" tapeworm). The proglottids mature, become gravid, detach from the tapeworm, and migrate to the anus or are passed in the stool ❶ (CDC).

Clinical Presentation

Most infections with *D. caninum* are asymptomatic. Severe diarrhea, urticaria, fever, and eosinophilia are occasionally encountered. The principal sign (in animals and children) consists of the passage of proglottids on the perianal region, feces, diapers, or occasionally on floor coverings and furniture. Proglottids are motile when freshly passed and might be mistaken for maggots or fly larvae.

Reference

Diplyidium caninum infection. Centers for Disease Control Web site. Available at: http://www.dpd.cdc.gov/dpdx/ HTML/Dipylidium.htm. Accessed April 15, 2005.

Further Reading

Chappell CL, Enos JP, Penn HM. Dipylidium caninum, an underrecognized infection in infants and children. *Pediatr Infect Dis J*. 1990;9:745-747.

Ferraris S, Reverso E, Parravicini LP, Ponzone A. Dipylidium caninum in an infant. *Eur J Pediatr*. 1993;152:702.

Molina CP, Ogburn J, Adegboyega P. Infection by Dipylidium caninum in an infant. *Arch Pathol Lab Med*. 2003;127: e157-e159.

Dirofilariasis

Dog Heartworm, Filaria Conjunctivae

Agent

Nematoda. Phasmidea, Filariae: *Dirofilaria (Nochtiella) immitis* (pulmonary); *D. tenuis* and *D. repens* (subcutaneous infection), and *D. reconditum* (eye), and *D. ursi.*

Reservoir
Dogs, wild carnivores (*D. tenuis* in raccoons; *D. ursi* in bears)

Vector
Mosquitoes

Vehicle
None

Geographic Distribution
Widespread. The precise distribution is unknown.

Incubation Period
60–90d

Diagnostic Tests
Identification of parasite in tissue (ie, lung biopsy)
Serologic tests available in some centers

Typical Therapy
Not available; excision is often diagnostic.

Background

- Human dirofilariasis was first reported in 1885 (eye infection in Italy).
- *D. repens* infection were reported 410 times from 30 countries in the world's literature to 1995—181 of these from Italy.
- During 1995 to 2000, 372 cases were reported from 25 countries—most from Italy, Sri Lanka, and the former Soviet Union.
- Pulmonary infection is usually due to *D. immitis*, a cosmopolitan parasite of dogs, found in North

America and South America, Australia, Japan, and Europe. Ten cases of human pulmonary dirofilariasis were reported in Europe during 1980 to 1995.

- *D. tenuis* is carried by raccoons in North America.
- *D. repens* is carried by dogs and is found in southern and eastern Europe, Asia Minor, central Asia, and Sri Lanka (but not the Americas).
- *D. ursi* is carried by bears and is found in North America and Japan.
- *D. striata* is carried by bobcats and feral cats and is found in North America and South America.
- *D. subdermata* is carried by porcupines in North America.
- Eye infections are caused by *D. tenuis*, *D. repens* and *D. immitis*.

Clinical Presentation

Pulmonary infestion usually presents as a well-circumscribed coin lesion. Occasionally the lesions are transient or multiple. Symptoms such as chest pain, dyspnea, fever, cough, and eosinophilia are present in only 50% of cases. Isolated infections have been reported in the mesentery, spermatic cord, peritoneal cavity, and liver.

Skin and subcutaneous infections are caused by *D. tenuis*, *D. repens*, *D. ursi*, *D. immitis*, and *D. striata*. Clinical manifestations are limited to a small (0.5 to 1.5 cm), discrete nodule which might appear on any area of the body. Local pain, inflammation, eosinophilia, and a sensation of motion could be present in some cases. Infections could involve the conjunctivae, anterior or posterior chambers.

Further Reading

Flieder DB, Moran CA. Pulmonary dirofilariasis: a clinico-pathologic study of 41 lesions in 39 patients. *Hum Pathol.* 1999;30:251-256.

Huynh T, Thean J, Maini R. Dipetalonema reconditum in the human eye. *Br J Ophthalmol.* 2001;85:1391-1392.

Muro A, Genchi C, Cordero M, Simon, F. Human dirofilariasis in the European Union. *Parasitol Today.* 1999;15:386-389.

Pampiglione S, Rivasi F. Human dirofilariasis due to Dirofilaria (Nochtiella) repens: an update of world literature from 1995 to 2000. *Parassitologia.* 2000;42:231-254.

Shah MK. Human pulmonary dirofilariasis: review of the literature. *South Med J.* 1999;92:276-279.

Dracunculus medinensis

Dracunculose, Dracontiasis, Filaria medinensis, Guinea Worm, Medina Worm, Fiery Serpent of the Israelites

Agent
Nematoda. Phasmidea, Filariae: *Dracunculus medinensis.*

Reservoir
Humans

Vector
None

Vehicle
Copepod (*Mesocyclops* and *Termocyclops*) in drinking water

Geographic Distribution

REGION VI—CAfr	BEN, BFA, CAF, CIV, CMR, ETH, GHA, KEN, MLI, MRT, NER, NGA, SDN, SEN, TCD, TGO, UGA
REGION IX—MidEast	YEM
REGION X—IndSub	IND, PAK

Incubation Period
12–18m

Diagnostic Tests
Identification of adult worm in situ; or identification of discharged larvae from wound

Typical Adult Therapy
Metronidazole 500 mg PO t.i.d. × 10d
Or thiabendazole 30 mg/kg PO b.i.d. × 3d
Worm removal

Typical Pediatric Therapy
Metronidazole 8 mg/kg PO t.i.d. × 10d
Or thiabendazole 30 mg/kg b.i.d. × 3d
Worm removal

Background

- Historically, dracunculiasis was known to occur in Egypt, Gambia, Guinea, Iraq, Brazil, Uzbekistan, and Iran. Isolated autochonous cases have also been reported in Japan, Korea, and Indonesia—presumably through ingestion of raw fish infested by zoonotic species of *Dracunculus*. Circulation of zoonotic *Dracunculus* among dogs and cats might persist in Uzbekistan, Tamil Nadu, Azerbaijan, China, Kazakhstan, and possibly Turkmenistan.
- As of 1996, human disease was reported from 17 countries (15 Africa, 2 Asia); 16 (Africa) in 1998; 13 (Africa) in 1999; and 13 (Africa) in 2003.
- Free-living larvae require ingestion by predatory copepods, measuring 1 to 2 mm—generally *Mesocyclops aequatorialis, M. kieferi, Metacyclops margaretae, Thermocyclops crassus, T. incisus, T. inopinus* and

T. oblongatus. Infective third-stage larvae develop in the cyclops body cavity within 14 days. Infection is usually acquired from water in ponds, step temples and other man-made sources of drinking water.

- When the copepod is ingested by a human, larvae are released and penetrate through the intestinal wall to the peritoneal cavity, and then to the wall of the thorax and abdomen within 15 days. Maturing worms mate, and the male dies; females migrate toward the legs, reaching mature size as gravid females after approximately 1 year. The female can attain a length of 100 cm; the smaller male dies in situ—a residual calcification can be seen on x-ray.

- The global burden of dracunculiasis was estimated at 48 million cases in 1947, and 10 million in 1976. An estimated 5 to 10 million cases occurred during the 1980s. In 1986, 3,500,000 cases were reported and 120 million persons were at risk. In 1990, 623,579 cases were reported; 229,773 (from 16,500 endemic villages) in 1993; 129,852 (8,902 villages) in 1995; 77,863 (9,522 villages) in 1997; and 75,223 in 2000. Only 54,638 cases were reported in 2002; 32,193 in 2003; and 15,413 in 2004.

- In 1995, Niger, Nigeria, and Sudan accounted for 73% of the world's cases. Sudan alone accounted for 77.6% in 1996; 61.7% in 1998; 68.6% in 1999; 73% in 2000; 78% in 2001; 76% in 2002.

Causal Agent

Dracunculiasis (guinea worm disease) is caused by the nematode (roundworm) *Dracunculus medinensis* (CDC).

Life Cycle

Humans become infected by drinking unfiltered water containing copepods (small crustaceans) which contain

larvae of *D. medinensis* ❶ [Figure 4-18]. Following ingestion, the copepods die and release the larvae, which penetrate the host stomach and intestinal wall and enter the
abdominal cavity and retroperitoneal space ❷. After maturation and copulation, the male worms die and the females (length: 70 to 120 cm) migrate in the subcutaneous
tissues towards the skin surface ❸. Approximately one year
after infection, the female worm induces a blister on the
skin, generally on the distal lower extremity, which rup-
tures. When this lesion comes into contact with water (ie,
when the patient seeks to relieve the local discomfort
through bathing), the female worm emerges and releases
larvae ❹. Larvae are ingested by a copepod ❺ and after two
weeks (and two molts) develop into infective larvae ❻.
Ingestion of the copepods closes the cycle ❶ (CDC).

Clinical Presentation

Symptoms consist of fever, urticaria and other allergic
phenomena, swelling, and local pain and burning. The
blister will eventually rupture, and the patient seeks relief
through immersing the affected skin in water. The resulting temperature change causes the blister to erupt, expos-
ing the worm, which then releases a milky white liquid
containing millions of larvae into the water. The process
of larval shedding continues for several days after it has
emerged from the ulcer.

More than 90% of the worms appear on the legs and
feet, but they can occur anywhere on the body. Ulcers can
take many weeks (8 weeks average) to heal and are sec-
ondarily infected with bacteria in approximately 50% of
cases. Permanent disabling scars and crippling could result. Each time a worm emerges, the patient might be un-
able to work and resume daily activities for an average of
3 months. This usually occurs during planting or harvest-
ing season, resulting in heavy crop losses.

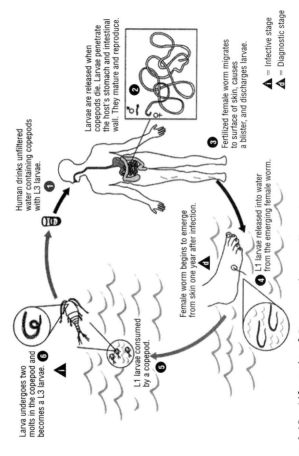

Human drinks unfiltered water containing copepods with L3 larvae. ❶

Larvae are released when copepods die. Larvae penetrate the host's stomach and intestinal wall. They mature and reproduce.

Fertilized female worm migrates to surface of skin, causes a blister, and discharges larvae. ❸

L1 larvae released into water from the emerging female worm. ❹

Female worm begins to emerge from skin one year after infection. ▲

L1 larvae consumed by a copepod. ❺

Larva undergoes two molts in the copepod and becomes a L3 larvae. ❻

▲ = Infective stage
▲ = Diagnostic stage

Figure 4-18 Life cycle of *Dracunculus medinensis.*

162

Reference

Dracunculiasis. Centers for Disease Control Web site. Available at: http://www.dpd.cdc.gov/dpdx/HTML/ Dracunculiasis.htm. Accessed April 15, 2005.

Further Reading

Anonymous. From the Centers for Disease Control and Prevention: progress toward global dracunculiasis eradication, June 2002. *JAMA.* 2002;288:817-2818.

Cairncross S, Muller R, Zagaria N. Dracunculiasis (Guinea worm disease) and the eradication initiative. *Clin Microbiol Rev.* 2002;15:223-246.

Cox FE. History of human parasitology. *Clin Microbiol Rev.* 2002;15:595-612.

Dracunculiasis: Guinea worm disease. Centers for Disease Control Web site. Available at: http://www.cdc.gov/ncidod/dpd/ parasites/guineaworm/default.htm. Accessed April 15, 2005.

Hopkins DR, Ruiz-Tiben E, Ruebush T II, Agle AN, Withers PC Jr. Dracunculiasis eradication: March 1994 update. *Am J Trop Med Hyg.* 1995;52:14-20.

Lymphatic filariasis. Centers for Disease Control Web site. Available at: http://www.cdc.gov/ncidod/dpd/parasites/ lymphaticfilariasis/default.htm. Accessed April 15, 2005.

Echinococcosis—American Polycystic

Echinococcus Oligarthus Infection, Echinococcus vogeli Infection, Human Polycystic Hydatid Disease, Polycystic Echinococcosis

Agent

Platyhelminthes, Cestoda, Cyclophyllidea, Taeniidae: *E. vogeli* and *E. oligarthus*

Reservoir

Bush dogs, pacas, rodents

Vector
None

Vehicle
Carnivore feces, soil

Geographic Distribution

REGION II—CAm	CRI, NIC, PAN
REGION III—SAm	ARG, BRA, CHL, COL, ECU, SUR, URY, VEN

Incubation Period
3–30y

Diagnostic Tests
Serology (might cross react with *E. granulosus*)
Identification of parasite in surgical specimens

Typical Adult Therapy
Albendazole 400 mg PO b.i.d. × 28d (not of proven benefit) followed by surgery as indicated

Typical Pediatric Therapy
Albendazole 10 mg/kg/day PO × 28d (not of proven benefit) followed by surgery as indicated

Background

- As of 1999, 42 cases of infection by *E. vogeli* and three by *E. oligarthus* had been published from 11 Latin American countries. Patient ages ranged from 6 to 78 years, with no difference by sex. The liver was involved, either alone or with other organs, in 80% of cases. As of 2002, 99 cases had been published in 11 countries, including 3 due to *E. oligarthus*, 39 *E. vogeli*, and 57 unspecified.

- *E. vogeli* is maintained primarily in a sylvatic predator-prey cycle which includes the bush dog (*Speothos venaticus*) and occasionally domestic dogs as definitive hosts. Pacas (*Agouti paca*) serve as intermediate hosts.
- *E. oligarthus* infects only felids as definitive hosts: cougars (*Felis concolor*), ocelots (*Felis pardalis*), jaguars (*Felis onca*), jaguarundi and Geoffroy's cat. Larvae are found in the muscles of large rodents (agoutis and pacas), which serve as intermediate hosts.
- The cyst lamella is thinner than that of *E. vogeli*, and secondary chambers are fewer in number.

Clinical Presentation

The signs and symptoms of American polycystic echino-coccosis are similar to those of hydatid disease due to *Echinococcus granulosis*. Right upper abdominal pain and hepatic mass are typical; jaundice and multiple cysts are reported in some cases.

Further Reading

D'Alessandro A. Polycystic echinococcosis in tropical America: Echinococcus vogeli and E. oligarthrus. *Acta Trop.* 1997;67:43-65.

Ferreira MS, Nishioka Sde A, Rocha A, D'Alessandro A. Echinococcus vogeli polycystic hydatid disease: report of two Brazilian cases outside the Amazon region. *Trans R Soc Trop Med Hyg.* 1995;89:286-287.

Kammerer WS, Schantz PM. Echinococcal disease. *Infect Dis Clin North Am.* 1993;7:605-618.

Oostburg BF, Vrede MA, Bergen AE. The occurrence of poly-cystic echinococcosis in Suriname. *Ann Trop Med Parasitol.* 2000;94:247-252.

Soares MC, Amaral IS. Images in hepatology. Polycystic echinococcosis by E. vogeli in the Amazon region. *J Hepatol.* 1998;28:908.

Echinococcus granulosis

Unilocular Hydatid

Agent
Platyhelminthes, Cestoda. Cyclophyllidea, Taeniidae:
Echinococcus granulosus.

Reservoir
Dogs, wolves, dingoes, sheep, horses

Vector
None

Vehicle
Soil, dogs, feces, flies

Geographic Distribution

REGION I—NAm	CAN, USA
REGION II—CAm	BLZ, CRI, GTM, HND, MEX, NIC, SLV
REGION III—SAm	ARG, BOL, BRA, CHL, ECU, FLK, PER, URY, VEN
REGION V—NAfr	DZA, EGY, LBY, MAR, TUN
REGION VI—CAfr	ERI, ETH, KEN, MLI, MOZ, MRT, NER, NGA, SDN, SOM, TCD, TZA, UGA, ZMB
REGION VII—SAfr	BWA, LSO, SWZ, ZAF
REGION VIII—Eur	ALB, AND, AUT, BEL, BGR, BIH, BLR, CHE, CYP, CZE, DEU, ESP, EST, FRA, FIN, GBR, GRC, HRV, HUN, IRL, LTU, LVA,

MCO, MDA, MKD, MLT,
NLD, POL, PRT, ROM,
SVK, SVN, SWE, UKR

REGION IX—MidEast   ARM, IRN, IRQ, ISR, JOR,
KWT, LBN, OMN, SAU,
SYR, YEM

REGION X—IndSub   IND, NPL, PAK
REGION XI—Asia   AFG, AZE, CHN, KAZ,
KGZ, MNG, RUS, TKM,
TJK, TWN, UZB

REGION XII—SEA   IDN, KHM, LAO, MMR,
MYS, PHL, THA, VNM

REGION XIII—Poly   NZL, SHN

Incubation Period
1–20y

Diagnostic Tests
Serology
Identification of parasite in surgical specimens

Typical Adult Therapy
Albendazole 400 mg b.i.d. × 28d. Repeat × 3, with
2-week hiatus between cycles.
Follow by surgery as indicated.
PAIR (puncture-aspiration-injection-reaspiration) is
also used.

Typical Pediatric Therapy
Albendazole 10 mg/kg/day × 28d. Repeat × 3, with
2-week hiatus between cycles.
Follow by surgery as indicated.
PAIR is also used.

Background

- Echinococcosis is most often associated with poor hygiene in areas contiguous to sheep farming and dogs. Childhood acquisition is usual; however, clinical disease might become manifest only after many years. The annual rate in some parts of western Europe approaches 40 per 100,000, with livestock infestation rates as high as 70% in some Mediterranean countries.
- Ova are passed in the feces of dogs and inadvertently ingested by humans or sheep. The eggshells are then digested and embryos can be found in the portal vein and liver within 8 hours of ingestion; visible larvae are present within 3 weeks. The cyst could attain a diameter of 10 cm within 10 weeks.
- More than 50% of cases involve the liver; 10 to 20% involve the lungs. Lung, brain, spinal, and orbital hydatid cysts are more commonly seen in younger patients, whereas hepatic cysts preferentially involve adults.

Clinical Presentation

Symptoms are often absent, even when large cysts are present, and cysts are often discovered incidentally on a routine x-ray or ultrasound study. Hepatic echinococcosis often presents as abdominal pain with or without a palpable mass in the right upper quadrant. Biliary compression or rupture of the cysts into a bile duct might mimic cholecystitis or cholelithiasis. Leakage from a cyst can produce fever, pruritus, urticaria, eosinophilia, or even anaphylactic shock.

Pulmonary cysts can rupture into the bronchial tree and produce cough, hemoptysis, and chest pain. Rupture of cysts can disseminate protoscolices to contiguous organs or into the vascular system, resulting in the formation of additional cysts. Rupture can occur spontaneously or as a result of trauma or surgery.

Extrahepatic cysts present as space-occupying lesions of brain, lung, bone, or virtually any other organ. In contrast to hepatic echinococcosis, extrahepatic cysts are often noncalcified.

Further Reading

Craig PS, Rogan MT, Campos-Ponce M. Echinococcosis: disease, detection and transmission. *Parasitology.* 2003; 127(suppl):S5-S20.

Eckert J, Deplazes P. Biological, epidemiological, and clinical aspects of echinococcosis, a zoonosis of increasing concern. *Clin Microbiol Rev.* 2004;17:107-135.

Torgerson PR, Heath DD. Transmission dynamics and control options for Echinococcus granulosus. *Parasitology.* 2003;127(suppl):S143-S158.

Echinococcus multilocularis

Alveolar Hydatid Disease, Small Fox Tapeworm

Agent
Platyhelminthes, Cestoda. Cyclophyllidea, Taeniidae: *E. multilocularis.*

Reservoir
Foxes, wolves, coyotes, dogs, cats, voles, lemmings, shrews, mice

Vector
None

Vehicle
Mammalian feces

Geographic Distribution

REGION I—NAm	CAN, USA
REGION V—NAfr	TUN
REGION VIII—Eur	AUT, BEL, BGR, CHE, CZE, DEU, ESP, FRA, GBR, ITA, LIE, LUX, NLD, NOR, POL, ROM, SVK
REGION IX—MidEast	IRN, IRQ, SYR, TUR
REGION X—IndSub	IND
REGION XI—Asia	AFG, CHN, JPN, MNG, RUS
REGION XIII—Poly	AUS

Incubation Period
Not known

Diagnostic Tests
Serology
Identification of parasite in surgical specimens

Typical Adult Therapy
Surgery (including liver transplantation in some cases)
Albendazole 400 mg PO b.i.d. × 28d—multiple courses
    advocated following wash-out periods

Typical Pediatric Therapy
Surgery (including liver transplantation in some cases)
Albendazole 10 mg/kg/d PO × 28d—multiple courses
    advocated following wash-out periods

Background

- *E. multilocularis* infection occurs only in the Northern Hemisphere. Although initially limited to Alaska and

Canada, the parasite has recently been described as far south as South Carolina. During the 1980s, four countries in Central Europe were considered endemic; 10 countries as of 1998. The annual incidence in western Europe is estimated at 0.5/100,000, increasing to as high as 80 to 100/100,000 in the Russian Federation and China.

- As of August 2001, 559 cases were identified in Europe—104 prior to 1980; 112 during 1981 to 1985; 127 during 1986 to 1990; 101 during 1991 to 1995; 115 during 1996 to 2000. In 28 cases, death was probably or definitely due to the parasite.
- More than 40 rodent species can serve as intermediate hosts, including microtine and arvicolid rodents, and occasionally muskrats and other small mammals. The usual definitive hosts are red foxes and arctic foxes (*Alopex lagopus*). Dogs and cats are also rarely implicated.

Causal Agent

Human echinococcosis (hydatidosis, or hydatid disease) is caused by the larval stages of cestodes (tapeworms) of the genus *Echinococcus*. *Echinococcus granulosus* causes cystic echinococcosis, the form most frequently encountered; *E. multilocularis* causes alveolar echinococcosis; *E. vogeli* causes polycystic echinococcosis; and *E. oligarthrus* is an extremely rare cause of human echinococcosis (CDC).

Life Cycle

Echinococcus granulosus adults (3 to 6 mm long) ❶ [Figure 4-19] reside in the small bowel of definitive hosts: dogs or other canids. Gravid proglottids release eggs ❷ [left section of Figure 4-19] which are passed in the feces. After ingestion by a suitable intermediate host (sheep, goat, swine, cattle, horses, camel), the egg hatches in the small bowel and releases an oncosphere ❸ [left section] which penetrates the intestinal wall and migrates through the circulatory system into various organs, notably the liver and lungs. Here, the oncosphere develops into a cyst ❹ [left section] that enlarges gradually, producing protoscolices and daughter cysts which fill the cyst interior. The definitive host becomes infected by ingesting the cyst-containing organs of the infected intermediate host. After ingestion, protoscolices ❺ evaginate, attach to the intestinal mucosa ❻, and develop into adult tapeworms ❶ in 32 to 80 days. *E. multilocularis* (1.2 to 3.7 mm) has a similar life cycle, with the following differences: the definitive hosts are foxes, and to a lesser extent dogs, cats, coyotes and wolves; the intermediate host[s] are small rodents; and larval growth (in the liver) continues indefinitely in the proliferative stage, resulting in invasion of the surrounding tissues. For *E. vogeli* (up to 5.6 mm long), the definitive hosts are bush dogs and dogs; the intermediate hosts are rodents; and the larval stage (in the liver, lungs and other organs) develops both externally and internally, resulting in multiple vesicles. *E. oligarthrus* (up to 2.9 mm long) has a life cycle that involves wild felids as definitive hosts and rodents as intermediate hosts. Humans become infected by ingesting eggs ❷ [right section], with resulting release of oncospheres ❸ [right section] in the intestine and the development of cysts ❹ [right section] in various organs (CDC).

Clinical Presentation

Humans acquire infection through ingestion of ova, which are excreted in the feces of definitive hosts.

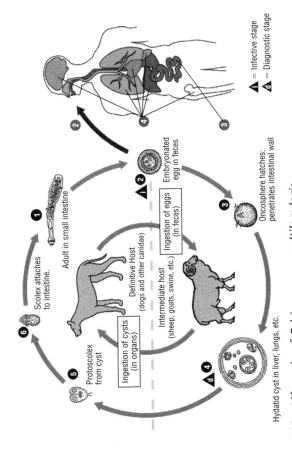

Figure 4-19 Life cycle of *Echinococcus multilocularis.*

▲ i = Infective stage
▲ d = Diagnostic stage

Adult in small intestine.
① Scolex attaches to intestine.

② Embryonated egg in feces

③ Oncosphere hatches; penetrates intestinal wall

Ingestion of eggs (in feces)

Definitive Host (dogs and other canidae)

Intermediate host (sheep, goats, swine, etc.)

④ Hydatid cyst in liver, lungs, etc.

⑤ Protoscolex from cyst

⑥

Ingestion of cysts (in organs)

173

Metacestodes develop in the liver and rarely in other organs. Following an incubation period of 5 to 15 years, infection might be manifest as epigastric pain or chronic cholestatic jaundice. The mean age at detection (Switzerland) is 52 years.

The liver is involved in 92 to 100% of patients. Metastatic lesions can involve the brain, spine, lungs, bones, and eyes. Fifteen percent of infections are asymptomatic. Spontaneous cure is rarely reported.

Reference
Echinococcosis. Centers for Disease Control Web site. Available at: http://www.dpd.cdc.gov/dpdx/html/Echinococcosis.htm. Accessed April 15, 2005.

Further Reading
Alveolar echinococcosis. Centers for Disease Control Web site. Available at: http://www.cdc.gov/ncidod/dpd/parasites/alveolarhydatid/factsht_alveolar_hydatid.htm. Accessed April 15, 2005.

Raether W, Hanel H. Epidemiology, clinical manifestations and diagnosis of zoonotic cestode infections: an update. *Parasitol Res.* 2003;91:412-438.

Eckert J, Deplazes P. Biological, epidemiological, and clinical aspects of echinococcosis, a zoonosis of increasing concern. *Clin Microbiol Rev.* 2004;17:107-135.

Vuitton DA, Zhou H, Bresson-Hadni S, et al. Epidemiology of alveolar echinococcosis with particular reference to China and Europe. *Parasitology.* 2003;127(suppl):S87-S107.

Echinostomiasis

Artyfechinostomomumiasis, Acanthoparyphiasis, Echinochasmus japonicus Infection, Echinoparyphium Infection, Episthmium Infection, Euparyphium Infection, Garrison's Fluke,

Himasthla Infection, Hypoderaeum Infection, Clinostomum complanatum, and marginatum, Neodiplostomum seoulensis

Agent
Platyhelminthes, Trematoda. At least 16 species—usually *Echinostoma ilocanum, E. malayanum, E. revolutum,* or *Echinoparyphium recurvatum, Artyfechinostomum malayanum* and *A. mehrai.*

Reservoir
Mammals, birds, humans, frogs, cats, snails

Vector
None

Vehicle
Land snails (*Pila*), clams, tadpoles, fish, water, water plants

Geographic Distribution
REGION II—CAm	MEX
REGION III—SAm	BRA
REGION VI—CAfr	KEN, TZA
REGION VIII—Eur	ROM
REGION X—IndSub	IND
REGION XI—Asia	CHN, JPN, KOR, PRK, RUS, SGP, TWN
REGION XII—SEA	IDN, KHM, MMR, MYS, PHL, THA, VNM

Incubation Period
Unknown

Diagnostic Tests
Identification of ova or adults in stool

Typical Therapy
Praziquantel 25 mg/kg t.i.d. × 1d (experimental)

Background

- Echinostomiasis is often widespread in endemic areas, but it tends to be clinically mild. The life cycle includes a first intermediate host (snail), second intermediate host (mollusc, fish, or amphibian larva) and definitive host (aquatic bird). The worldwide prevalence is estimated at 150,000 cases.
- At least sixteen species of *Echinostoma* have been reported to cause human infection. The more important forms include:
  ○ *E. malayanum*—found in Malaya, Thailand, India, and the Sino-Tibetan border. First intermediate host: *Lymnaea leuteola*. Second intermediate hosts: *Lymnaea leuteola, Gyraulus convexiusculus, Indoplanorbis,* and fish (*Barbus stigma*). *Echinostoma sufrartyfex* appears to be synonymous with *E. malayanum*.
  ○ *E. lindoensis*—formerly common in the area of Lake Lindoe, Celebes (Sulawesi). First intermediate hosts: *Anisus sarasinorum, Gyraulus convexiusculus.* Second intermediate hosts: *Vivipara javanica*, mussels.
  ○ *Euparyphium jassyense*—found in mink and trout. First intermediate host: *Stagnicola emargilatus.* Second intermediate host: tadpoles (Romania).
  ○ *Euparyphium* (*Echinostoma*) *ilocanum*—found in the Philippines, Celebes (Sulawesi), and Indonesia. First intermediate hosts: *Gyraulus convexiusculus* in the Philippines and Indonesia, *G. prashadi and Hippeutis umbilicalis* in the Philippines. Second intermediate host: *Gyraulus prashadi, Vivipara*

Burranghina, Planorbis umbilicatus, Vivipara rudipellis, and other snail species.

○ *Echinostoma revolutum*—found in ducks and geese. Human infection described in Thailand. First intermediate hosts: at least 14 snail species. Second intermediate hosts: bivalves, tadpoles, various snails.

○ *Echinostoma hortense*—found in rats and mice. Human infection described in China, Korea, and Japan. First intermediate hosts: *Lymnaea japonica, L. pervia* and *L. ollula.* Second intermediate hosts: tadpoles and fish.

○ *Echinostoma cinetorchis*—found in Japan, Taiwan, and Korea. First intermediate hosts: *Hippeutis cantori, Segmentina nitidella,* and various snails (*Cipangopaludina* spp.).

○ *Echinostoma macrochis*—found in rats. Human infection described in Japan. The snail hosts are *Cipangopaludina malleata, C. japonica, Segmentina nitidella,* and *Viviparus malleatus.*

○ *Echinostoma agustitestis* infection—has been reported from Fujian, China.

○ *Echinochasmus perfoliatus*—found in cats and dogs in Hungary, Italy, Romania, and Asia. Human infection described in Japan and Taiwan.

○ *Echinostoma japonicus*—found in birds. Human infection described in Japan, China, and Taiwan.

○ *Echinostoma jiufoensis*—Human infection described in China.

○ *Echinoparyphium recurvatum (E. paraulum)*— found in ducks, geese, swans, and doves. Human infection described in Taiwan and Yunnan (China).

○ *Episthmium caninum*—found in dogs. Human infection, acquired from freshwater fish, has been described in Thailand.

- *Euparyphium melis*—Human infection described in China and Romania.
- *Hypoderueum conideum*—found in birds. Human infection described in Thailand and Taiwan.
- *Clinostomum* spp.—found in freshwater fish. Has been associated with laryngitis and pharyngolaryngitis after eating freshwater fish.
- *Artyfechinostomosis*—has caused bowel perforation in India. *A. malayanum* has been recently recognized in the Philippines and is reported in humans and pigs.
- *Acanthoparyphium tyosenense*—has been recovered from humans in Korea; clinical significance unknown.
- *F. seoulensis*—was found in Korean males in their twenties who had acquired infection from roasted or raw snakes or frogs. Clinical significance unknown.
- *Echinochasmus japonicus* infection—has been associated with ingestion of cyprinoid or sweetfish.
- *Echinochasmus liliputanus*—is a parasite of dogs, cats, foxes, and badgers. Human infection has been reported from Anhui Province, China.
- *Echinochasmus fujianensis*—infests dogs, cats, pigs, and rats. Human infection is fairly common in Fujian Province, China.
- *Himasthla muehlensi*—a single human infection might have been acquired from infested clams in New York.

Clinical Presentation

Most infestations are either asymptomatic or limited to mild abdominal pain. Bloating, diarrhea, and eosinophilia are reported in some cases. The parasite is thought to survive for less than 1 year in the human intestine.

Clinostomum infestation can present as a foreign object in the pharynx and as laryngitis and pharyngitis.

Further Reading

Bangs MJ, Purnomo-Anthony RL. Echinostomiasis in the highlands of Irian Jaya, Indonesia. *Ann Trop Med Parasitol.* 1993;87:417-419.

Chung DI, Kong HH, Moon CH. Demonstration of the second intermediate hosts of Clinostomum complanatum in Korea. *Korean J Parasitol.* 1995;33:305-312.

Chung DI, Moon CH, Kong HH, Choi DW, Lim DK. The first human case of Clinostomum complanatum (Trematoda: Clinostomidae) infection in Korea. *Korean J Parasitol.* 1995;33:219-223.

Dzikowski R, Levy MG, Poore MF, Flowers JR, Paperna I. Clinostomum complanatum and Clinostomum marginatum (Rudolphi, 1819) (Digenea: Clinostomidae) are separate species based on differences in ribosomal DNA. *J Parasitol.* 2004;90:413-414.

Graczyk TK, Fried B. Echinostomiasis: a common but forgotten food-borne disease. *Am J Trop Med Hyg.* 1998;58:501-504.

Hong ST, Shoop WL. Neodiplostomum seoulensis n. comb. (Trematoda: Neodiplostomidae). *J Parasitol.* 1994;80: 660-663.

Huffman JE, Fried B. Echinostoma and echinostomiasis. *Adv Parasitol.* 1990;29:215-269.

Jueco NL, Monzon RB. Cathaemasia cabrerai sp.N. (Trematoda: Cathaemasiidae) a new parasite of man in the Philippines. *Southeast Asian J Trop Med Public Health.* 1984;15:427-429.

Kaul BK, Singhal GD, Pillai PN. Artyfechinostomum mehrai infestation with bowel perforation. *J Indian Med Assoc.* 1974;63:263-265.

Liu LX, Harinasuta KT. Liver and intestinal flukes. *Gastroenterol Clin North Am.* 1996;25:627-636.

Monzon RB, Kitikoon V. Lymnaea (Bullastra) cumingiana Pfeiffer (Pulmonata: Lymnaeidae): second intermediate host of Echinostoma malayanum in the Philippines. *Southeast Asian J Trop Med Public Health.* 1989;20:453-460.

Radomyos P, Bunnag D, Harinasuta T. Report of Episthmium caninum (Verma, 1935) Yamaguti, 1958 (Digenea: Echinostomatidae) in man. *Southeast Asian J Trop Med Public Health.* 1985;16:508-511.

Reddy DB, Ranganaykamma I. Artyfechinostomum maehari infestation in man. *J Trop Med Hyg.* 1964;67:58-59.

Seo BS, Lee SH, Chai JY, Hong SJ. Studies on intestinal trematodes in Korea XX. Four cases of natural human infection by Echinochasmus japonicus. *Kisaengchunghak Chapchi.* 1985;23:214-220.

Shirai R, Matsubara K, Ohnishi T, et al. A case of human infection with Clinostomum sp. *Kansenshogaku Zasshi.* 1998;72:1242-1245.

Tiewchaloern S, Udomkijdecha S, Suvouttho S, Chunchamsri K, Waikagul J. Clinostomum trematode from human eye. *Southeast Asian J Trop Med Public Health.* 1999;30:382-384.

Entamoeba histolytica

Agent
Protozoa. Sarcomastigota, Entamoebidea: *E. histolytica* (must be distinguished from noninvasive, *E. dispar*).

Reservoir
Humans

Vector
Flies (*Musca*)—occasionally

Vehicle
Food, water, sexual contact, flies

Geographic Distribution
Worldwide

Diagnostic Tests
Fresh stool/aspirate for microscopy
Stool antigen assay
Stool PCR
Note: serological tests usually negative.

Typical Adult Therapy
Metronidazole 750 mg t.i.d. $\times$ 10d, or tinidazole 600 mg b.i.d. $\times$ 5d

Typical Pediatric Therapy
Metronidazole 15 mg/kg t.i.d. $\times$ 10d

Background

- It is estimated that 10% of all humans are infested by *E. histolytica*, and 50 million develop clinical amebiasis annually, with 40,000 to 110,000 deaths.
- Amebiasis ranks second (malaria is first) as a cause of death due to parasites.
- *E. histolytica* can coexist with the nonpathogenic *E. dispar*. *E. dispar* accounts for 90% of *Entamoeba* infection in humans and is rarely associated with disease. *E. dispar* is morphologically indistinguishable from *E. histolytica*; however, the two can be differentiated using lectin analysis, monoclonal antibodies and ELISA-based diagnostic kits. Furthermore, unlike *E. histolytica*, *E. dispar* is difficult to culture in axenic culture.
- *Entamoeba moshkovskii* has been associated with asymptomatic colonization of the human colon in Bangladesh, North America, Italy, and South Africa.

Causal Agent

Several protozoan species in the genus *Entamoeba* infect humans, but not all of them are associated with disease. *Entamoeba histolytica* is well recognized as a pathogenic amoeba, associated with intestinal and extraintestinal infections. The other species are important because they may be confused with *E. histolytica* in diagnostic investigations (CDC).

Life Cycle

Cysts are passed in feces ❶ [Figure 4-20]. Infection by *Entamoeba histolytica* occurs through ingestion of mature cysts ❷ in fecally contaminated food, water, or hands. Excystation ❸ occurs in the small intestine and released trophozoites ❹ migrate to the large intestine. Trophozoites multiply by binary fission and produce cysts ❺, which are passed in feces ❶. Cysts can survive days to weeks in the external environment. (Trophozoites are rapidly destroyed once outside the body, and if ingested would not survive exposure to the gastric environment.) In many cases, the trophozoites remain confined to the intestinal lumen (🅐: noninvasive infection) of asymptomatic carriers. In some patients the trophozoites invade the intestinal mucosa (🅑: intestinal disease), or, through the bloodstream, extraintestinal sites such as the liver, brain, and lungs (🅒: extraintestinal disease). It is now known that the invasive and noninvasive forms represent two separate species, respectively *E. histolytica* and *E. dispar*, however not all persons infected with *E. histolytica* will have invasive disease. These two species are morphologically indistinguishable. Transmission can also occur through fecal exposure during sexual contact

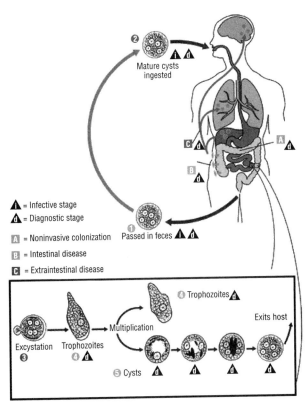

Figure 4-20   Life cycle of *Entamoeba histolytica*.

(in which case not only cysts, but also trophozoites could prove infective) (CDC).

Clinical Presentation

Patients with noninvasive infection might present with nonspecific gastrointestinal complaints such as chronic, in-termittent diarrhea, mucus, abdominal pain, flatulence, and weight loss. The onset of invasive infection is usually gradual (more than 1 to 3 weeks) and characterized by abdominal pain, tenderness, and bloody stools. Fever is present in one third of cases, and the abdomen could be enlarged and tender. Signs of fluid loss and electrolyte loss might be seen in severe infections. In children, colitis can present as rectal bleeding alone and without diarrhea. Fecal leukocytes might not be present, but are not as numerous as in shigellosis. Charcot-Leyden crystals are often seen in the stool.

Fulminant colitis is rare and carries a very high mortality. Predisposing factors include malnourishment, pregnancy, and corticosteroid treatment. Such patients are severely ill with fever, leukocytosis, profuse bloody and mucoid diarrhea, and generalized abdominal pain. Hypotension and peritonitis might be evident. Intestinal perforation and necrosis, or hepatic abscess could ensue.

Other complications include toxic megacolon (complicates 0.5% of amoebic colitis cases); annular ameboma of the colon, which could mimic carcinoma. Chronic, irritative bowel syndromes, ulcerative postdysenteric colitis or perianal amebiasis might also follow acute amoebic colitis.

Extraintestinal amebiasis might involve a wide variety of organs. Liver abscess presents as severe right sided abdominal or chest pain and tenderness, accompanied by fever and chills. Serological tests are positive (ie, negative in patients with amoebic dysentery) and the abscess is seen on ultrasound and other imaging studies. Other forms of amebiasis include brain abscess; rectovaginal fistulae, and penile infection.

Reference

Amebiasis. Centers for Disease Control Web site. Available at: http://www.dpd.cdc.gov/dpdx/HTML/Amebiasis.htm. Accessed April 15, 2005.

Further Reading

Amebiasis (Entamoeba histolytica infection or E. histolytica infection). Centers for Disease Control Web site. Available at: http://www.cdc.gov/ncidod/dpd/parasites/amebiasis/default.htm. Accessed April 15, 2005.

Espinosa Cantellano M, Martinez-Palomo A. Pathogenesis of intestinal amebiasis: from molecules to disease. *Clin Microbiol Rev.* 2000;13:318-331.

Jackson TF, Ravdin JI. Differentiation of Entamoeba histolytica and Entamoeba dispar infections. *Parasitol Today.* 1996;12:406-409.

Partners for Parasite Control (PPC). World Health Organization Web site. Available at: http://www.who.int/ctd/intpara/. Accessed April 15, 2005.

Stauffer W, Ravdin JI. Entamoeba histolytica: an update. *Curr Opin Infect Dis.* 2003;16:479-485.

Entamoeba polecki

Agent
Protozoa. Sarcomastigota, Entamoebidea: *E. polecki, E. chattoni.*

Reservoir
Pigs, monkeys

Vector
None

Vehicle
Contaminated food

Geographic Distribution
To date, *E. polecki* infection has been reported in scattered areas of Europe, Asia, Oceania, and South America.

REGION III—SAm	VEN
REGION X—IndSub	IND, BGD, PAK
REGION XII—SEA	IDN, KHM, THA, VNM
REGION XIII—Poly	AUS, PNG

Incubation Period
Unknown

Diagnostic Tests
Identification of cysts in stool

Typical Adult Therapy
Metronidazole 750 mg PO t.i.d. × 10d (investigational)

Typical Pediatric Therapy
Metronidazole 15 mg/kg t.i.d. × 10d (investigational)

Background
- Most cases of *E. polecki* infection have been reported from Southeast Asia and Papua New Guinea.
- The parasite is found in pigs, monkeys, and other animals, and humans are infected through ingestion of fecally contaminated material.
- Concurrent infection by other parasites is common.

Clinical Presentation
Most infections are mild or subclinical. Symptoms could include mucoid diarrhea and abdominal pain. Severe disease is unusual and should suggest another etiology.

Further Reading
Barnish G, Ashford RW. Occasional parasitic infections of man in Papua New Guinea and Irian Jaya (New Guinea). *Ann Trop Med Parasitol.* 1989;83:121-135.

Boles JM, Masure O. Entamoeba polecki infection in France. *Mayo Clin Proc.* 1986;61:226.

Chacin-Bonilla L. Entamoeba polecki: human infections in Venezuela. *Trans R Soc Trop Med Hyg.* 1992;86:634.

Gay JD, Abell TL, Thompson JH Jr, Loth V. Entamoeba polecki infection in Southeast Asian refugees: multiple cases of a rarely reported parasite. *Mayo Clin Proc.* 1985;60:523-530.

Sargeaunt PG, Patrick S, O'Keeffe D. Human infections of Entamoeba chattoni masquerade as Entamoeba histolytica. *Trans R Soc Trop Med Hyg.* 1992;86(6):633-634.

Verweij JJ, Polderman AM, Clark CG. Genetic variation among human isolates of uninucleated cyst-producing Entamoeba species. *J Clin Microbiol.* 2001;39:1644-1646.

Wiwanitkit V. Entamoeba polecki as a cause of human infection. *Rev Med Microbiol.* 2004;15:41-43.

Enterobius vermicularis

Pinworm, Oxyuriasis, Seatworm

Agent
Nematoda. Phasmidea: *E. vermicularis* (controversy exists as to the existence of *E. gregorii*).

Reservoir
Humans

Vector
None

Vehicle
Fecal–oral contact, air, clothing, sexual contact (rare)

Geographic Distribution
Worldwide

Incubation Period
28–42d

Diagnostic Tests
Apply cellophane tape to anal verge in a.m. and paste onto glass slide for microscopy

Typical Adult Therapy
Albendazole 400 mg PO as single dose—repeat in 2w
Or mebendazole 100 mg PO as single dose—repeat in 2w
Or pyrantel pamoate 11 mg/kg (max 1 g) PO as single dose

Typical Pediatric Therapy
Mebendazole 100 mg PO as single dose (> age 2)—
   repeat in 2w
Or pyrantel pamoate 11 mg/kg (max 1 g) PO × 1

Background

- It is estimated that 400 million persons are infested by pinworm worldwide. The highest prevalence occurs among children ages 5 to 10 years. The disease is equally common among males and females.
- *E. vermicularis* could be the most prevalent nematode parasite in the United States and Europe. Humans are the only host, and transmission is maintained through fecal–oral spread and uncommonly by inhalation or ingestion of eggs from fomites. In temperate climates, transmission is facilitated by decreased washing, increased clothing and contact, and prolonged survival of eggs.
- The short-lived female worm resides in the cecum but wanders out into the perineal area to oviposit eggs (4,000 to 16,000 per worm). Rarely, adult worms

migrate to other sites such as the vulva, peritoneum, and appendix. Ova mature rapidly, and remain viable for as long as 13 days—with a potential for wide transmission. Retroinfection occurs when larvae hatch from eggs and return to the cecum.

- Transmission of an unrelated protozoan parasite, *Dientamoeba fragilis*, might occur via the ova of *E. vermicularis*. *D. fragilis* has been found to persist in the intestinal canal of pinworms for more than 84 days.
- Cellophane tape applied to the perineum on awakening is used to detect eggs deposited on skin. Eggs are not usually seen on stool examination. Adult worms can also be seen but are quite small (10 by 0.5 mm).

Causal Agent

The nematode (roundworm) *Enterobius vermicularis* (previously *Oxyuris vermicularis*) also called human pinworm. (Adult females: 8 to 13 mm, adult male: 2 to 5 mm.). Humans are considered to be the only hosts of *E. vermicularis*. A second species, *Enterobius gregorii*, has been described and reported from Europe, Africa, and Asia. For all practical purposes, the morphology, life cycle, clinical presentation, and treatment of *E. gregorii* are identical to those of *E. vermicularis* (CDC).

Life Cycle

Eggs are deposited on perianal folds ❶ [Figure 4-21]. Self-infection occurs by transferring infective eggs to the mouth ❷ with hands that have scratched this area. Person-to-person transmission can also occur through handling of contaminated clothes or bed linens. Enterobiasis may also

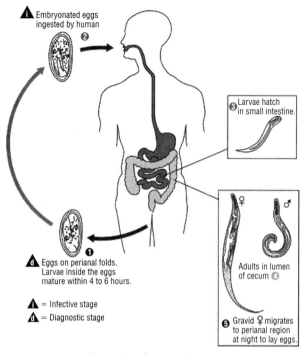

Figure 4-21   Life cycle of *Enterobius vermicularis*.

be acquired through surfaces in the environment that are contaminated with pinworm eggs (eg, curtains, carpeting). Some small number of eggs may become airborne, inhaled and swallowed. Following ingestion of infective eggs, larvae hatch in the small intestine ❸ and adults establish themselves in the colon ❹. The time interval from ingestion of infective eggs to oviposition by adult females is one month.

The life span of adults is two months. Gravid females migrate nocturnally and oviposit while crawling on the skin of the perianal area ❺. Larvae develop (ie, the eggs become infective) in 4 to 6 hours under optimal conditions ❶. Retro-infection, or the migration of newly hatched larvae from the anal skin back into the rectum, may occur (CDC).

Clinical Presentation

The typical manifestation of enterobiasis is nocturnal pruritus ani related to hypersensitivity to worm antigens. Local dermal tingling is also encountered. Migration of adult females to the vulva can result in vulvovaginitis or predispose to urinary tract infection. Eosinophilia is occasionally present. Complications are rare, and they include appendicitis, salpingitis, and urethritis.

Reference

Enterobiasis. Centers for Disease Control Web site. Available at: http://www.dpd.cdc.gov/dpdx/HTML/Enterobiasis.htm. Accessed April 15, 2005.

Further Reading

Hasegawa H, Takao Y, Nakao M, Fukuma T, Tsuruta O, Ide K. Is Enterobius gregorii Hugot, 1983 (Nematoda: Oxyuridae) a distinct species? *J Parasitol.* 1998;84:131-134.

Kucik CJ, Martin GL, Sortor BV. Common intestinal parasites. *Am Fam Physician.* 2004;69:1161-1168.

Pinworm infection. Centers for Disease Control Web site. Available at: http://www.cdc.gov/ncidod/dpd/parasites/pinworm/default.htm. Accessed April 15, 2005.

Totkova A, Klobusicky M, Holkova R, Valent M. Enterobius gregorii—reality or fiction? *Bratisl Lek Listy.* 2003;104:130-133.

Fasciola hepatica

Lederegelbefall, Sheep Liver Fluke

Agent
Parasite—Platyhelminthes, Trematoda. Echinostomatida, Fasciolidae: *F. hepatica* or *F. gigantica. Eurytrema pancreaticum.*

Reservoir
Sheep, cattle, snails (*Lymnaea, Fossaria*)

Vector
None

Vehicle
Food, aquatic plants, watercress (*Nasturtium officinale*)

Geographic Distribution
Worldwide

Incubation Period
2w–3m

Diagnostic Tests
Identification of ova in stool or duodenal aspirates
    (adult parasites in surgical specimens)
Serology; cholangiography; CT scan

Typical Therapy
Triclabendazole 10 mg/kg PO × 2 doses
Or bithionol 50 mg/kg every other day × 10 doses

Background

- Fascioliasis is a disease of sheep, cattle, and goats—with humans representing an accidental host.
- Infection occurs when humans consume uncooked aquatic vegetables, such as watercress, which are contaminated with encysted parasite larvae. The larvae escape from the cysts in the small intestine soon after ingestion and migrate across the intestinal wall into the abdominal cavity. Within 24 hours of infection, the larvae have transformed into immature worms. Once they reach the liver, they feed on hepatic tissue until they reach the bile ducts, where they mature into adults. As hermaphroditic trematodes, each worm produces eggs which are released via the biliary tree into the feces.
- Immature eggs reach fresh water, mature within two weeks, and release miracidia. The latter must encounter suitable snail intermediate hosts within 24 hours of hatching. Suitable vectors are aquatic or amphibious snails of the Lymnaeidae family. Within the snail, miracidia undergo asexual multiplication, producing several thousand cercariae over several weeks. The latter are released into fresh water, eventually encysting as metacercariae on aquatic plants (ie, watercress and water caltrop).
- More than 300,000 cases of fascioliasis were reported from more than 61 countries during 1970 to 1994—most from Bolivia, Cuba, Egypt, France, Iran, Peru, Portugal, the former Soviet Union, Spain, and the United Kingdom. The true number of human infestations is estimated at 2.4 to 17 million.
- Of reported cases, 5.1% occur in Africa, 17.3% in Latin America, and 74.1% from Europe. France

accounted for 37.1% of the world's cases during 1969 to 1989, and Portugal for 20.7%.

- It is estimated that 180 million humans, 250 million sheep and 350 million cattle are at risk worldwide.
- Human infection with *F. gigantica* is encountered in Zimbabwe, Uganda, Russia (Tashkent), Iraq, Vietnam, Thailand, the Philippines, and the United States (Hawaii).
- The snail hosts are *L. truncatula* (Europe, western Asia, African highlands), *L. viator* and *L. diaphana* (South America), *L. bulmoides* and *L. humilis* (North America), *L. columella* (worldwide), *L. cubensis* (Caribbean), *L. tomentosa* (Australia).
- *E. pancreaticum,* as an asymptomatic infection, has been found in humans in Japan.

Causal Agents

The trematodes *Fasciola hepatica* (the sheep liver fluke) and *Fasciola gigantica*, parasites of herbivores that can infect humans accidentally (CDC).

Life Cycle

Immature eggs are discharged in the biliary ducts and pass into the stool ❶ [Figure 4-22]. Eggs become embryonated in water ❷, and release miracidia ❸ which invade a suitable snail intermediate host ❹, notably several species of the *Lymnae*. In the snail the parasites undergo several developmental stages (sporocysts ❹a, rediae ❹b, and cercariae ❹c). Cercariae are released from the snail ❺ and encyst as metacercariae on aquatic vegetation or other surfaces. Mammals acquire infection by eating vegetation containing metacercariae. Humans can become

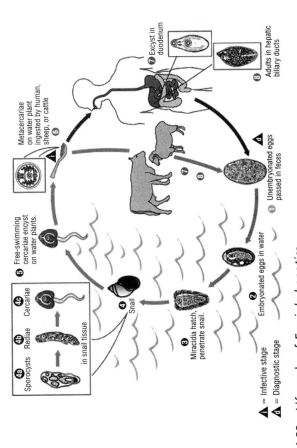

1 Excyst in duodenum

8 Adults in hepatic biliary ducts

6 Metacercariae on water plant ingested by human, sheep, or cattle

5 Free-swimming cercariae encyst on water plants.

4a Sporocysts **4b** Rediae **4c** Cercariae

in snail tissue

4 Snail

3 Miracidia hatch, penetrate snail.

2 Embryonated eggs in water

1 Unembryonated eggs passed in feces

▲ = Infective stage

△ = Diagnostic stage

Figure 4-22 Life cycle of *Fasciola hepatica*.

195

infected by ingesting metacercariae on freshwater plants, especially watercress ❻. After ingestion, the metacercariae excyst in the duodenum ❼ and migrate through the intestinal wall, the peritoneal cavity, and the liver parenchyma into the biliary ducts, where they develop into adults ❽. In humans, maturation into adults takes approximately 3 to 4 months. The adult flukes (*Fasciola hepatica*: up to 30 mm by 13 mm; *F. gigantica*: up to 75 mm) reside in the larger biliary ducts of the mammalian host. *Fasciola hepatica* infects various animal species, primarily herbivores (CDC).

Clinical Presentation

The presence and severity of disease depend on the intensity of infection and the host. Symptoms can appear a few days after ingestion of larvae, when the immature worms reach the abdominal cavity and begin migrating across or within the liver. Typical early symptoms include fever, abdominal pain, gastrointestinal disturbances, and urticaria. Hepatomegaly, anemia, and jaundice might also be present. A latent phase follows, during which the only finding is prominent eosinophilia. Eventually, the patient enters a chronic phase characterized by biliary colic, epigastric pain, jaundice, hepatomegaly, and abdominal tenderness.

Reference

Fascioliasis. Centers for Disease Control Web site. Available at: http://www.dpd.cdc.gov/dpdx/HTML/Fascioliasis.htm. Accessed April 15, 2005.

Further Reading

Fasciola infection. Centers for Disease Control Web site. Available at: http://www.cdc.gov/ncidod/dpd/parasites/ fasciola/default.htm. Accessed April 15, 2005.

Ishii Y, Koga M, Fujino T, et al. Human infection with the pancreas fluke, Eurytrema pancreaticum. *Am J Trop Med Hyg.* 1983;32:1019-1022.

Mas Coma MS, Esteban JG, Bargues MD. Epidemiology of human fascioliasis: a review and proposed new classification. *Bull World Health Organ.* 1999;77:340-346.

Sezgin O, Altintas E, Disibeyaz S, Saritas U, Sahin B. Hepatobiliary fascioliasis: clinical and radiologic features and endoscopic management. *J Clin Gastroenterol.* 2004;38:285-291.

Fasciolopsis buski

Agent
Platyhelminthes, Trematoda. Echinostomatida, Fasciolidae: *F. buski*.

Reservoir
Pigs, humans, dogs, snails (*Hippeutis, Segmentina*)

Vector
None

Vehicle
Food, aquatic plants, water chestnut (*Eliocharis tuberosa*), water caltrop (*Trapa natans*), water fern (*Salvinia natans*)

Geographic Distribution

REGION X—IndSub	BGD, IND, PAK
REGION XI—Asia	CHN, JPN, KOR, PRK, TWN
REGION XII—SEA	IDN, KHM, LAO, MMR, MYS, THA, VNM

Incubation Period
1–3m

Diagnostic Tests
Identification of ova in stool; passage (vomiting) of adult worm

Typical Adult Therapy
Praziquantel 25 mg/kg t.i.d. $\times$ 3 doses
Or niclosamide 2 g chewed thoroughly

Typical Pediatric Therapy
Praziquantel 25 mg/kg t.i.d. $\times$ 3 doses
Or niclosamide 1 g (for weight $\leq$ 34 kg) to 1.5 g (weight
   > 34 kg)

Background

- An estimated 17 million are infested by *Fasciolopis*. The parasite was first described in 1843 and is found in the Far East.
- Worms grow to a length of 75 mm and can survive for more than 6 months in humans.
- Pigs and dogs can act as reservoirs. The snail reservoirs are *Hippeutis umbilicalis*, *H. cantori*, *Segmentina hemisphaerula* and *S. trochoideus*.
- The vehicles are water calthrop (*Trapa natans* in China, *T. bicornis* in India, *T. bisponosa* in Taiwan); water chestnut (*E. tuberosa*, in southern China); water bamboo (*Zigania aquatica*, in Chekiang and Canton); water morning glory (*Ipomoea aquatica*), lotus (*Nymphaea lotus*) and water hyacinth (*Eichornia crassipes*, in Taiwan).

Causal Agent

The trematode *Fasciolopsis buski,* the largest intestinal fluke of humans (CDC).

Life Cycle

Immature eggs are discharged into the intestine and stool ❶ [Figure 4-23]. Eggs become embryonated in water ❷, and release miracidia ❸ which invade a suitable snail intermediate host ❹. In the snail the parasites undergo several developmental stages (sporocysts ❹ⓐ, rediae ❹ⓑ, and cercariae ❹ⓒ). Cercariae are released from the snail ❺ and encyst as metacercariae on aquatic plants ❻. Mammalian hosts become infected by ingesting metacercariae attached to aquatic plants. After ingestion, metacercariae excyst in the duodenum ❼ and attach to the intestinal wall. Adult flukes (20 to 75 mm by 8 to 20 mm) appear in approximately 3 months, attached to the intestinal wall of the mammalian hosts (humans and pigs) ❽. Adults have a life span of one year (CDC).

Clinical Presentation

Most infections are asymptomatic or subclinical. Symptoms can mimic peptic ulcer and include epigastric pain, nausea, eosinophilia, and diarrhea. Generalized edema and prostration have been described in heavy infections.

Reference

Fasciolopsiasis. Centers for Disease Control Web site. Available at: http://www.dpd.cdc.gov/dpdx/HTML/Fasciolopsiasis. htm. Accessed April 15, 2005.

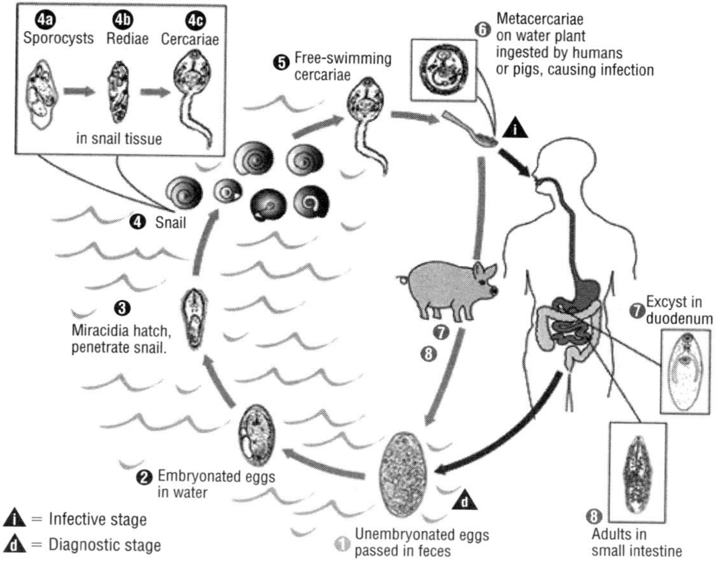
4a Sporocysts
4b Rediae
4c Cercariae
in snail tissue
4 Snail
5 Free-swimming cercariae
6 Metacercariae on water plant ingested by humans or pigs, causing infection
i
7 Excyst in duodenum
8 Adults in small intestine
7
8
d
1 Unembryonated eggs passed in feces
2 Embryonated eggs in water
3 Miracidia hatch, penetrate snail.
i = Infective stage
d = Diagnostic stage

Figure 4-23 Life cycle of *Fasciolopsis buski*.

Further Reading

Fasciolopsis infection. Centers for Disease Control Web site. Available at: http://www.cdc.gov/ncidod/dpd/parasites/fasciolopsis/default.htm. Accessed April 15, 2005.

Graczyk TK, Gilman RH, Fried B. Fasciolopsiasis: is it a controllable food-borne disease? *Parasitol Res.* 2001;87:80-83.

Liu LX, Harinasuta KT. Liver and intestinal flukes. *Gastroenterol Clin North Am.* 1996;25:627-636.

Rabbani GH, Gilman RH, Kabir I, Mondel G. The treatment of Fasciolopsis buski infection in children: a comparison of thiabendazole, mebendazole, levamisole, pyrantel pamoate, hexylresorcinol and tetrachloroethylene. *Trans R Soc Trop Med Hyg.* 1985;79:513-515.

Waikagul J. Intestinal fluke infections in Southeast Asia. *Southeast Asian J Trop Med Public Health.* 1991;22(suppl):158-162.

Filariasis

General Description

Filariasis can be caused by roundworms, of which generally eight species are important for human infection, resulting in lymphatic and tissue damage. Three predominant organisms lead to most of the human morbidity: *Brugia malayi*, *Wuchereria bancrofti* (resulting in lymphedema syndromes), and *Onchocerca volvulum* (resulting in river blindness). Other species include *Brugia timori*, *Loa loa*, and *Mansonella* spp. (*M. perstans*, *M. streptocerca*, and *M. ozzardi*).

The infectious cycle begins with the bite of an arthropod that transmits infective larvae that then migrate to various parts of the host, such as lymphatic and subcutaneous tissues, where adults develop and produce microfilariae. The adult worms will generally lead to chronic infection and, with a few exceptions, the female worms produce microfilariae that invade the circulatory system. As outlined in the following pages, the worms primarily differ in associated vector(s), geographic distribution, and clinical syndromes.

Filariasis—*Brugia malayi*

Malayan Filariasis

Agent
Nematoda. Phasmidea, Filariae: *B. malayi*

Reservoir
Humans, nonhuman primates, cats, civet cats

Vector
Mosquito (*Mansonia, Aedes, Anopheles*)

Vehicle
None

Geographic Distribution

REGION X—IndSub	BGD, IND, LKA
REGION XI—Asia	CHN, JPN, KOR, PRK
REGION XII—SEA	BRN, IDN, MMR, MYS, PHL, THA, VNM

Incubation Period
5–18m (range 1m–2y)

Diagnostic Tests
Identification of microfilariae in nocturnal blood
    specimen.
Nucleic acid amplification.
Serology can be helpful.

Typical Therapy
Diethylcarbamazine:
50 mg day 1; 50 mg t.i.d. day 2; 100 mg t.i.d. day 3
Then 2 mg/kg t.i.d. × 18 days.
Or ivermectin 200 ug/kg PO as single dose

Background

- The worldwide prevalence of *B. malayi* infection as of 1996 was estimated at 12.91 million (0.47% of the population of Asia).
- Microfilaremia can be nocturnally periodic or semiperiodic.
- *Brugia malayi* and *Brugia timori* do not coexist in a given population; however, *Wuchereria bancrofti* can coexist with either.
- The principal vectors for periodic *B. malayi* are *Anopheles barbirostris, A. campestris, A. donaldi, Mansonia annulata, M. annulifera,* and *M. uniformis.* Local or subsidiary vectors include *A. anthrophagus, A. kweiyangensis, A. nigerrimus, A. sinensis, M. bonneae, M. dives, M. indiana, Ochlerotatus kiangsiensis,* and *O. togoi.*
- The principal vectors of subperiodic *B. malayi* are *Mansonia annulata, M. bonneae,* and *M. dives.* Local or subsidiary vectors include *Coquillettidia crassipes* and *Mansonia uniformis.*

Life Cycle

The typical vector for *Brugia malayi* filariasis are mosquito species from the genera *Mansonia* and *Aedes.* During a blood meal, an infected mosquito introduces third-stage filarial larvae onto the skin of the human host, where they penetrate into the bite wound ❶ [Figure 4-24]. They

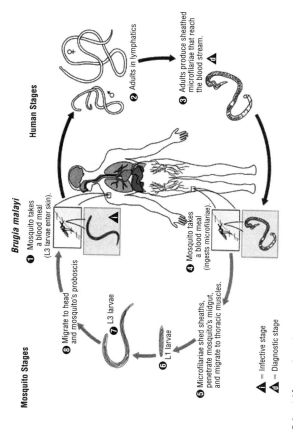

Human Stages

① Mosquito takes
a blood meal
(L3 larvae enter skin).

② Adults in lymphatics

③ Adults produce sheathed
microfilariae that reach
the blood stream.

Brugia malayi

④ Mosquito takes
a blood meal
(ingests microfilariae).

Mosquito Stages

⑧ Migrate to head
and mosquito's proboscis.

⑦ L3 larvae

⑥ L1 larvae

⑤ Microfilariae shed sheaths,
penetrate mosquito's midgut,
and migrate to thoracic muscles.

▲ = Infective stage
◭ = Diagnostic stage

Figure 4-24 Life cycle of *Brugia malayi*.

develop into adults that commonly reside in the lymphatics ❷. The adult worms resemble those of *Wuchereria bancrofti* but are smaller. Female worms measure 43 to 55 mm in length by 130 to 170 μm in width, and males measure 13 to 23 mm in length by 70 to 80 μm in width. Adults produce microfilariae, measuring 177 to 230 μm in length and 5 to 7 μm in width, which are sheathed and have nocturnal periodicity. The microfilariae migrate into lymph and enter the bloodstream reaching the peripheral blood ❸. A mosquito ingests the microfilariae during a blood meal ❹. After ingestion, the microfilariae lose their sheaths and work their way through the wall of the proventriculus and cardiac portion of the midgut to reach the thoracic muscles ❺. There the microfilariae develop into first-stage larvae ❻ and subsequently into third-stage larvae ❼. The third-stage larvae migrate through the hemocoel to the mosquito's proboscis ❽, and can infect another human when the mosquito takes a blood meal ❶ (CDC).

Clinical Presentation

The main clinical features which differentiate Bancroftian from brugian filariasis are the rarity of genital lesions (hydrocoele) and chyluria in the latter. Edema extending above the knee is also primarily a feature of Bancroftian disease. Abscess formation is often encountered with brugian filariasis in Malaysia, Indonesia, and Thailand; but not in India or other countries.

Reference

Filariasis. Centers for Disease Control Web site. Available at: http://www.dpd.cdc.gov/dpdx/HTML/Filariasis.htm. Accessed April 15, 2005.

Further Reading

Brown KR, Ricci FM, Ottesen EA. Ivermectin: effectiveness in lymphatic filariasis. *Parasitology.* 2000;121(suppl):S133-S146.

The Global Alliance to Eliminate Lymphatic Filariasis Web site. Available at: http://www.filariasis.org. Accessed April 15, 2005.

Kron M, Walker E, Hernandez L, Torres E, Libranda-Ramirez B. Lymphatic filariasis in the Philippines. *Parasitol Today.* 2000;16:329-333.

Lymphatic Filariasis. Centers for Disease Control Web site. Available at: http://www.cdc.gov/ncidod/dpd/parasites/lymphaticfilariasis/default.htm. Accessed April 15, 2005.

Meyrowitsch DW, Nguyen DT, Hoang TH, Nguyen TD, Michael E. A review of the present status of lymphatic filariasis in Vietnam. *Acta Trop.* 1998;70:335-347.

Taylor MJ, Hoerauf A. Wolbachia bacteria of filarial nematodes. *Parasitol Today.* 1999;15:437-442.

Filariasis—*Brugia timori*

Timor Filariasis

Agent
Nematoda. Phasmidea, Filariae: *B. timori.*

Reservoir
Humans

Vector
Mosquito (*Anopheles barbirostris, Aedes oceanicus, Aedes samoanus*)

Vehicle
None

Geographic Distribution
REGION XII—SEA   IDN

Incubation Period
5–18m (range 1m–2y)

Diagnostic Tests
Identification of microfilariae in blood specimen

Typical Adult Therapy
Diethylcarbamazine:
50 mg day 1; 50 mg t.i.d. day 2; 100 mg t.i.d. day 3; 2 mg/
kg t.i.d. days 4 to 21

Typical Pediatric Therapy
Diethylcarbamazine:
25 mg day 1; 25 mg t.i.d. day 2; 50 mg t.i.d. day 3; 2 mg/
kg t.i.d. days 4 to 21

Background
- The disease is limited to East Timor and islands of the Lesser Sunda Archipelago: Flores, Alor, Sumba, Roti, and Savu.
- Clinical disease on Flores occurs in coastal (but not highland) areas, and it is more common among males than females. Disease rates on the island double between the first and second decades of life.
- In the highland population of Alor Island, 25% of the population is microfilaremic and 13% has lymphedema (2001).
- *B. malayi* and *B. timori* do not coexist in a given population; however, *Wuchereria bancrofti* can coexist with either.

Clinical Presentation

Clinical and pathological features are similar to those of Bancroftian filariasis. Scarring over thick, hard, cordlike lymphatics are a hallmark of the disease. Elephantiasis is rare.

Further Reading

Davis BR. Filariases. *Dermatol Clin.* 1989;7:313-321.

Ottesen EA. Efficacy of diethylcarbamazine in eradicating infection with lymphatic-dwelling filariae in humans. *Rev Infect Dis.* 1985;7:341-356.

Partono F, Maizels RM. Towards a filariasis-free community: evaluation of filariasis control over an eleven-year period in Flores, Indonesia. *Trans R Soc Trop Med Hyg.* 1989;83:821-826.

Supali T, Wibowo H, Ruckert P, et al. High prevalence of Brugia timori infection in the highland of Alor Island, Indonesia. *Am J Trop Med Hyg.* 2002;66:560-565.

Filariasis—*Brugia*—Other

Zoonotic Brugia

Zoonotic *Brugia* species are carried by a variety of carnivores and rodents, particularly in the United States, Colombia, Brazil, Peru, and Ethiopia.

Possible agents include *B. beaveri* (raccoon) and *B. leporis* (rabbits) in the United States; *B. guyanensis* (coatimundi) in South America; *B. tupaie* (tree shrews), *B. pahangi* (dogs, cats, slow loris, monkeys, wildcats) in Malaysia; *B. patei* (dogs, cats, bush babies) in Africa; *B. ceylonensis* (dogs) and *B. guckley* (hares) in Sri Lanka.

The species which infect humans have not been identified. Human infection usually involves lymphatics of the neck, groin, or axilla. Most cases present as painful regional lymphadenopathy, occasionally with eosinophilia.

Geographic Distribution

REGION I—NAm	USA
REGION III—SAm	ARG, BOL, BRA, CHL, COL, ECU, GUF, GUY, PER, PRY, SUR, URY, VEN
REGION VI—CAfr	ETH
REGION X—IndSub	LKA
REGION XII—SEA	MYS

Filariasis—*Loa Loa*

Calabar Swellings, Filaria Lacrimalis, Filaria Loa, Filaria Oculi Humani, Filaria Subconjunctivalis, Fugitive Swellings, Microfilaria Diurna

Agent
Nematoda. Phasmidea, Filariae: *L. loa*

Reservoir
Humans

Vector
Fly (deer fly = *Chrysops)*

Vehicle
None

Geographic Distribution

REGION VI—CAfr	AGO, BEN, CAF, CIV, CMR, COD, COG, GAB, GHA, GIN, GNB, GNQ, MLI, NGA, SDN, TCD, UGA

Incubation Period
4m–3y

Diagnostic Tests
Microfilariae in blood (take during daylight hours)
Adult worm recovered
Serology
Nucleic acid amplification

Typical Therapy
Diethylcarbamazine:
50 mg PO day 1; 50 mg PO t.i.d. day 2; 100 mg PO t.i.d.
  day 3; 3 mg/kg PO t.i.d. days 4 to 21
  Note: Ivermectin can cause encephalopathy if dual
infection with *Onchocerca* is present.

Background

- Loiasis occurs only in Africa, and an estimated 20 to 30
  million people live in endemic areas.
- Human infection by *Loaina* spp., zoonotic parasites of
  rabbits and kangaroos, have been reported in South
  America and Australia.
- The disease is most often acquired during daylight in
  proximity to streams or ponds in parts of west and
  central Africa. Highest transmission takes place during
  the wet season.
- Microfilaria rates are highest among males, with adults
  affected more often than children.

Life Cycle

The vector[s] for *Loa loa* filariasis are flies from two
species of the genus *Chrysops*, *C. silacea* and *C. dimidiata*.
During a blood meal, an infected fly (genus *Chrysops*,

day-biting flies) introduces third-stage filarial larvae onto the skin of the human host, where they penetrate into the bite wound ❶ [Figure 4-25]. The larvae develop into adults that commonly reside in subcutaneous tissue ❷. The female worms measure 40 to 70 mm in length and 0.5 mm in diameter, while the males measure 30 to 34 mm in length and 0.35 to 0.43 mm in diameter. Adults produce microfilariae measuring 250 to 300 μm by 6 to 8 μm, which are sheathed and have diurnal periodicity. Microfilariae have been recovered from spinal fluids, urine, and sputum. During the day they are found in peripheral blood, but during the noncirculation phase, they are found in the lungs ❸. The fly ingests microfilariae during a blood meal ❹. After ingestion, the microfilariae lose their sheaths and migrate from the fly's midgut through the hemocoel to the thoracic muscles of the arthropod ❺. There the microfilariae develop into first-stage larvae ❻ and subsequently into third-stage infective larvae ❼. The third-stage infective larvae migrate to the fly's proboscis ❽ and can infect another human when the fly takes a blood meal ❶ (CDC).

Clinical Presentation

In many cases, infected patients are asymptomatic, with eosinophilia as their sole clinical finding. Transient areas of localized subcutaneous edema (Calabar swellings) are preceded by pain and itching for several hours. The lesions are nonerythematous, measure 10 to 20 cm, and last for days to weeks. Calabar swellings are most common around joints. Accompanying pruritus or urticaria might be noted.

Often, an adult worm will pass beneath the conjunctiva, resulting in local swelling, pain, and inflammation. Complications include endomyocardial fibrosis, retino-

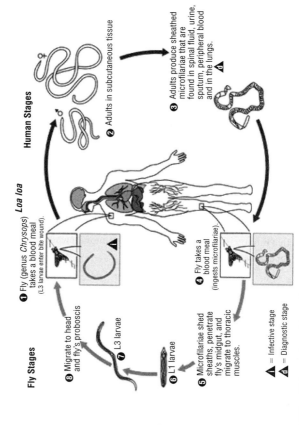

Human Stages

② Adults in subcutaneous tissue

③ Adults produce sheathed microfilariae that are found in spinal fluid, urine, sputum, peripheral blood and in the lungs. ◢

① Fly (genus *Chrysops*) takes a blood meal (L3 larvae enter bite wound). ▲

④ Fly takes a blood meal (ingests microfilariae).

Fly Stages

⑧ Migrate to head and fly's proboscis.

⑦ L3 larvae

⑥ L1 larvae

⑤ Microfilariae shed sheaths, penetrate fly's midgut, and migrate to thoracic muscles.

▲ = Infective stage
◢ = Diagnostic stage

Loa loa

Figure 4-25 Life cycle of *Loa loa*.

pathy, encephalopathy, peripheral neuropathy, arthritis, pleural effusion, and breast calcification.

Reference

Filariasis. Centers for Disease Control Web site. Available at: http://www.dpd.cdc.gov/dpdx/HTML/Filariasis.htm. Accessed April 15, 2005.

Further Reading

Boussinesq M, Gardon J. Prevalences of Loa loa microfila-raemia throughout the area endemic for the infection. *Ann Trop Med Parasitol.* 1997;91:573-589.

Cook GC. Discovery and clinical importance of the filariases. *Infect Dis Clin North Am.* 2004;18:219-230.

Filariasis. Centers for Disease Control Web site. Available at: http://www.dpd.cdc.gov/dpdx/HTML/Filariasis.htm. Accessed April 15, 2005.

Nutman TB, Kradin RL. Case records of the Massachusetts General Hospital, weekly clinicopathological exercises. Case 1-2002: a 24-year-old woman with paresthesias and muscle cramps after a stay in Africa. *N Engl J Med.* 2002;346:115-122.

Filariasis—*Mansonella ozzardi*

Filaria Ozzardi, Microfilaria Bolivarensis, Tetrapetalonema Ozzardi

Agent

Nematoda. Phasmidea, Filariae: *M. ozzardi.*

Reservoir

Humans

Vector

Fly (black fly = *Simulium* spp.) or gnats/midges (*Culicoides* spp.)

Vehicle
None

Geographic Distribution

REGION II—CAm	GTM, MEX, PAN
REGION III—SAm	ARG, BOL, BRA, COL, GUF, GUY, PER, SUR, VEN
REGION IV—Carib	ATG, DMA, GLP, HTI, KNA, LCA, PRI, TCA, TTO, VCT
REGION VI—CAfr	MRT

Incubation Period
5–18m (range 1m–2y)

Diagnostic Tests
Identification of microfilariae in skin snips or blood

Typical Therapy
Ivermectin 150 ug/kg PO as single dose

Background

- *M. ozzardi* is found in Central America, northern South America (Brazil and Venezuela) and the Caribbean.
- Microfilaria rates in endemic foci increase with age.
- Vectors include *Simulium amazonicum* and possibly *Culicoides insinuatus* (Amazon region), *C. furens* (St. Vincent and Haiti), *C. phlebotomus* (Trinidad) and *C. parensis* (Antigua and northern Argentina).
- Natural infection has not been reported in animals.

- Microfilaria of a similar species, *M. bolivarensis*, have been found in the blood of Amerindians in Bolivar State, Venezuela.

Life Cycle

During a blood meal, an infected arthropod (midges, genus *Culicoides*, or blackflies, genus *Simulium*) introduces third-stage filarial larvae onto the skin of the human host, where they penetrate into the bite wound ❶ [Figure 4-26]. They develop into adults that commonly reside in subcutaneous tissues ❷. Adult worms are rarely found in humans. The size range for female worms is 65 to 81 mm in length and 0.21 to 0.25 mm in diameter but unknown for males. Adult worms recovered from experimentally infected Patas monkeys measured 24 to 28 mm in length and 70 to 80 μm in diameter (males) and 32 to 62 mm in length and .130 to .160 mm in diameter (females). Adults produce unsheathed and non-periodic microfilariae that reach the blood stream ❸. The arthropod ingests microfilariae during a blood meal ❹. After ingestion, the microfilariae migrate from the arthropod's midgut through the hemocoel to the thoracic muscles ❺. There the microfilariae develop into first-stage larvae ❻ and subsequently into third-stage infective larvae ❼. The third-stage infective larvae migrate to arthropod's proboscis ❽ and can infect another human when the arthropod takes a blood meal ❶ (CDC).

Clinical Presentation

Clinical features are mild and are limited to any combination of pruritus, bronchospasm, rash, headache, arthralgias, fever, eosinophilia, and lymphadenopathy.

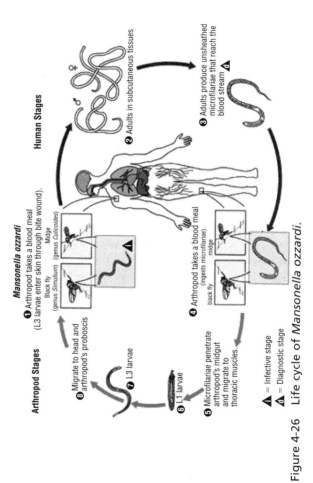

Figure 4-26 Life cycle of *Mansonella ozzardi*.

Mansonella ozzardi

Human Stages

❶ Arthropod takes a blood meal (L3 larvae enter skin through bite wound).

Black fly (genus *Simulium*)   Midge (genus *Culicoides*)

❷ Adults in subcutaneous tissues

❸ Adults produce unsheathed microfilariae that reach the blood stream ◬

❹ Arthropod takes a blood meal (ingests microfilariae). black fly   midge

Arthropod Stages

❺ Microfilariae penetrate arthropod's midgut and migrate to thoracic muscles.

❻ L1 larvae

❼ L3 larvae

❽ Migrate to head and arthropod's proboscis.

◬ = Infective stage
◬ = Diagnostic stage

216

Reference

Filariasis. Centers for Disease Control Web site. Available at:
http://www.dpd.cdc.gov/dpdx/HTML/Filariasis.htm.
Accessed April 15, 2005.

Further Reading

Bartoloni A, Cancrini G, Bartalesi F, et al. Mansonella ozzardi infection in Bolivia: prevalence and clinical associations in the Chaco region. *Am J Trop Med Hyg.* 1999;61:830-833.

Weller PF, Simon HB, Parkhurst BH, Medrek TF. Tourism-acquired Mansonella ozzardi microfilaremia in a regular blood donor. *JAMA.* 1978;240:858-859.

Yangco BG, Vincent AL, Vickery AC, Nayar JK, Sauerman DM. A survey of filariasis among refugees in south Florida. *Am J Trop Med Hyg.* 1984;33:246-251.

Filariasis—*Mansonella perstans*

Agent
Nematoda. Phasmidea, Filariae: *Mansonella* (*Esslingeria*) *perstans.*

Reservoir
Humans

Vector
Midge (*Culicoides* spp.)

Vehicle
None

Geographic Distribution
REGION II—CAm   MEX, PAN

REGION III—SAm	ARG, BRA, COL, GUY, SUR, VEN
REGION IV—Carib	DOM, GLP, KNA, LCA, TTO, VCT
REGION V—NAfr	DZA, TUN
REGION VI—CAfr	AGO, BDI, BEN, BFA, CAF, CIV, CMR, COD, COG, ERI, ETH, GAB, GHA, GIN, GMB, GNQ, KEN, LBR, MLI, MOZ, MWI, NER, NGA, RWA, SDN, SEN, SLE, TCD, TGO, TZA, UGA, ZMB, ZWE

Incubation Period
5–18m (range 1m–2y)

Diagnostic Tests
Identification of microfilariae in blood

Typical Adult Therapy
Mebendazole 100 mg PO b.i.d. × 10d
Or ivermectin 150 ug/kg PO as single dose

Typical Pediatric Therapy
Ivermectin 150 ug/kg PO as single dose

Background

- The parasite currently classified as *M. perstans* has had several names in the past: *Acanthocheilonema perstans, Dipetalonema berghei, D. perstans, D. semiclarum, Esslingeria perstans, Filaria perstans, Tetrapetalonema berghei* and *T. perstans*.

- *M. perstans* is found in tropical Africa, central and eastern South America, and the Caribbean.
- Infection has been documented in monkeys, gorillas, chimpanzees, and other animals.
- The principal vector in Africa is *Culicoides grahami.* The New World vectors have not been identified.

Life Cycle

During a blood meal, an infected midge (genus *Culicoides*) introduces third-stage filarial larvae onto the skin of the human host, where they penetrate into the bite wound ❶ [Figure 4-27]. They develop into adults that reside in body cavities, most commonly the peritoneal cavity or pleural cavity, but less frequently in the pericardium ❷. The size range for female worms is 70 to 80 mm in length and 120 μm in diameter, and the males measure approximately 45 mm by 60 μm. Adults produce unsheathed and subperiodic microfilariae, measuring 200 by 4.5 μm, that reach the blood stream ❸. A midge ingests microfilariae during a blood meal ❹. After ingestion, the microfilariae migrate from the midge's midgut through the hemocoel to the thoracic muscles of the arthropod ❺. There the microfilariae develop into first-stage larvae ❻ and subsequently into third-stage infective larvae ❼. The third-stage infective larvae migrate to the midge's proboscis ❽ and can infect another human when the midge takes a blood meal ❶ (CDC).

Clinical Presentation

Patients develop recurrent pruritic subcutaneous swellings, fever, headache, joint pain, abdominal or chest pain, and eosinophilia. Hepatosplenomegaly and intraocular lesions are occasionally seen.

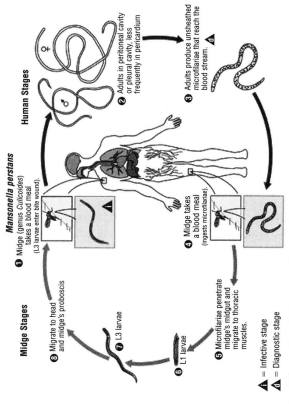

Human Stages

❷ Adults in peritoneal cavity or pleural cavity, less frequently in pericardium

❸ Adults produce unsheathed microfilariae that reach the blood stream. △

Mansonella perstans

❶ Midge (genus *Culicoides*) takes a blood meal (L3 larvae enter bite wound).

❹ Midge takes a blood meal (ingests microfilariae)

Midge Stages

❽ Migrate to head and midge's proboscis

❼ L3 larvae

❻ L1 larvae

❺ Microfilariae penetrate midge's midgut and migrate to thoracic muscles.

△ = Infective stage
△ = Diagnostic stage

Figure 4-27   Life cycle of *Mansonella perstans*.

Reference

Filariasis. Centers for Disease Control Web site. Available at:
    http://www.dpd.cdc.gov/dpdx/HTML/Filariasis.htm.
    Accessed April 15, 2005.

Further Reading

Baird JK, Neafie RC, Connor DH. Nodules in the conjunctiva,
    bung-eye, and bulge-eye in Africa caused by Mansonella
    perstans. *Am J Trop Med Hyg.* 1988;38:553-557.

Baird JK, Neafie RC, Lanoie L, Connor DH. Adult Mansonella
    perstans in the abdominal cavity in nine Africans. *Am J Trop
    Med Hyg.* 1987;37:578-584.

Gardon J, Kamgno J, Gardon-Wendel N, Demanga-Ngangue,
    Duke BO, Boussinesq M. Efficacy of repeated doses of iver-
    mectin against Mansonella perstans. *Trans R Soc Trop Med
    Hyg.* 2002;96:325-326.

Noireau F, Itoua A, Carme B. Epidemiology of Mansonella per-
    stans filariasis in the forest region of south Congo. *Ann Trop
    Med Parasitol.* 1990;84:251-254.

Filariasis—*Mansonella streptocerca*

Agent

Nematoda. Phasmidea, Filariae: *M. (Esslingeria) streptocerca.*

Reservoir

Nonhuman primates

Vector

Midge (*Culicoides grahami* and *C. milnei*)

Vehicle

None

Geographic Distribution

REGION VI—CAfr   AGO, BEN, CAF, CIV, CMR,
                           COD, COG, GAB, GHA,
                           GNQ, NER, NGA, TCD,
                           TGO, UGA

Incubation Period

5–18m (speculative)

Diagnostic Tests

Identification of microfilariae in skin snips

Typical Therapy

Ivermectin 150 ug/kg PO (single dose)
Or diethylcarbamazine:
50 mg PO day 1; 50 mg PO t.i.d. day 2; 100 mg PO t.i.d.
   day 3; then 2 mg/kg PO t.i.d. × 18 days

Background

- In the past, *M. streptocerca* has been variously classified as *Acanthocheilonema streptocerca, Agamofilaria streptocerca, Dipetalonema streptocerca,* and *Esslingeria streptocerca.*
- *M. streptocerca* is found in central and western Africa.
- The principal vector appears to be *C. grahami*, and transmission is diurnal.

Life Cycle

During a blood meal, an infected midge (genus *Culicoides*) introduces third-stage filarial larvae onto the skin of the human host, where they penetrate into the bite wound ❶ [Figure 4-28]. They develop into adults that reside in the dermis, most commonly less than 1 mm from the skin surface ❷. The females measure approximately 27 mm in length. Their diameter is 50 μm at the level of the vulva (anteriorly) and ovaries (near the posterior end), and up to 85 μm at the mid-body. Males measure 50 μm in diameter. Adults produce unsheathed and non-periodic microfilariae, measuring 180 to 240 μm by 3 to 5 μm, which reside in the skin but can also reach the peripheral blood ❸. A midge ingests the microfilariae during a blood meal ❹. After ingestion, the microfilariae migrate from the midge's midgut through the hemocoel to the thoracic muscles ❺. There, the microfilariae develop into first-stage larvae ❻ and subsequently into third-stage larvae ❼. The third-stage larvae migrate to the midge's proboscis ❽ and can infect another human when the midge takes another blood meal ❶ (CDC).

Clinical Presentation
Infection is rare and limited to pruritic and hypopigmented macules and papules, principally over the thorax and shoulders. Regional edema might occur in some cases. Recurrent pruritic subcutaneous lesions, arthralgia, and eosinophilia, headache, fever, or abdominal pain might also be present.

Reference
Filariasis. Centers for Disease Control Web site. Available at: http://www.dpd.cdc.gov/dpdx/HTML/Filariasis.htm. Accessed April 15, 2005.

Further Reading
Fischer P, Bamuhiiga J, Buttner DW. Occurrence and diagnosis of Mansonella streptocerca in Uganda. *Acta Trop.* 1997;63:43-55.

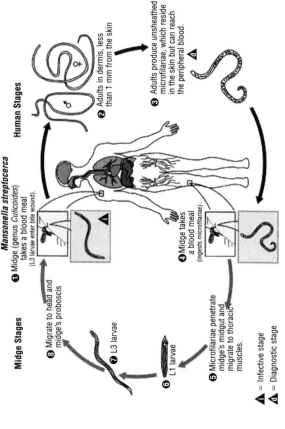

Mansonella streptocerca

Human Stages

1. Midge (genus *Culicoides*) takes a blood meal (L3 larvae enter bite wound).

2. Adults in dermis, less than 1 mm from the skin.

3. Adults produce unsheathed microfilariae, which reside in the skin but can reach the peripheral blood. ◭

4. Midge takes a blood meal (ingests microfilariae).

Midge Stages

5. Microfilariae penetrate midge's midgut and migrate to thoracic muscles.

6. L1 larvae

7. L3 larvae

8. Migrate to head and midge's proboscis.

◭ = Infective stage

◭ = Diagnostic stage

Figure 4-28 Life cycle of *Mansonella streptocerca*.

224

Fischer P, Bamuhiiga J, Buttner DW. Treatment of human
Mansonella streptocerca infection with ivermectin. *Trop
Med Int Health.* 1997;2:191-199.

Okelo GB, Kyobe J, Gatiri G. Mansonella streptocerca in the
Central African Republic. *Trans R Soc Trop Med Hyg.*
1988;82:464.

Filariasis—Mansonelliasis—Other

Mansonella, Zoonotic

Background

- Human infection by *M. rhodhaini,* a parasite of
  chimpanzees, has been reported in Gabon. Human
  cerebral infection by *Meningonema peruzzii,* a related
  parasite that infests monkeys, has been reported in the
  Democratic Republic of Congo and Zimbabwe.
- Human infection by *Dipetalonema (Mansonella)
  semiclarum* has also been reported in Africa.
- Related zoonotic parasites known as Dipetalonema-
  like have been found in rare cases of eye and
  subcutaneous infection in North America. A single
  case of blood infection by *M. interstitium* (a squirrel
  parasite) was reported from the United States.
- *Wuchereria lewisi* sp. were recovered from a man in
  Brazil.

Geographic Distribution

REGION I—NAm   USA
REGION VI—CAfr   GAB, COD, ZWE

Further Reading

Boussinesq M, Bain O, Chabaud AG, Gardon-Wendell N,
Kamgo J, Chippeaux JB. M. Mesocestoides (Cestoda) infec-

tion in a California child. *Pediatr Infect Dis J.* April 1992;11:
332-334.

Fain A. Dipetalonema semiclarum sp. nov. from the blood of
man in the Republic of Zaire (Nematoda: Filarioidea). *Ann
Soc Belg Med Trop.* 1974;54:195-207.

Schacher JF. Intraspecific variation in microfilariae, with description of Wuchereria lewisi sp. nov. (Nematoda,
Filarioidea) from man in Brazil. *Ann Trop Med Parasitol.*
1969;63:341-351.

Oriehel TC, Eberhard ML. Zoonotic filariasis. *Clin Microbiol
Rev.* 1998;11:366-381.

Filariasis—*Onchocerca volvulus*

Aswad, Craw-craw, Erysipelas de la Costa, Flussblindheit, Jur Blindness, Lichenified Onchodermatitis, Nakalanga Syndrome, Onchozerkose, River Blindness, Robles' Disease, Sowda

Agent
Nematoda. Phasmidea, Filariae: *O. volvulus.*

Reservoir
Humans

Vector
Fly (blackfly = *Simulium* spp.)

Vehicle
None

Geographic Distribution

REGION II—CAm	CRI, GTM, MEX
REGION III—SAm	BRA, COL, ECU, VEN

| REGION VI—CAfr | AGO, BDI, BEN, BFA, CAF, CIV, CMR, COD, COG, ERI, ETH, GAB, GHA, GIN, GNB, GNQ, LBR, MLI, MWI, NER, NGA, SDN, SEN, SLE, TCD, TGO, TZA, UGA |
| REGION IX—MidEast | SAU, YEM |

Incubation Period
12–18m

Diagnostic Tests
Identification of microfilariae in skin snips or on oph-thalmoscopy

Typical Therapy
Excision of nodules.
Ivermectin 150 ug/kg PO once.
Repeat every 6 months.

Background

- *O. volvulus* can live for up to 14 years in the human body. Each adult female worm (thin, but more than a half meter in length) produces millions of microfilariae that migrate throughout the body and give rise to visual impairment (punctate keratitis), rashes, intense pruritis, and depigmentation of the skin; lymphadenitis; and hanging groin and elephantiasis of the genitals.
- Clinical manifestations begin 1 to 3 years after the injection of infective larvae by a blackfly (*Simulium*). After mating, the female blackfly seeks a blood meal and might ingest microfilariae if the meal is taken from a person infected with onchocerciasis.

- Recent studies suggest that the host reaction and eye damage are actually directed at bacteria (*Wolbachia* spp.) found in the parasite. In fact, the Mazzotti reaction (fever, tachycardia, hypotension, adenitis, pruritis, and arthralgia following administration of therapy) can represent a reaction to *Wolbachia* rather than parasite antigens.
- The World Health Organization (WHO) recognizes five forms of skin disease for purposes of survey and control: acute papular onchodermatitis, chronic papular onchodermatitis, lichenified onchodermatitis, atrophy, and depigmentation.
- The disease is responsible for 0.9% of all blindness and is the second leading cause of infectious blindness. It appears that savanna strains of *O. volvulus* are more likely to produce ocular disease than are rain-forest strains.
- Onchocerciasis has been implicated in the etiology of Nakalanga syndrome (hyposexual dwarfism) in Sudan; and sowda (a form of endemic filarial limb dermatosis with adenopathy) on the Arabian Peninsula. It has been suggested that sowda might be caused by a zoonotic species rather than *O. volvulus*.
- Of the 50.4 million people at risk for onchocerciasis as of 2003, 96% reside in Africa (Africa accounts for 30 of the 36 endemic countries).
- As of 2003, 17.7 million were infested in Africa and Yemen (including 6.5 million with dermatitis, 500,000 visually impaired and 270,000 blind); and 140,455 were infested in Latin America.
- In Latin America, 4.7 million persons were considered at risk in 1995; 1,574,470 in 1996; 659,618 in 1999; and 503,285 in 2002.

- A mass treatment program was initiated in west Africa in 1974, resulting in 1.5 million cured and 400,000 cases of blindness prevented to 1998.
- African disease primarily occurs between latitudes 15°N and 14°S, with four main clinical patterns: blinding type in the savanna woodland belt or northern tropics; less-blinding type in the west and equatorial rain forest; mixed pattern of blinding and less-blinding in the Zaire basin; less-blinding in the east African highlands from Ethiopia to Malawi.
- American vectors tend to bite above waist level and African vectors in lower areas, and onchocercal nodules follow similar anatomic distribution.

Life Cycle

During a blood meal, an infected blackfly (genus *Simulium*) introduces third-stage filarial larvae onto the skin of the human host, where they penetrate into the bite wound ❶ [Figure 4-29]. In subcutaneous tissues the larvae ❷ develop into adult filariae, which commonly reside in nodules in subcutaneous connective tissues ❸. Adults can live in the nodules for approximately 15 years. Some nodules may contain numerous male and female worms. Females measure 33 to 50 cm in length and 270 to 400 μm in diameter, while males measure 19 to 42 mm by 130 to 210 μm. In the subcutaneous nodules, the female worms are capable of producing microfilariae for approximately 9 years. The microfilariae, measuring 220 to 360 μm by 5 to 9 μm and unsheathed, have a life span that may reach 2 years. They are occasionally found in peripheral blood, urine, and sputum but are typically found in the skin and in the lymphatics of connective tissues ❹. A blackfly ingests the microfilariae during a

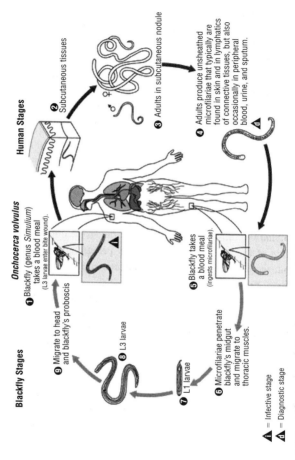

Figure 4-29 Life cycle of *Onchocerca volvulus*.

blood meal ❺. After ingestion, the microfilariae migrate from the blackfly's midgut through the hemocoel to the thoracic muscles ❻. There, the microfilariae develop into first-stage larvae ❼ and subsequently into third-stage infective larvae ❽. The third-stage infective larvae migrate to the blackfly's proboscis ❾ and can infect another human when the fly takes a blood meal ❶ (CDC).

Clinical Presentation
Adult worms live in firm nodules located over bony prominences and can survive for 15 years in the human host. Microfilaria migrate through the subcutaneous tissues, producing macular, papular, or dyschromic skin lesions; pruritus; lymphadenopathy; and eosinophilia. Upon entering the eye, the microfilaria produce punctate keratitis or uveitis.

Reference
Filariasis. Centers for Disease Control Web site. Available at: http://www.dpd.cdc.gov/dpdx/HTML/Filariasis.htm. Accessed April 15, 2005.

Further Reading
Hougard JM, Yameogo L, Seketeli A, Boatin B, Dadzie KY. Twenty-two years of blackfly control in the onchocerciasis control programme in west Africa. *Parasitol Today.* 1997;13:425-431.

Little MP, Basanez MG, Breitling LP, Boatin BA, Alley ES. Incidence of blindness during the Onchocerciasis control programme in western Africa, 1971-2002. *J Infect Dis.* 2004;189:1932-1941.

Onchocerciasis/River Blindness. Centers for Disease Control Web site. Available at: http://www.cdc.gov/ncidod/dpd/parasites/riverblindness/default.htm. Accessed April 15, 2005.

Onchocerciasis (river blindness). World Health Organization Web site. Available at: http://www.who.int/ocp/. Accessed April 15, 2005.

Thylefors B. Eliminating onchocerciasis as a public health problem. *Trop Med Int Health.* April 2004;9(4):A1-A3.

Filariasis—Onchocerciasis—Zoonotic

A cattle parasite, *Onchocerca guttarosa*, has been found to occasionally cause dermal nodules in humans (zoonotic onchocerciasis). Eight cases of human infection by zoonotic *Onchocerca* species were reported to 2000—from Albania, the United States, Canada, Switzerland, Japan and the Crimea. Presumed pathogens in these cases were the cattle parasite, *O. gutturosa;* and the horse parasites, *O. cervicalis* and *O. retuculata. Onchocerca lupi* is suspected as a possible cause of conjunctival infection in humans.

Clinical Presentation

A 21-mm filarial worm was recovered from the anterior chamber of the right eye of a 32-year-old man in western Oregon; the worm was identified as a female *Dipetalonema* in the fourth stage of development. It was the third such case to be reported from western Oregon. In this and one other case the worms were morphologically similar to adult worms identified as *D. arbuta* Highby 1943 from the body cavity of the porcupine (*Erethizon dorsatum*) and a similar species, *D. sprenti* Anderson 1953, from the body cavity of the beaver (*Castor canadensis*).

Further Reading

Beaver PC, Meyer EA, Jarroll EL, Rosenquist RC. Dipetalonema from the eye of a man in Oregon, USA. A case report. *Am J Trop Med Hyg.* 1980;29:369-372.

Filariasis—*Wuchereria bancrofti*

Bancroftian Filariasis

Agent
Nematoda. Phasmidea, Filariae: *W. bancrofti.*

Reservoir
Humans

Vector
Mosquitoes (*Anopheles, Aedes, Culex*)

Vehicle
None

Geographic Distribution
Bancroftian filariasis is endemic to over 100 countries, primarily in the developing world.

REGION II—CAm	CRI, PAN
REGION III—SAm	BRA, COL, GUF, GUY, SUR, VEN
REGION IV—Carib	ATG, BRB, CUB, DOM, GLP, KNA, LCA, MTQ, PRI, TTO, VIR, VCT, VGB
REGION V—NAfr	EGY, MAR
REGION VI—CAfr	AGO, BDI, BEN, BFA, CAF, CIV, CMR, COD, COG, COM, CPV, DJI, ERI, ETH, GAB, GHA, GIN, GMB, GNQ, KEN, LBR, MDG, MLI, MOZ, MRT, MUS, MWI, NER, NGA, REU, RWA, SDN, SEN, SLE, SOM, STP, SYC, TCD, TGO, TON, TZA, UGA, ZMB

REGION VII—SAfr	BWA, LSO
REGION IX—MidEast	OMN, SAU, TUR, YEM
REGION X—IndSub	BDG, IND, LKA, MDV, NPL, PAK
REGION XI—Asia	CHN, KOR, MNG, PRK, TWN
REGION XII—SEA	BRN, IDN, LAO, PHL, THA, VNM
REGION XIII—Poly	ASM, COK, FJI, KIR, NCL, NIU, NRU, PNG, SLB, TKL, TUV, VUT, WLF

Incubation Period

5–18m (range 1m–2y)

Diagnostic Tests

Identification of microfilariae in nocturnal blood
    specimen.
Nucleic acid amplification.
Serology can be helpful.

Typical Therapy

Diethylcarbamazine:
50 mg day 1; 50 mg t.i.d. day 2; 100 mg t.i.d. day 3
Then 2 mg/kg t.i.d. × 18 days
Or ivermectin 200 ug/kg PO as single dose

Background

- In 2001, it was estimated that 1,114,663,580 persons
  were at risk: 62.9% in Southeast Asia, 29.4% in Africa,
  4.4% in the western Pacific, 2.7% in the eastern
  Mediterranean and 0.6% in the Americas. It is
  estimated that 75 to 119 million people are infested by
  W. bancrofti (3% of the world's population). Of those

infected, 70% live in India, Bangladesh, Nigeria, and Myamar. As of 2003, an estimated 643,556,600 persons were at risk worldwide.

- India accounts for 47% of chronic filariasis and 39% of the at-risk population, worldwide.

- As of 2000, almost 25 million men suffer from genital disease caused by Bancroftian filariasis; 15 million (mostly women) from elephantiasis or lymphedema; 76 million from microfilaremia.

- Filariasis is the second leading cause of permanent and long-term disability in the world.

- The first three WHO National Lymphatic Elimination Programs were launched in 1999. By the end of 2002, 54,689,600 persons in 32 countries had received treatment.

- Patterns of microfilaremia can occur in three forms: a nocturnal periodic form (peak densities close to midnight) found in Africa, Asia, and Latin America; a nonperiodic or diurnal form (peak densities at approximately 16:30) found in the South Pacific; a nocturnal subperiodic form (peak densities at approximately 20:30) found in some foci in western Thailand. Nonperiodic filaremia occurs in Oceania.

Life Cycle

Different species of the following genera of mosquitoes are vectors of *W. bancrofti* filariasis depending on geographical distribution: *Culex* (*C. annulirostris*, *C. bitaeniorhynchus*, *C. quinquefasciatus*, and *C. pipiens*); *Anopheles* (*A. arabinensis*, *A. bancroftii*, *A. farauti*, *A. funestus*, *A. gambiae*, *A. koliensis*, *A. melas*, *A. merus*, *A. punctulatus* and *A. wellcomei*); *Aedes* (*A. aegypti*, *A. aquasalis*, *A. bellator*, *A. cooki*, *A. darlingi*, *A. kochi*, *A. polynesiensis*,

A. pseudoscutellaris, A. rotumae, A. scapularis, and *A. vigilax*); *Mansonia* (*M. pseudotitillans, M. uniformis*); *Coquillettidia* (*C. juxtamansonia*). During a blood meal, an infected mosquito introduces third-stage filarial larvae onto the skin of the human host, where they penetrate into the bite wound ❶ [Figure 4-30]. They develop in adults that commonly reside in the lymphatics ❷. The female worms measure 80 to 100 mm in length and 0.24 to 0.30 mm in diameter, while the males measure about 40 mm by .1 mm. Adults produce microfilariae measuring 244 to 296 μm by 7.5 to 10 μm, which are sheathed and have nocturnal periodicity, except the South Pacific microfilariae which have the absence of marked periodicity. The microfilariae migrate into lymph and blood channels moving actively through lymph and blood ❸. A mosquito ingests the microfilariae during a blood meal ❹. After ingestion, the microfilariae lose their sheaths and some of them work their way through the wall of the proventriculus and cardiac portion of the mosquito's midgut and reach the thoracic muscles ❺. There the microfilariae develop into first-stage larvae ❻ and subsequently into third-stage infective larvae ❼. The third-stage infective larvae migrate through the hemocoel to the mosquito's proboscis ❽ and can infect another human when the mosquito takes a blood meal ❶ (CDC).

Clinical Presentation

Clinical manifestations reflect either acute inflammation or lymphatic obstruction. Repeated episodes of lymphangitis, lymphadenitis, fever, headache, backache, and nausea could occur; and funiculitis, epididymitis, or orchitis are common. In long-standing cases, lymphedema or persistent adenopathy might develop.

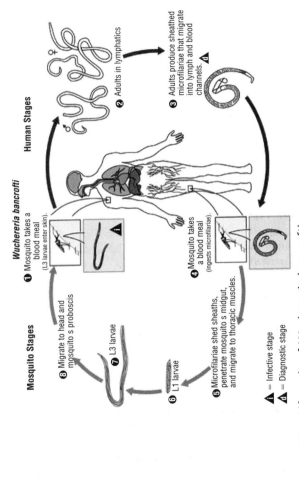

Wuchereria bancrofti

Human Stages

❶ Mosquito takes a blood meal (L3 larvae enter skin).

❷ Adults in lymphatics

❸ Adults produce sheathed microfilariae that migrate into lymph and blood channels. ◭

❹ Mosquito takes a blood meal (ingests microfilariae).

Mosquito Stages

❺ Microfilariae shed sheaths, penetrate mosquito's midgut, and migrate to thoracic muscles.

❻ L1 larvae

❼ L3 larvae

❽ Migrate to head and mosquito's proboscis.

▲ = Infective stage
◭ = Diagnostic stage

Figure 4-30 Life cycle of *Wuchereria bancrofti*.

Hydrocele is the most common clinical manifestation of lymphatic filariasis, and it causes sexual disability. Hydrocoelectomy accounts for 25% of all surgical procedures performed in endemic areas of Ghana and Kenya. Lower limb involvement is characterized by initial pretibial pitting edema, which eventually becomes nonpitting and involves the entire leg. The skin of the leg or scrotum becomes thick, fissured, and warty; and ulceration and secondary infection could occur. Chyluria reflects rupture of swollen lymphatics into the urinary tract.

Microfilariae can be found in properly timed blood specimens, hydrocele fluid or chylous urine; and adult worms can be found in biopsy material. Eosinophilia usually appears only during acute episodes of inflammation.

Reference

Filariasis. Centers for Disease Control Web site. Available at: http://www.dpd.cdc.gov/dpdx/HTML/Filariasis.htm. Accessed April 15, 2005.

Further Reading

de-Almeida AB, Freedman DO. Epidemiology and immunopathology of bancroftian filariasis. *Microbes Infect.* 1999;1:1015-1022.

The Global Alliance to Eliminate Lymphatic Filariasis Web site. Available at: http://www.filariasis.org. Accessed April 15, 2005.

Hoerauf A. Control of filarial infections: not the beginning of the end, but more research is needed. *Curr Opin Infect Dis.* 2003;16:403-410.

Molyneux DH, Taylor MJ. Current status and future prospects of the Global Lymphatic Filariasis Programme. *Curr Opin Infect Dis.* 2001;14:155-159.

Gastrodiscoides hominis

Agent
Platyhelminthes, Trematoda. Echinostomatida, Zygocotylidae: *G. hominis*.

Reservoir
Pigs, herbivores, snails (*Helicorbis coenosis*)

Vector
None

Vehicle
Freshwater plants

Geographic Distribution
REGION III—SAm	GUY
REGION X—IndSub	BGD, IND
REGION XI—Asia	CHN, KAZ
REGION XII—SEA	IDN, MMR, MYS, PHL, THA, VNM

Incubation Period
Unknown

Diagnostic Tests
Identification of ova or adult parasite in stool

Typical Therapy
Praziquantel 25 mg/kg t.i.d. $\times$ 1d (experimental)

Background
- *G. hominis* is found primarily in Malaysia, India, the former Soviet Union, Pakistan, Myanmar, Vietnam, and the Philippines.

- The natural reservoirs are pigs, deer, and humans. Humans acquire the disease through ingestion of metacercariae on vegetables.
- Adult parasites are found in the cecum and colon. Eggs are in the feces and embryonate within 17 days. Although the life cycle is not well known, but by analogy with related species, we can deduce that the miracidia invade intermediate snail hosts (*Helicorbis*), giving rise to two generations of redia, and then cercaria 28 to 150 days after infection. These then leave the snail and encyst on vegetation such as the water caltrop, which are then eaten by humans.
- A single case of human intestinal infection by a related baboon parasite, *Watsonius watsoni*, has been reported in an African man who had died of severe diarrhea. *Fischoederius elongatus*, a parasite of ruminants acquired by eating aquatic plants, was implicated as the cause of epigastric pain and vomiting in a woman in Guangdong, China.

Clinical Presentation

Human infection is usually asymptomatic, or, at most, limited to diarrhea.

Further Reading

Dutt SC, Srivastava HD. The life history of Gastrodiscoides hominis (Lewis and McConnel, 1876) Leiper, 1913—the amphistome parasite of man and pig. *J Helminthol.* 1972;46:35-46.

Kumar V. The digenetic trematodes, Fasciolopsis buski, Gastrodiscoides hominis and Artyfechinostomum malayanum, as zoonotic infections in South Asian countries. *Ann Soc Belg Med Trop.* 1980;60:331-339.

Murty CV, Reddy CR. A case report of Gastrodiscoides hominis infestation. *Indian J Pathol Microbiol.* 1980;23:303-304B.

Giardia lamblia

Beaver Fever, Lambliaisis

Agent
Protozoa. Archezoa, Metamonada, Trepomonadea. Flagellate: *Giardia lamblia* (*G. intestinalis, G. duodenalis*).

Reservoir
Humans, beavers

Vector
None

Vehicle
Food, water, fecal–oral contact, flies

Geographic Distribution
Worldwide

Incubation Period
1–3w (range 3d–6w)

Diagnostic Tests
String test (gelatin capsule containing string)
Stool microscopy or antigen assay
Nucleic acid amplification

Typical Adult Therapy
Metronidazole 250 mg t.i.d. × 5d
Or tinidazole 2 g × 1
Or furazolidone 100 mg q.i.d. × 7d
Or paromomycin 10 mg/kg t.i.d. × 7d

Typical Pediatric Therapy
Metronidazole 5 mg/kg t.i.d. × 5d
Or tinidazole 50 mg × 1 (maximum 2 g)
Or furazolidone 1.5 mg/kg q.i.d. × 7d

Background

- Giardiasis occurs worldwide, with peak prevalence below age 10 years in developing world countries (15 to 20% infected). In developed countries, 6 to 8% of adults and 2% of children are infected at least once.
- Acquisition from surface water (including in cold climates) and person-to-person spread (including fecal–oral and heterosexual contact) occur.
- Giardia can survive for 2 to 3 months in cool water, and routine chlorination is not effective against cysts. The minimal infective dose is 10 to 25 cysts. In nature, the parasite is found in dogs, cats, beavers, and cattle.

Causal Agent

Giardia intestinalis, is a protozoan flagellate (Diplomonadida). This protozoan was initially named *Cercomonas intestinalis* by Lambl in 1859 and renamed *Giardia lamblia* by Stiles in 1915, in honor of Professor A. Giard of Paris and Dr. F. Lambl of Prague. However, many consider the name, *Giardia intestinalis*, to be the correct name for this protozoan. The International Commission on Zoological Nomenclature is reviewing this issue (CDC).

Life Cycle

Cysts are resistant forms responsible for transmission of giardiasis. Both cysts and trophozoites are found in the feces ❶ [Figure 4-31]. The cysts are hardy, and can survive several months in cold water. Infection occurs through ingestion of cysts in water or food, or by the fecal–oral route (hands or fomites) ❷. In the small intestine, excystation releases trophozoites (each cyst produces two trophozoites) ❸. Trophozoites multiply by

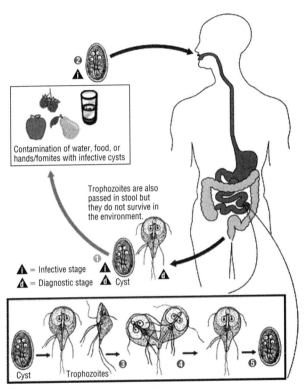

Contamination of water, food, or hands/fomites with infective cysts

Trophozoites are also passed in stool but they do not survive in the environment.

▲ = Infective stage

▲d = Diagnostic stage   ▲d Cyst

Cyst   Trophozoites   ❸   ❹   ❺

Figure 4-31   Life cycle of *Giardia lamblia*.

longitudinal binary fission remaining in the lumen of the proximal small bowel, either free or attached to the mucosa by a ventral sucking disk ❹. Encystation occurs as the parasites transit toward the colon. The cyst is the stage found most commonly in non-diarrheal feces ❺. Because the cysts are infectious when passed in the stool or shortly afterward, person-to-person transmission is possible. Although animals are infected with *Giardia*, their importance as a reservoir is unclear (CDC).

Clinical Presentation

The usual interval between infection and the onset of acute symptoms ranges from 1 to 2 weeks. In most instances, the individual will experience sudden, explosive, watery, foul-smelling diarrhea; excessive gas; abdominal pain; bloating; nausea; asthenia; and anorexia. Upper gastrointestinal symptoms such as vomiting could predominate. Fever is unusual.

Asymptomatic infection is common. Blood or mucus in the stool is rare, and there is neither leucocytosis nor eosinophilia. Occasionally, the illness could last for months or even years, causing recurrent episodes of impaired digestion, lactose intolerance, diarrhea, asthenia, and weight loss. Severe and prolonged infections are reported among patients with IgA deficiency and malnutrition.

Reference

Giardiasis. Centers for Disease Control Web site. Available at: http://www.dpd.cdc.gov/dpdx/HTML/Giardiasis.htm. Accessed April 15, 2005.

Further Reading

Ali SA, Hill DR. Giardia intestinalis. *Curr Opin Infect Dis.* 2003; 16:453-460.

Giardiasis. Centers for Disease Control Web site. Available at: http://www.cdc.gov/ncidod/dpd/parasites/giardiasis/default.htm. Accessed April 15, 2005.

Rose JB, Slifko TR. Giardia, Cryptosporidium, and Cyclospora and their impact on foods: a review. *J Food Prot.* 1999;62:1059-1070.

Vesy CJ, Peterson WL. Review article: the management of Giardiasis. *Aliment Pharmacol Ther.* 1999;13:843-850.

Gnathostomiasis

Wandering Swelling, Yangtze Edema

Agent
Nematoda. Phasmidea: *Gnathostoma spinigerum* (rarely *G. hispidum, G. doloresi* and *G. nipponicum*).

Reservoir
Cats, dogs, poultry, frogs, fish

Vector
None

Vehicle
Fish, amphibians, reptiles

Geographic Distribution
REGION II—CAm	MEX
REGION III—SAm	ECU
REGION VI—CAfr	TZA, ZMB
REGION X—IndSub	BGD, IND, LKA
REGION XI—Asia	CHN, JPN, TWN
REGION XII—SEA	IDN, KHM, LAO, MMR, MYS, PHL, THA, VNM

Incubation Period
3–4w (range 2d–1y)

Diagnostic Tests
Identification of larva in tissue
Serological testing in specialized laboratories

Typical Adult Therapy
Albendazole 400 mg daily for 21 days has been recommended as an adjunct to surgical excision.

Typical Pediatric Therapy
Mebendazole 100 mg b.i.d. × 5d has been recommended as an adjunct to surgical excision.

Background

- Most cases of gnathostomiasis are reported from Asia, with sporadic reports from the Americas, Africa, Europe, and Australia.
- Four species are known to cause human infection: *G. hispidum, G. doloresi, G. nipponicum* and *G. spinigerum*. A fifth species, *G. malaysiae*, has been suspected to cause infection following ingestion of freshwater shrimp in Myanmar.
- The adult nematode lives in the stomach wall of the definitive host (usually carnivore) and passes ova into the feces. First-stage larvae hatch in water and are ingested by copepods (*Cyclops*) where they develop into second-stage larvae. Four species of *Cyclops* have been implicated.
- The third-stage larvae develop in a second intermediate host: snakes (rock python or cobra in India; freshwater fish in the Philippines), frogs, crayfish, crabs, amphibia, reptiles, mammals, or chickens. These are, in turn, eaten by the definitive host; 28 vertebrate species have been implicated as second intermediate hosts: 2 fish, 3 amphibian, 5 reptile, 3 bird, 2 crab, and 13 rodent or monkey.
- Humans can also act as host to the third-stage larva, which are acquired through ingestion of the skin or meat of the second intermediate host.

Causal Agent

The nematodes (roundworm) *Gnathostoma spinigerum* and *Gnathostoma hispidum*, which infect vertebrate ani-

mals. Human gnathostomiasis is due to migrating immature worms (CDC).

Life Cycle

In the natural definitive host (pigs, cats, dogs, wild animals) adult worms reside in a tumor which they induce
in the gastric wall. Eggs are unembryonated when passed
in the feces ❶ [Figure 4-32], and become embryonated in
water, to release first-stage larvae ❷. If ingested by a small
crustacean (*Cyclops*, first intermediate host), first-stage
larvae develop into second-stage larvae ❸. Following ingestion of the *Cyclops* by a fish, frog, or snake (second intermediate host), the second-stage larvae migrate into
the flesh and develop into third-stage larvae ❹. When the
second intermediate host is ingested by a definitive host,
the third-stage larvae develop into adult parasites in the
stomach wall ❺. Alternatively, the second intermediate
host may be ingested by the paratenic host (animals such
as birds, snakes, and frogs) in which the third-stage larvae do not develop further but remain infective to the
next predator ❻. Humans become infected by eating undercooked fish or poultry containing third-stage larvae,
or reportedly by drinking water containing infective
second-stage larvae in *Cyclops* ❼ (CDC).

Clinical Presentation

Initial symptoms include nausea, abdominal pain, or urticaria. The presence of worms in skin or soft tissue results
in migratory, pruritic or painful swellings which can be
erythematous and attain a size of several centimeters.
Swellings can last for 1 to 4 weeks in a given area and then
reappear in a new location—a pattern which can continue
for months or years. Central nervous system infection
(less than 1% of patients with subcutaneous gnathostomi-

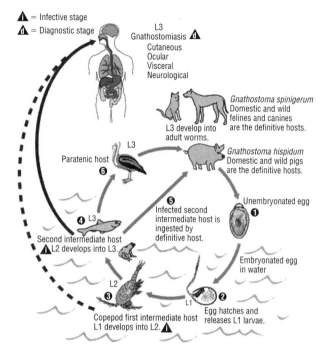

▲ = Infective stage
🄳 = Diagnostic stage

L3
Gnathostomiasis 🄳
Cutaneous
Ocular
Visceral
Neurological

Gnathostoma spinigerum
Domestic and wild
felines and canines
are the definitive hosts.

L3 develop into
adult worms.

L3

Paratenic host
❻

Gnathostoma hispidum
Domestic and wild pigs
are the definitive hosts.

❺
Infected second
intermediate host is
ingested by
definitive host.

Unembryonated egg
❶

❹ L3
Second intermediate host
▲ L2 develops into L3.

Embryonated egg
in water

L2
❸

L1
❷

Egg hatches and
releases L1 larvae.

Copepod first intermediate host
L1 develops into L2. ▲

Figure 4-32   Life cycle of gnathostomiasis.
Source: Some of the elements in this figure are based
on an illustration by Dr. Sylvia Paz Díaz Camacho,
Universidade Autónoma de Sinaloa, Mexico.

asis) is associated with radiculopathy or paralysis. Other
syndromes include eye infestation, persistent abdominal
pain, or pneumonitis. Eosinophilia is prominent.

Reference

Gnathostomiasis. Centers for Disease Control Web site.
    Available at: http://www.dpd.cdc.gov/dpdx/HTML/
    gnathostomiasis.htm. Accessed April 15, 2005.

Further Reading

Chai JY, Han ET, Shin EH, et al. An outbreak of gnathostomiasis among Korean emigrants in Myanmar. *Am J Trop Med Hyg.* 2003;69:67-73.

McCarthy J, Moore TA. Emerging helminth zoonoses. *Int J Parasitol.* 2000;30:1351-1360.

Moore DA, McCroddan J, Dekumyoy P, Chiodini PL. Gnathostomiasis: an emerging imported disease. *Emerg Infect Dis.* 2003;9:647-650.

Ogata K, Nawa Y, Akahane H, et al. Short report: gnathostomiasis in Mexico. *Am J Trop Med Hyg.* 1998;58:316-318.

Rusnak JM, Lucey DR. Clinical gnathostomiasis: case report and review of the English-language literature. *Clin Infect Dis.* 1993;16:33-50.

Gongylonema pulchrum

Filaria Labialis Infection, Scutate Threadworm

Agent
Nematoda. Phasmidea: *G. pulchrum.*

Reservoir
Sheep, cattle, pigs, bears, monkeys

Vector
None

Vehicle
Insect (ingestion)

Geographic Distribution

REGION I—NAm	USA
REGION V—NAfr	MAR
REGION VII—SAfr	ZAF

REGION VIII—Eur	BGR, DEU, ESP, HUN
REGION IX—MidEast	IRN
REGION X—IndSub	LKA
REGION XI—Asia	CHN, JPN, RUS
REGION XII—SEA	LAO
REGION XIII—Poly	NZL

Incubation Period
Unknown—presumed 60 to 80 days

Diagnostic Tests
Identification of worm following extraction

Typical Therapy
None proven; albendazole is recommended in addition to extraction of the parasite.

Background

- *Gongylonema* was first recovered from a human in 1864.
- Sporadic cases of human gongylonemiasis have been reported in several countries including Bulgaria, Hungary, Spain, China, Laos, Morocco, the former Soviet Union, New Zealand, Sri Lanka, and the United States. As of 2000, 40 to 50 cases had been reported in the world's literature.
- *G. pulchrum* is a nematode parasite of sheep, cattle, pigs, other ungulates, bears, and monkeys. Adult worms live in tunnels within the esophageal mucosa, tongue, and oral cavity of infected animals. Humans are infected through accidental ingestion of the intermediate hosts—small cockroaches and dung beetles (*Apodius* and *Onthophagus* species) or their body parts in food). To date, all infections have been inadvertent.

- After ingestion of ova by the intermediate insect host, infective stage nematodes develop over a period of 20 to 30 days. Adults develop in the mammal host 60 to 80 days following ingestion. Male worms are 62 × 0.15 to 0.3 mm, and females 145 × 0.2 to 0.5 mm.

Clinical Presentation

Human gongylonemiasis is limited to development of tunnels in the buccal mucosa, lips, tonsils, hard and soft palate, or jaw. Actively migrating threadlike structures are seen by the patient or health worker, without additional systemic symptoms. Occasional reports of soft tissue mass and spitting of blood have also been reported. Infection is chronic, with some cases persisting more than one year. No drug has been proven effective, however albendazole is suggested as an adjunct to extraction of the worm.

Further Reading

Jelinek T, Loscher T. Human infection with Gongylonema pulchrum: a case report. *Trop Med Parasitol*. 1994;45:329-330.

Wilde H, Suankratay C, Thongkam C, Chaiyabutr N, Chaiyabutr N. Human gongylonema infection in Southeast Asia. *J Travel Med*. 2001;8:204-206.

Wilson ME. Worms that cause lumps in the mouth. *Lancet*. 2001;357:1888.

Gordiid Worms

Gordiid Worms

The adult Gordiid worm (hair snake) is found in fresh water, while larvae are parasitic to various insect species. Adults measure 10 to 50 cm. Sporadic human infections have followed inadvertant ingestion of insects or contaminated water. Most infections have been asymptomatic; however, cases of outer ear and genital infection have been reported. Species involved include *Gordius aquaticus*, *G. villoti*, *G. robustus*, *Chordodes capensis* and *Parachrododes tricuspidatus*.

Further Reading

Cowen WW, Williams RK. Horse hair worms or untying the gordian knot. *Cent Afr J Med*. December 1965;11:359-360.

Smith DR, Watson DD, Clevenger RR, McBride RC. Paragordius varius. *Arch Pathol Lab Med*. September 1990;114:981-983.

Heterophyid Infections

Agent

Platyhelminthes, Trematoda. Plagiorchiida, Heterophyidae: *Heterophyes heterophyes*, *H. nocens*, *H. dispar*, *Ascocotyle coleostoma*, *et al*, *Prosthodendrium molenkampi*, *Phaneropsolus bonnie*, *P. spinicirrus*.

Reservoir

Snails (*Cerithidea cingulata*, *Pirenella conica*), fish

Vector

None

Vehicle

Fish (mullet and tilapia [*Oreochromis nilo*])

Geographic Distribution

REGION V—NAfr	EGY, TUN
REGION VI—CAfr	SDN
REGION VIII—Eur	ALB, BGR, BIH, ESP, GRC, HRV, MKD, SVN

REGION IX—MidEast	SAU, IRN
REGION X—IndSub	IND
REGION XI—Asia	AZE, CHN, JPN, KAZ, KGZ, KOR, PRK, RUS, TJK, TKM, TWN, UZB
REGION XII—SEA	IDN, MYS, PHL, THA, VNM

Incubation Period
7–14d

Diagnostic Tests
Identification of ova or adults in stool

Typical Therapy
Praziquantel 25 mg/kg t.i.d. × 3 doses

Background

- A large number of heterophyid fluke species parasitize humans, other mammals, and birds and share similar epidemiological and clinical features.
- Species of *Heterophyes* (*H. heterophyes, H. nocens, H. continua, H. katsuradai*), *Metagonimus* (*M. yokogawai*), *Haplorchis* (*H. taichui, H. vanissimus* and *H. pumilio*), *Stellantchasmus* (*S. falcatus*), *Procerovum* (*P. calderon*), *Pygidiopsis, Centrocestus, Stictodora, Heterophyopsis, Diochitrema, Phagicola, Appophalus, Cryptocotyle, Plagiorchis. Brachylaima, Cotylurus,* and *Carneophallus* can cause disease in humans.
- Following ingestion by freshwater snails, larvae develop into metacercariae which later encyst in fish or shrimp. The latter infect humans following ingestion. Intestinal lesions produced by *Heterophyes* are somewhat distal to those of *Metagonimus*. In

addition to local symptoms (diarrhea, abdominal pain) produced by adult flukes, ova may spread via lymphatics to distant sites such as the myocardium, spinal cord, or brain and produce granulomata and fibrosis.

- *Heterophyes heterophyes* is found in the rat, fox, dog, wolf, jackal, cat, black kite (*Milvus migrans aegyptius*) and bat (*Rhinolophus divosus acrotis*—in Yemen). Snail hosts include *Pirinella conica* (Middle East), *Cerithidea cingulata*, and *Tympanotomus micropterus* (Far East). *Melanoides tuberculata* and *Cleopatra bulimoides* are also infected on occasion. The usual intermediate hosts are mullet (*Mugil cephalus*) or *Acanthogobius* (in Japan). Minnows (*Gambusia affinis*), goby (*Acanthogobius* spp), and tilapia (*Oreochromis nilo*) might also be infected.

- *Gymnophalloides seoi* is a common intestinal trematode transmitted from oysters (*Crassostrea gigas*) to humans in Korea. The natural host is the Palearctic oystercatcher (*Haematopus ostralegus*). Human infection was first reported in Korea in 1988, and presents as fever, abdominal pain, anorexia, weight loss, diarrhea, or pancreatitis.

- *Centrocestus formosanus* infection is reported from China, Taiwan, and the Philippines. *C. cuspidatus* is found in Taiwan and Egypt, *C. caninus*, a parasite of dogs, cats, and rats in Thailand and Taiwan, is acquired by eating freshwater fish or frogs. *C. kurokawi* infection has been reported in Japan, and *C. longus* infection in Taiwan.

- *Plagiorchis* species emerge from snails and pass through insects in order to become infective. *Plagiorchis philippinensis* has been identified in cases of human infection in Ilocos, Philippines; *P. muris* in

Japan and Republic of Korea; *P. javensis* in Indonesia; and *P. harinasutai* in Thailand.

- *Phaneropsolus bonnie* and *Phaneropsolus spinicirrus* infestations have been limited to Thailand. *Prosthdendrium molemkampi* is acquired through consumption of small fish contaminated with the water nymphs of dragonflies.

- *Haplorchis pumilio (Monorchotrema taihokui)*, a parasite of dogs, cats, and night herons, has been acquired from eating fish in the Philippines, Taiwan, and Egypt. *H. yokogawi* has been acquired from eating mullet or shrimp in Thailand, the Philippines and southern China. Additional species include *H. pleurolophocerca* (Egypt), *H. taichui* (Bangladesh, Thailand, Laos, Philippines, and Taiwan), *H. microrchis* (Japan), and *H. vanissimus* (Japan).

- *Carneophallus brevicaeca* is found in shrimps *(Macrobrachium* sp.*)* and infects humans in the Philippines. In fatal cases, ova have been identified in the heart, brain and spinal cord.

- *Cotylurus japonicus* is normally found in the intestines of aquatic birds. A single case of human intestinal infection was reported in Hunan, China.

- *Brachylaima ruminae* is found in the intestines of rats and poultry which feed on snail intermediates *(Rumina decollata)*. Rare cases of human infection, characterized by abdominal pain and diarrhea, have been reported in Australia.

- Summary of reservoirs and vehicles: Freshwater fish harbor the metacercarial stage of *M. yokogawai, M. takahashii, M. miyatai, C. armatus, E. hortense, E. cinetorchis, E. japonicus,* or *P. muris*. Brackish water fish serve as the second intermediate hosts for *H. nocens, H. continua, P. summa, S. falcatus, S. fuscata,* and *S. lari*. Brackish water bivalves are the source of infection with *A. tyosenense*. Tadpoles and frogs are the second intermediate hosts for *N. seoulense*, but the major source of human infection is the grass snake *Rhabdophis tigrina*, a paratenic host. The metacercariae of *G. seoi* are observed in oysters.

- The natural definitive hosts are, in most cases, mammals such as rats, cats, and dogs. However, several species (*C. armatus, S. lari, E. japonicus, A. tyosenense,* and *G. seoi*) have birds as natural definitive hosts.

Causal Agent

The trematode *Heterophyes heterophyes*, a minute intestinal fluke (CDC).

Life Cycle

Adults release embryonated eggs, which are passed in the host's feces ❶ [Figure 4-33]. After ingestion by a suitable snail (first intermediate host), the eggs hatch and release miracidia which penetrate the snail's intestine ❷. Genera *Cerithidia* and *Pironella* are important snail hosts in Asia and the Middle East respectively. The miracidia undergo several developmental stages in the snail, ie, sporocysts ❷ₐ, rediae ❷ᵦ, and cercariae ❷꜀. Many cercariae are produced from each redia. The cercariae are released from the snail ❸ and encyst as metacercariae in the tissues of a suitable fresh or brackish water fish (second intermediate host) ❹. The definitive host becomes infected by ingesting undercooked or salted fish containing metacercariae ❺. After ingestion, the metacercariae excyst, attach to the mucosa of the small intestine ❻ and mature into adults (measuring 1.0 to 1.7 mm by 0.3 to 0.4 mm) ❼. In addi-

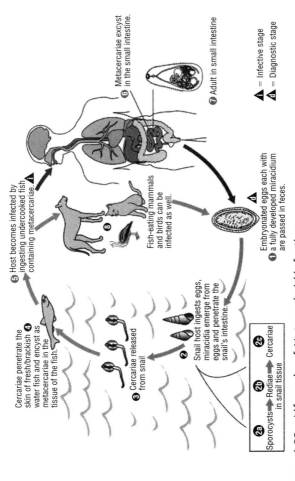

- Metacercariae excyst in the small intestine. ⑥
- Adult in small intestine ⑦

▲ = Infective stage
△ = Diagnostic stage

- Host becomes infected by ingesting undercooked fish containing metacercariae. ⑤ ▲

- Fish-eating mammals and birds can be infected as well. ⑧

- Embryonated eggs each with a fully developed miracidium are passed in feces. ① △

- Cercariae penetrate the skin of fresh/brackish water fish and encyst as metacercariae in the tissue of the fish. ④

- Snail host ingests eggs, miracidia emerge from eggs and penetrate the snail's intestine. ②

- Cercariae released from snail ③

⑳ Sporocysts → ② Rediae → ② Cercariae in snail tissue

Figure 4-33   Life cycle of *Heterophyid* infections.

257

tion to humans, various fish-eating mammals (eg, cats and dogs) and birds can be infected by *Heterophyes heterophyes* ❽ (CDC).

Clinical Presentation

Patients typically present with abdominal pain and mucous diarrhea, which may persist for days to weeks. Infestation resolves spontaneously within two months. Symptoms of metagonimiasis may follow ingestion of a single sweetfish and consist of severe abdominal pain, prostration, and watery diarrhea. In endemic areas, chronically infested patients rarely suffer from diarrhea or abdominal pain.

Reference

Heterophyiasis. Centers for Disease Control Web site. Available at: http://www.dpd.cdc.gov/dpdx/HTML/heterophyiasis. htm. Accessed April 15, 2005.

Further Reading

Belizario VY Jr, Bersabe MJ, de Leon WU, et al. Intestinal heterophyidiasis: an emerging food-borne parasitic zoonosis in southern Philippines. *Southeast Asian J Trop Med Public Health.* 2001;32(suppl 2):36-42.

Chai JY, Lee SH. Food-borne intestinal trematode infections in the Republic of Korea. *Parasitol Int.* 2002;51:129-154.

Liu LX, Harinasuta KT. Liver and intestinal flukes. *Gastroenterol Clin North Am.* 1996;25:627-636.

Rousset JJ, Baufine-Ducrocq H, Rabia M, Benoit A. Ascocotyle coleostoma colic distomiasis. The 1st world case or the follow-up of a tropical pathology congress in Egypt. *Presse Med.* 1983;12:2331-2332.

Wiwanitkit V, Nithiuthai S, Suwansaksri J, Chongboonprasert C, Tangwattakanont K. Survival of heterophyid metacercariae in uncooked Thai fish dishes. *Ann Trop Med Parasitol.* 2001;95:725-727.

Hirudinae

Leeches

Agent
Parasite—Class Hirudinea, Order Arhynchobdellida (Families: Haemopidae, Hirudinidae, and Erpobdellidae, and Order Rhynchobdellida. Families: Glossiphoniidae and Piscicolidae). There are 500 species worldwide; 42 species in the United States.

Reservoir
Fresh, shallow water

Vector
None

Vehicle
Water and arboreal (in rain forests)

Geographic Distribution
Worldwide temperate and tropical shallow freshwaters (pH > 7); some marine examples; moist terrestrial environments

Incubation Period
1h–3w

Clinical Hints
Unexplained anemia; unexplained bleeding from a body orifice; obstruction of the nasopharynx.

Diagnostic Tests
Direct examination

Typical Therapy
Removal of the worm

Background

Leeches are large (1 to 20 cm), free-living, segmented worms having highly contractile, flattened, muscular bodies with two suckers at each end of the body. The head is at the narrower end and has anywhere between two and ten small dark eyespots which can be used for identification. Attachment is painless, and a person might not realize he has been bitten.

Clinical Presentation

External parasitism is usually obvious, but small, unengorged leeches might not be appreciated at first; or leeches that have attached to the mucosa of the upper respiratory, genitourinary, and gastrointestinal tracts might not be obvious until bleeding or obstruction occurs days or weeks later. A history of seeing leeches while bathing in fresh water might alert the clinician that the person has been parasitized.

Further Reading

Alcelik T, Cekic O, Totan Y. Ocular leech infestation in a child. *Am J Ophthalmol.* 1997;124:110-112.

Boye ES, Joshi EC. Occurrence of the leech Limnatis paluda as a respiratory parasite in man: case report from Saudi Arabia. *J Trop Med Hyg.* 1994;97:18-20.

Cundall DB, Whitehead SM, Hechtel FO. Severe anaemia and death due to the pharyngeal leech Myxobdella africana. *Trans R Soc Trop Med Hyg.* 1986;80:940-944.

Mohammad Y, Rostrum M, Dubaybo BA. Laryngeal hirudinia-
     sis: an unusual cause of airway obstruction and hemoptysis.
     Pediatr Pulmonol. 2002;33:224-226.

Prasad SB, Sinha MR. Vaginal bleeding due to leech. *Postgrad
     Med J.* 1983;59:272.

Hookworm

Ancylostomiasis, Hakenwurmer-Befall, Miner's Anemia, Necatoriasis, Uncinariasis

Agent
Nematoda. Phasmidea: *Necator americanus, Ancylostoma duodenale, A. ceylonicum* (in Calcutta and the Philippines), and *Cyclodontostom* spp.

Reservoir
Humans

Vector
None

Vehicle
Soil—contact

Geographic Distribution
Worldwide

Incubation Period
7d–2y

Diagnostic Tests
Examination of stool for ova

Typical Therapy

Albendazole 400 mg × 1 dose

Or mebendazole 100 mg b.i.d. × 3d

Or pyrantel pamoate 11 mg/kg (max 3 g) × 3d

Background

- Hookworm is most commonly associated with walking barefoot in rural areas having moist soil and poor sanitation.
- It is estimated that 1.28 billion are infested (as compared to 457 million in 1947).
- The prevalence in sub-Saharan Africa is estimated at 33.0% (192 million cases).
- Approximately 44 million pregnant women have hookworm at any point in time.
- In 1985, 65,000 fatal cases were estimated; 8,000 in 1998; 7,000 in 1999.
- *Ancylostoma duodenale* is found in southern Europe, India, China, Japan, Paraguay, Chile, Peru, Western Australia, Malaysia, Myanmar, Philippines, Indonesia, Oceania, and west Africa.
- *Necator americanus* is found in western, southern, and central Africa, southern Asia, the southern United States, Oceania, the Caribbean, Central America, and South America.

Causal Agents

The human hookworms include two nematode (roundworm) species, *Ancylostoma duodenale* and *Necator americanus.* (Adult females: 10 to 13 mm (*A. duodenale*), 9 to 11 mm (*N. americanus*); adult males: 8 to 11 mm

(*A. duodenale*), 7 to 9 mm (*N. americanus*). A smaller group of hookworms infecting animals can invade and parasitize humans (*A. ceylanicum*) or can penetrate the human skin (causing cutaneous larva migrans), but do not develop any further (*A. braziliense, Uncinaria stenocephala*) (CDC).

Life Cycle

Eggs are passed in the stool ❶ [Figure 4-34], and under favorable conditions (moisture, warmth, shade), larvae hatch in 1 to 2 days. The released rhabditiform larvae grow in the feces and/or the soil ❷, and after 5 to 10 days (and two moults) they become infective filariform (third-stage) larvae ❸. These infective larvae can survive for 3 to 4 weeks in favorable environmental conditions. On contact with the human host, larvae penetrate the skin and are carried through the veins to the heart and then to the lungs. They penetrate into the pulmonary alveoli, ascend the bronchial tree to the pharynx, and are swallowed ❹. Larvae then reach the small intestine, where they reside and mature into adults. Adult worms live in the lumen of the small intestine, where they attach to the intestinal wall with resultant blood loss by the host ❺. Most adult worms are eliminated in 1 to 2 years, but longevity records can reach several years. Some *A. duodenale* larvae, following penetration of the host skin, can become dormant (in the intestine or muscle). In addition, infection by *A. duodenale* may also occur by the oral and transmammary route. In contrast, *N. americanus* requires a transpulmonary migration phase (CDC).

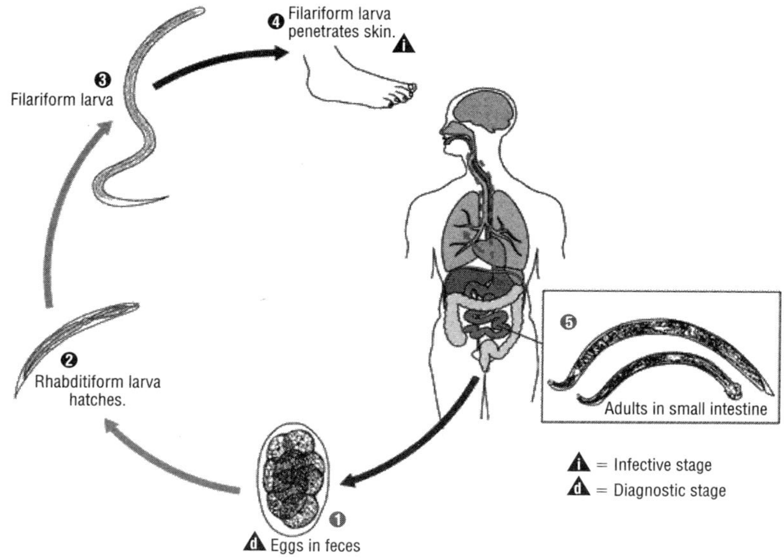

Figure 4-34   Life cycle of hookworm.

① Eggs in feces
▲ = Diagnostic stage

② Rhabditiform larva hatches.

③ Filariform larva

④ Filariform larva penetrates skin.
▲ = Infective stage

⑤ Adults in small intestine

▲ = Infective stage
▲ = Diagnostic stage

Clinical Presentation

Initial manifestations of hookworm consist of pruritus, erythema, and a papular or vesicular rash at the site of larval penetration (ground itch). Migration of larvae through the lungs can result in a Loeffler-like syndrome with transitory cough, wheezing, diffuse opacities on x-ray and eosinophilia in sputum and blood. Migration of *A. duodenale* larvae to the breast, with infection of nursing infants (hypobiosis) has been described. The major finding in overt infection is iron-deficiency anemia. Heavy intestinal infection can also produce local symptoms of abdominal pain, diarrhea, and occasionally malabsorption with weight loss (most commonly in children).

A. caninum is a leading cause of eosinophilic enteritis in humans and is found in dogs, foxes, and other canids worldwide. Most human infections are asymptomatic; however, some may experience abdominal pain and eosinophilia.

Reference

Hookworm. Centers for Disease Control Web site. Available at: http://www.dpd.cdc.gov/dpdx/HTML/Hookworm.htm. Accessed April 15, 2005.

Further Reading

Partners for Parasite Control (PPC). World Health Organization Web site. Available at: http://www.who.int/ctd/intpara/. Accessed April 15, 2005.

Bhaibulaya M, Indrangarm S. Man, an accidental host of Cyclodontostomum purvisi (Adams, 1933), and the occurrence in rats in Thailand. *Southeast Asian J Trop Med Public Health*. 1975;6:391-394.

de-Silva NR. Impact of mass chemotherapy on the morbidity due to soil-transmitted nematodes. *Acta Trop.* 2003;86:197-214.

Horton J. Albendazole: a broad spectrum anthelminthic for treatment of individuals and populations. *Curr Opin Infect Dis.* 2002;15:599-608.

Grover JK, Vats V, Uppal G, Yadav S. Anthelmintics: a review. *Trop Gastroenterol.* 2001;22:180-189.

Hymenolepis diminuta

Rat Tapeworm

Agent
Platyhelminthes, Cestoda. Cyclophyllidea, Hymeno-lepididae: *H. diminuta.* Similar to Anoplocephalidea, *Mathevotaenia*: *M. symmetrica.*

Reservoir
Rodents, various insects

Vector
None

Vehicle
Arthropod—ingestion

Geographic Distribution
Rat tapeworm infection appears to have a worldwide distribution.

Incubation Period
2–4w

Diagnostic Tests
Identification of ova in stool

Typical Adult Therapy
Praziquantel 25 mg/kg as single dose
Or niclosamide 2 g, then 1 g/d × 6d

Typical Pediatric Therapy
Praziquantel 25 mg/kg as single dose
Or niclosamide 1 g, then 0.5 g/d × 6d (1.5 g, then 1 g for
  weight > 34 kg)

Background

- Rats (*Rattus norvegicus, R. alexandrinus*) and mice (*Mus
  musculus, Apodemus sylvaticus*) are the definitive hosts;
  they become infected through ingestion of arthropod
  intermediates—fleas (*Nosopsyllus fasciatus, Xenopsylla
  cheopis, Leptopsylla segnis, Pulex irritans*), grain beetles
  (*Oryzaephilus sarinamensis*), or cockroaches (*Blattella
  germanica* and *Periplaneta americana*).
- Tapeworms of the genus *Mathevotaenia symmetrica*, a
  cosmopolitan parasite of rats, not previously reported
  in humans, were recovered from a girl in Bangkok.

Clinical Presentation
Rat tapeworm infestation is most often seen in children,
and is characterized by mild abdominal pain, nausea, diarrhea, and eosinophilia.

Further Reading
Hamrick HJ, Bowdre JH, Church SM. Rat tapeworm
  (Hymenolepis diminuta) infection in a child. *Pediatr Infect
  Dis J.* 1990;9:216-219.

Hymenolepiasis. Centers for Disease Control Web site. Available at: http://www.dpd.cdc.gov/dpdx/HTML/Hymenolepiasis.htm. Accessed April 15, 2005.

Lamon C, Greer GJ. Human infection with an anoplocephalid tapeworm of the genus Mathevotaenia. *Am J Trop Med Hyg*. July 1986;35:824-826.

Tena D, Perez Simon M, Gimeno C, et al. Human infection with Hymenolepis diminuta: case report from Spain. *J Clin Microbiol*. 1998;36:2375-2376.

Verghese SL, Sudha P, Padmaja P, Jaiswal PK, Kuruvilla T. Hymenolepis diminuta infestation in a child. *J Commun Dis*. 1998;30:201-203.

Hymenolepis nana

Dwarf Tapeworm, Rodentolepsiasis, Vampirolepis Nana

Agent
Platyhelminthes, Cestoda. Cyclophyllidea, Hymenolepididae: *Hymenolepis (Rodentolepis) nana.*

Reservoir
Humans, rodents (notably hamsters)

Vector
None

Vehicle
Food, water, fecal–oral contact

Geographic Distribution
Worldwide

Incubation Period
2–4w

Diagnostic Tests
Identification of ova in stool

Typical Adult Therapy
Praziquantel 25 mg/kg once
Or niclosamide 2 g/d × 1, then 1 g/d × 6d

Typical Pediatric Therapy
Praziquantel 25 mg/kg once
Or niclosamide 1 g/d × 1, then 0.5 g/d × 6d (1.5 g, then
    1g for weight > 34 kg)

Background

- *Hymenolepis nana* infestation is most often
  encountered as pediatric infestation in crowded, urban
  areas where hygiene is poor.
- This is the most common cestode infection of the
  southeastern United States and Latin America—
  because the parasite is transmitted human-to-human
  through the fecal–oral route, and it does not require
  an animal intermediate for replication.

Causal Agents

Hymenolepiasis is caused by two cestodes (tapeworm)
species, *Hymenolepis nana* (the dwarf tapeworm, adults
measuring 15 to 40 mm in length) and *Hymenolepis dim-
nuta* (rat tapeworm, adults measuring 20 to 60 cm in
length). *Hymenolepis diminuta* is a cestode of rodents

infrequently seen in humans and frequently found in rodents (CDC).

Life Cycle

Eggs of *Hymenolepis nana* are immediately infective when passed with the stool and cannot survive for more than 10 days in the external environment ❶ [Figure 4-35]. When eggs are ingested by an arthropod intermediate host ❷ (various species of beetles and fleas) they develop into cysticercoids, which are ingested by humans or rodents ❸ and develop into adults in the small intestine. A morphologically identical variant, *H. nana* var. *fraterna*, infects rodents and uses arthropods as intermediate hosts. When eggs are ingested ❹ (in contaminated food or water, or from hands contaminated with feces), oncospheres contained in the eggs are released. The oncospheres (hexacanth larvae) penetrate the intestinal villus and develop into cysticercoid larvae ❺. Upon rupture of the villus, the cysticercoids return to the intestinal lumen, evaginate their scoleces ❻, attach to the intestinal mucosa and develop into adults that reside in the ileal portion of the small intestine producing gravid proglottids ❼. Eggs are passed in the stool when released from proglottids through their genital atria, or when proglottids disintegrate in the small intestine ❽. An alternate mode of infection consists of internal autoinfection, in which hexacanth embryo released from eggs, penetrates intestinal villi, thus continuing the infective cycle without passage through the external environment ❾. The life span of adult worms is 4 to 6 weeks, but internal autoinfection allows the infection to persist for years (CDC).

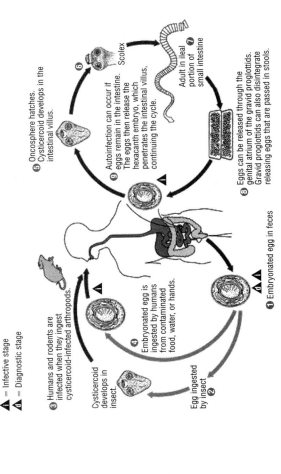

Figure 4-35 Life cycle of *Hymenolepis nana*.

△ = Infective stage
▲ = Diagnostic stage

❶ Embryonated egg in feces

❷ Egg ingested by insect

❸ Cysticercoid develops in insect

❸ Humans and rodents are infected when they ingest cysticercoid-infected arthropods.

❹ Embryonated egg is ingested by humans from contaminated food, water, or hands.

❺ Oncosphere hatches. Cysticercoid develops in the intestinal villus.

❻ Scolex

❼ Adult in ileal portion of small intestine

❽ Eggs can be released through the genital atrium of the gravid proglottids. Gravid proglottids can also disintegrate releasing eggs that are passed in stools.

❾ Autoinfection can occur if eggs remain in the intestine. The eggs then release the hexacanth embryo, which penetrates the intestinal villus, continuing the cycle.

271

Clinical Presentation

Symptoms are most common among children, and include nausea, abdominal pain, diarrhea, irritability, and weight loss. Pruritis ani and sleep and behavioral disturbances are occasionally encountered. Eosinophilia is present in 5 to 10% of patients. Infection is maintained by autoinfection (worm reproduces within the intestinal lumen).

Reference

Hymenolepiasis. Centers for Disease Control Web site. Available at: http://www.dpd.cdc.gov/dpdx/HTML/ Hymenolepiasis.htm. Accessed April 15, 2005.

Further Reading

Goncalves ML, Araujo A, Ferreira LF. Human intestinal parasites in the past: new findings and a review. *Mem Inst Oswaldo Cruz.* 2003;98(suppl 1):103-118.

Sirivichayakul CC, Radomyos PP, Praevanit RR, Pojjaroen-Anant CC, Wisetsing PP. Hymenolepis nana infection in Thai children. *J Med Assoc Thai.* 2000; 83:1035-1038.

Isospora belli

Agent

Protozoa. Sporozoa, Apicomplexa: *I.* (*Cystoisospora*) *belli.*

Reservoir

Humans

Vector

None

Vehicle

Food, liquids, fecal–oral contact, sexual (homosexual) contact

Geographic Distribution
Worldwide

Incubation Period
7–10d

Diagnostic Tests
Microscopy of stool or duodenal contents.
Advise laboratory when this organism is suspected.

Typical Adult Therapy
Trimethoprim/sulfamethoxazole 160/800 mg q.i.d. × 10d
Then b.i.d. × 3 weeks (can be indefinite in AIDS patients)

Typical Pediatric Therapy
Trimethoprim/sulfamethoxazole 2 mg/kg to 10 mg/kg
    q.i.d. × 10d
Then b.i.d. × 3 weeks

Background

- Infection by *I. belli* is most common in tropical and
  subtropical areas, especially sub-Saharan Africa, Brazil,
  El Salvador, Mexico, Haiti, the Middle East, and
  Southeast Asia.
- *I. natalensis* and *I. chilensis* infections have been rarely
  reported in humans.

Causal Agent

The coccidian parasite, *Isospora belli*, infects the epithelial
cells of the small intestine, and is the least common of the
three intestinal coccidia that infect humans (CDC).

Life Cycle

At time of excretion, the immature oocyst usually contains one sporoblast (rarely two) ❶ [Figure 4-36]. After excretion, the sporoblast divides in two (the oocyst now contains two sporoblasts). The sporoblasts secrete a cyst wall to become sporocysts; and the sporocysts divide twice to produce four sporozoites each ❷. Infection occurs by ingestion of sporocysts-containing oocysts. Sporocysts excyst in the small intestine and release their sporozoites, which invade the epithelial cells and initiate schizogony ❸. Upon rupture of the schizonts, merozoites are released, invade new epithelial cells, and continue the cycle of asexual multiplication ❹. Trophozoites develop into schizonts which contain multiple merozoites. After a minimum of one week, the sexual stage begins with the development of male and female gametocytes ❺. Fertilization results in the development of oocysts, which are excreted in the stool ❶. *Isospora belli* infects both humans and animals (CDC).

Clinical Presentation

Isosporiasis is characterized by abdominal cramps, watery diarrhea, headache, weight loss, and myalgias. Fever and vomiting might also be present. A low-grade eosinophilia is present in 50% of patients; and fecal leucocytes are not seen.

Infection in AIDS patients could cause significant weight loss and dehydration, requiring hospitalization. Disease is also more severe among patients with lymphoma and leukemia. Chronic and severe infection could occasionally affect immunocompetent patients as well,

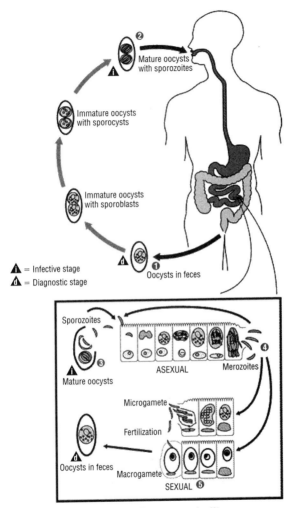

Figure 4-36   Life cycle of *Isospora belli*.

and infants and young children are most likely to suffer severe disease. Disseminated extraintestinal infection has rarely been reported.

Reference
Isosporiasis. Centers for Disease Control Web site. Available at: http://www.dpd.cdc.gov/dpdx/HTML/isosporiasis.htm. Accessed April 15, 2005.

Further Reading
Isospora infection. Centers for Disease Control Web site. Available at: http://www.cdc.gov/ncidod/dpd/parasites/ isospora/default.htm. Accessed April 15, 2005.

Leclerc H, Schwartzbrod L, Dei-Cas E. Microbial agents associated with waterborne diseases. *Crit Rev Microbiol.* 2002;28:371-409.

Lindsay DS, Blagburn BL. Biology of mammalian isospora. *Parasitol Today.* 1994;10:214-220.

Ribes JA, Seabolt JP, Overman SB. Point prevalence of Cryptosporidium, Cyclospora, and Isospora infections in patients being evaluated for diarrhea. *Am J Clin Pathol.* 2004;122:28-32.

Lagochilascaris minor

Agent
Nematoda. Phasmidea: *L. minor.*

Reservoir
Unknown

Vector
None

Vehicle
Ingestion of ova—details not known

Geographic Distribution
REGION II—CAm	CRI, MEX
REGION III—SAm	BOL, BRA, COL, SUR, VEN
REGION IV—Carib	TTO

Incubation Period
>30d

Diagnostic Tests
Identification of ova or adult parasites in tissue and exudates

Typical Therapy
There is no proven therapy.
Albendazole has been used with some success.

Background
- Sporadic cases are reported from Latin America and the Caribbean.
- Adult worms live in the intestine of opossums, from which larva pass in stool to be ingested by mice and other small mammals. Larvae hatch and migrate to the muscle tissue of these animals.
- Humans (an accidental host for this infection) are infected through ingestion of soil or small mammals.

Clinical Presentation
Lagochilascariasis is characterized by slowly developing soft tissue masses of the head, neck, nasopharynx, or

tonsils. Initially, the patients may complain of a sensation of "something crawling" in the back of the mouth. Lesions become fluctuant, forming sinuses and fistulae, which discharge pus that contains worms, larvae and eggs. Worms can also exit through the nose or mouth or involve the paranasal sinuses and, rarely, the brain or lungs.

Further Reading

Botero D, Little MD. Two cases of human Lagochilascaris infection in Colombia. *Am J Trop Med Hyg.* 1984;33:381-386.

de Aguilar-Nascimento JE, Silva GM, Tadano T, Valadares Filho M, Akiyama AM, Castelo A. Infection of the soft tissue of the neck due to Lagochilascaris minor. *Trans R Soc Trop Med Hyg.* 1993;87:198.

Vargas-Ocampo F, Alvarado-Aleman FJ. Infestation from Lagochilascaris minor in Mexico. *Int J Dermatol.* 1997;36: 56-58.

Leishmaniasis—Cutaneous

Aleppo Button, Baghdad Boil, Bay Sore, Bejuco, Biskra Button, Bolho, Bush Yaws, Chiclero Ulcer, Cutaneous Leishmaniasis, Delhi Ulcer, Domal, El-Mohtafura, Forest Yaws, Granuloma Endemicum, Hashara, Jericho Boil, Kandahar Sore, Leishmaniose—Kutane, Leishmaniosi Cutanea, Lepra de Montana, Liana, Okhet, Oriental Sore, Pendjeh Sore, Pian Bois, Saldana, Ulcera de Bejuco, Uta, Yatevi

Agent

Neozoa, Euglenozoa, Kenetoplastea. Flagellate: *Leishmania tropica, et al.*

Reservoir
Humans, hyraces, rodents, marsupials, dogs, sloths, anteaters, armadillos.

Vector
Fly (sandfly = *Phlebotomus* spp. for Old World; *Lutzomyia* spp. or *Psychodopygus* spp. for New World)

Vehicle
None

Geographic Distribution
Various forms of cutaneous leishmaniasis are found in nearly 80 countries:

REGION II—CAm	BLZ, CRI, GTM, HND, MEX, NIC, PAN, SLV
REGION III—SAm	ARG, BOL, BRA, COL, ECU, GUF, GUY, PER, PRY, SUR, VEN
REGION IV—Carib	ES-CN, SCG
REGION V—NAfr	DZA, EGY, LBY, MAR, TUN
REGION VI—CAfr	BEN, BFA, CAF, CIV, CMR, DJI, ETH, ERI, GIN, GMB, KEN, MLI, MRT, MWI, NER, NGA, SDN, SEN, SOM, TCD, TGO, TZA, UGA
REGION VII—SAfr	NAM, ZAF
REGION VIII—Eur	ALB, BGR, ESP, FRA, GIB, GRC, ITA, MLT, PRT
REGION IX—MidEast	IRN, IRQ, ISR, JOR, KWT, LBN, SAU, SYR, TUR, YEM
REGION X—IndSub	IND, PAK

REGION XI—Asia   AFG, CHN, TKM, TWN,
                        UZB
REGION XII—SEA   IDN, KHM

Incubation Period
2–8w (range 1w–months)

Diagnostic Tests
Identification of organism on smear or specialized
   culture
Nucleic acid amplification

Typical Therapy
If deep/extensive:

Stibogluconate 10 mg/kg/d i.v. or IM × 10d (max 600
   mg/d).

Ketoconazole effective against *L. mexicana.*

Topical paromomycin in methlybenzethonium can be
   used for superficial infections.

Background

- The genus *Leishmania* is divided into two subgenera:
  Leishmania (Leishmania) and *Leishmania (Viannia).*
- Species of *Leishmania (Viannia)* are restricted to the
  New World and include: *L. braziliensis* complex
  (*L. braziliensis* and *L. peruviana*), *L. guyansis* complex
  (*L. guyanensis, L. panamensis* and *L. shawi*), *L. naiffi*
  complex (*L. naiffi*), and *L. lainsoni* complex (*L. lainsoni*).
- Species of *Leishmania (Leishmania)* are found in both
  the Old World and New World and include: *L
  donovani* complex *(L. donovani* and *L. archibaldi), L.
  infantum* complex *(L. infantum*—note that *L. chagasi*

is synonymous with *L. infantum*), *L. tropica* complex,
L. killicki complex, *L. aethiopica* complex, *L. major*
complex, *L. turanica* complex, *L. gerbilli* complex,
L. arabica complex, *L. mexicana* complex, *L.
amazoensis* complex *(L. amazoensis* and *L. aristidesi)*—
note that *L. garnhami* is synonymous with
L. amazonensis, L. enriettii complex, *L. hertigi* complex
(L. hertigi and *L. deanei).*

- Old World infection is caused by *L. major (rural)*,
  L. tropica (urban) or *L. aethiopica* (limited to Ethiopia
  and Kenya). New World infection is caused by *L.
  guyanensis, L. panamensis, L. peruviana, L. naiffi,
  L. shawi, L. lainsoni, L. mexicana* complex, *L.
  amazonensis (L. garnhami)*, and *L. venezuelensis.*
- Worldwide, 1 million to 1.5 million new cases are
  estimated per year.

Causal Agent

Leishmaniasis is a vector-borne disease that is transmitted by sandflies and caused by obligate intracellular protozoa of the genus *Leishmania*. Human infection is
caused by approximately 21 of 30 species that infect
mammals. These include the *L. donovani* complex with 3
species (*L. donovani, L. infantum,* and *L. chagasi*); the
L. mexicana complex with 3 main species (*L. mexicana, L.
amazonensis,* and *L. venezuelensis*); *L. tropica; L. major;
L. aethiopica;* and the subgenus *Viannia* with 4 main
species (*L. (V.) braziliensis, L. (V.) guyanensis, L. (V.)
panamensis,* and *L. (V.) peruviana*). The various species
are morphologically indistinguishable, but can be differentiated by isoenzyme analysis, molecular methods, or
monoclonal antibodies (CDC).

Life Cycle

Leishmaniasis is transmitted by the bite of female phle-
botomine sandflies, which inject the infective stage (promastigote), during blood meals ❶ [Figure 4-37].
Promastigotes that reach the puncture wound are phagocytized by macrophages ❷ and transform into amastigotes ❸. Amastigotes multiply in infected cells and invade
different tissues, depending in part on the *Leishmania*
species ❹. Sandflies become infected during blood meals
on an infected host, as they ingest macrophages infected
with amastigotes (❺,❻). In the sandfly's midgut, parasites
differentiate into promastigotes ❼, which multiply and
migrate to the proboscis ❽ (CDC).

Clinical Presentation

Typically, a nodule develops at the site of a sandfly bite
following a few days to several months. The lesion can be
erythematous or covered by a thin yellow crust. The nodule reaches a diameter of 1 to 5 cm over a period of weeks
or months and is not painful. The crust may thicken and
even replace the nodule; or it can fall away to reveal an
ulcer with a raised edge. Satellite papules are common.
The lesion could heal over a period of months or even
years, leaving a depressed scar. Secondary infection is not
prominent, and the major residua are scarring and disability.

Lesions caused by *L. major* evolve and heal most rapidly, and are often inflamed or exudative (wet sore or
rural sore). Lesions caused by *L. tropica* are less inflamed
(dry sore or urban sore). Lesions due to *L. infantum* appear only after several months, and are small, nodular,
and persist for years. Lesions of *L. aethiopica* are typically
single, and they often involve the face. Satellite papules

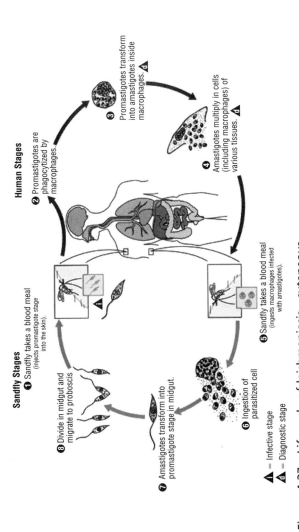

Sandfly Stages

❶ Sandfly takes a blood meal (injects promastigote stage into the skin).

❽ Divide in midgut and migrate to proboscis

❼ Amastigotes transform into promastigote stage in midgut.

❻ Ingestion of parasitized cell

❺ Sandfly takes a blood meal (ingests macrophages infected with amastigotes).

Human Stages

❷ Promastigotes are phagocytized by macrophages.

❸ Promastigotes transform into amastigotes inside macrophages.

❹ Amastigotes multiply in cells (including macrophages) of various tissues.

▲ = Infective stage
△ = Diagnostic stage

Figure 4-37   Life cycle of leishmaniasis—cutaneous.

283

evolve to produce a slowly growing, shiny tumor or plaque that might not crust nor ulcerate. If the site borders an area of mucosa, mucocutaneous leishmaniasis could develop, with swelling of the lips and enlargement of the nose over many years.

L. brasiliensis produces deep, usually single, ulcers with a granulomatous base. Fifteen percent of patients will relapse after spontaneous recovery or therapeutic improvement. The lesions of *L. guyanensis* are multiple, fleshy, and protuberant, and involve the limbs. Unlike other *Leishmania* species, *L. braziliensis* and *L. panamensis* are commonly associated with metastatic lesions along the path of draining lymphatics. The lesions of *L. mexicana* (chiclero ulcer) are commonly located on the side of the face or behind the ears. Destruction of the pinna is common.

Three forms of cutaneous leishmaniasis do not heal spontaneously: Disseminated cutaneous leishmaniasis, Leishmaniasis recidivans, and American mucosal leishmaniasis. Diffuse cutaneous leishmaniasis is often seen with *L. amazoensis* infections, and also occurs in about 0.01% of *L. aethiopica* infections. The nodule spreads locally without ulceration, while secondary hematogenous lesions appear on other body sites. These are often symmetrical, and they involve the face and extensor surfaces of the limbs. The external genitalia might also be affected, but the eye, mucosae and peripheral nerves are not infected (in contrast to lepromatous leprosy). The infection evolves gradually over many years.

Leishmaniasis recidivans (lupoid leishmaniasis) is a rare complication of *L. tropica* infection. After initial healing, papules reappear in the edge of the scar and the lesion spreads slowly over many years. The condition most commonly involves the face, and could be quite disfiguring.

Reference

Leishmaniasis. Centers for Disease Control Web site. Available at: http://www.dpd.cdc.gov/dpdx/HTML/Leishmaniasis. htm. Accessed April 15, 2005.

Further Reading

Berman J. Current treatment approaches to leishmaniasis. *Curr Opin Infect Dis.* 2003;16:397-401.

Lawn SD, Yardley V, Vega-Lopez F, Watson J, Lockwood DN. New World cutaneous leishmaniasis in returned travellers: treatment failures using intravenous sodium stibogluconate. *Trans R Soc Trop Med Hyg.* 2003;97:443-445.

Leishmaniasis. World Health Organization/Communicable Disease Surveillance and Response Web site. Available at: http://www.who.int/emc/diseases/leish/index.html. Accessed April 15, 2005.

Leishmania infection. Centers for Disease Control Web site. Available at: http://www.cdc.gov/ncidod/dpd/parasites/ leishmania/default.htm. Accessed April 15, 2005.

Vega Lopez F. Diagnosis of cutaneous leishmaniasis. *Curr Opin Infect Dis.* 2003;16:97-101.

Leishmaniasis—Mucocutaneous

Agla, Espundia

Agent
Protozoa. Neozoa, Euglenozoa, Kenetoplastea. Flagellate: *Leishmania braziliensis, et al.*

Reservoir
Rodents, Humans, sloths, marsupials

Vector
Fly (sandfly = *Lutzomyia* or *Psychodopygus*)

Vehicle
None

Incubation Period
2–8w (range 1w–6m)

Geographic Distribution
This disease is found in Mexico and most countries of Central and South America. A form of the disease has also been reported in Sudan.

REGION II—CAm	BLZ, CRI, GTM, HND, MEX, NIC, PAN
REGION III—SAm	ARG, BOL, BRA, COL, ECU, GUF, PRY, PER, VEN
REGION VI—CAfr	SDN

Diagnostic Tests
Microscopy (culture in specialized laboratories)
Serology
Nucleic acid amplification

Typical Therapy
Stibogluconate 20 mg/kg/d (max. 800 mg) i.v./IM × 20d
Or amphotericin B 0.5 mg/kg/d × 4–8w

Background

- The current taxonomy of *Leishmania* species is discussed under "Leishmaniasis—Cutaneous."
- Mucocutaneous leishmaniasis is limited to Latin America, with the rare exception of Sudan. *Leishmania* (*Viannia*) *braziliensis* is the most widely distributed Leishmania species in the New World. Its principal

habitats are forests, coffee, and cocoa plantations and cities–suburbs. *L. panamensis* is also implicated in mucosal infection.

- The principal vectors are *Lutzomyia (Psychodopygus) wellcomei* and *Lu. whitmani* in forest areas, and *Lu. intermedia* in houses. Parasites are also found in *Lu. carrerai carrerai, Lu. llanos martinsi, Lu. migonei, Lu. spincrasa, Lu. yucumensis, Lu. squamiventris, Lu. ovallesi, Lu. Lichyi,* and *Lu. pessoai.*

- Proven and suspected reservoirs include rodents (*Akodon arviculoides, Rattus rattus, Oryzomys nigripes, Or. capito, Or. concolor, Rhipidomys leucodactylus,* and *Proechimys* spp.*), marsupials (*Didelphis marsupialis*), edentates (*Choloepus didactylus*), carnivores (*Canis familiaris*) and horses (*Equus caballus and Equus asinus*).

- A form of mucocutaneous disease (Sudanese mucosal leishmaniasis) has been reported. It is not preceded or accompanied by cutaneous lesions, and it presents as either nasal obstruction, discharge and bleeding; oral fullness, loss of teeth, and bleeding gums; or perforation of the hard palate. The mucocutaneous form is found almost exclusively in Sudanese adult males.

Clinical Presentation

As many as 40% of patients with cutaneous ulcers due to *L. brasiliensis* will develop mucosal involvement; 50% of these will occur within 2 years of the original infection, and 90% within 10 years (cases appearing after as many as 35 years have been reported). 15% of patients give no history of a previous primary skin lesion.

In virtually all cases the nasal mucosa is affected, and in 33% a second site is also involved—the pharynx, palate, larynx, or upper lip, in order of frequency. The initial presentation is typically nasal obstruction associated with a nodule or polyp on the inferior turbinate. The process evolves slowly to perforate the nasal septum, and could ultimately destroy the entire mouth and nose.

Death could result from secondary sepsis, starvation or laryngeal obstruction. Extensive lesions are less common in infection by *Leishmania panamensis* and *Leishmania guyanensis.*

Further Reading

Communicable Disease Surveillance and Response/World Health Organization Web site. Available at: http://www.who.int/emc/diseases/leish/index.html. Accessed April 15, 2005.

Leishmania infection. Centers for Disease Control Web site. Available at: http://www.cdc.gov/ncidod/dpd/parasites/leishmania/default.htm. Accessed April 15, 2005.

Marsden PD. Clinical presentations of Leishmania braziliensis braziliensis. *Parasitol Today.* 1985;1:129-133.

Silveira FT, Lainson R, Corbett CE. Clinical and immuno-pathological spectrum of American cutaneous leishmaniasis with special reference to the disease in Amazonian Brazil: a review. *Mem Inst Oswaldo Cruz.* 2004;99:239-251.

Leishmaniasis—Visceral

Burdwan Fever, Cachectic Fever, Dum Dum Fever, Kala-Azar, Ponos

Agent

Protozoa. Neozoa, Euglenozoa, Kenetoplastea. Flagellate: *Leishmania donovani, L. infantum, L. cruzi;* rarely, *L. tropica.*

Reservoir

Humans, rodents, dogs, foxes

Vector
Fly (sandfly = *Phlebotomus* for Old World; *Lutzomyia* for New World)

Vehicle
Blood

Geographic Distribution
Visceral leishmaniasis is reported from over 100 countries.

REGION II—CAm	CRI, GTM, HND, MEX, NIC, PAN, SLV
REGION III—SAm	ARG, BOL, BRA, COL, ECU, GUY, PER, PRY, SUR, VEN
REGION IV—Carib	SCG
REGION V—NAfr	DZA, EGY, LBY, MAR, TUN
REGION VI—CAfr	AGO, BFA, CAF, CIV, CMR, COD, COG, DJI, ERI, ETH, GAB, GHA, GIN, GMB, GNB, GNQ, KEN, MLI, MOZ, MWI, NER, NGA, RWA, SDN, SEN, SLE, SOM, TCD, TZA, UGA, ZMB
REGION VIII—Eur	ALB, AND, AUT, BIH, BGR, BLR, ESP, EST, FRA, GIB, GRC, HRV, HUN, ITA, LTU, LVA, MDA, MKD, MLT, PRT, ROM, UKR, SVK
REGION IX—MidEast	ARE, ARM, IRN, IRQ, ISR, JOR, KWT, LBN, OMN, QAT, SAU, TUR, YEM

REGION X—IndSub	BGD, IND, LKA, NPL, PAK
REGION XI—Asia	AFG, AZE, CHN, KAZ, KGZ, KOR, MNG, RUS, TJK, TKM, PRK, UZB
REGION XII—SEA	IDN, KHM, LAO, MMR, THA, VNM

Incubation Period
2–6m (10d–12m)

Diagnostic Tests
Smear / culture of bone marrow, splenic aspirate, lymph nodes
Serology
Nucleic acid amplification

Typical Adult Therapy
Miltefosine 50 to 150 mg PO daily × 4–6 weeks
Or stibogluconate 20 mg/kg/d (max 800 mg) × 20d
Or amphotericin B 1 mg/kg/QOD × 8w (or lipid complex 3 mg/kg/d × 5d)

Typical Pediatric Therapy
Stibogluconate 20 mg/kg/d (max 800 mg) × 20d
Or amphotericin B 1 mg/kg/QOD × 8w (or lipid complex 3 mg/kg/d × 5d)

Background

- Visceral leishmaniasis is widely distributed. Worldwide, 500,000 new cases and 75,000 to 80,000 deaths per year are estimated. The ongoing prevalence is estimated at 2.5 million. More than 90% of the world's cases are reported from India, Bangladesh, Brazil, and Sudan.

- The case-fatality rate for untreated disease approaches 90% (3.4 to 15% in treated infection). As many as 20% of infections are subclinical.
- 75,000 deaths were attributed to leishmaniasis in 1991; 57,000 in 1999.
- The current taxonomy of *Leishmania* species is discussed under "Leishmaniasis—Cutaneous." *L. infantum* causes visceral leishmaniasis (and occasionally cutaneous leishmaniasis) in the Mediterranean basin, western Asia, and eastern China between 30°N and 45°N. Most human infections occur under the age of 5 years. The disease is enzootic in domestic dogs, but it is also encountered in wild dogs, jackals, and foxes. The principal vectors are *Phlebotomus perniciosus* and *P. ariasi.*
- *L. donovani* causes anthroponotic visceral leishmaniasis (kala-azar) in India and some parts of China, and enzootic visceral leishmaniasis in sub-Saharan Africa. India and Sudan account for more than 50% of the world's cases. Humans are the only known reservoir in Asia. Highest rates are found in the age group 10 to 29 years, with a male/female ratio of 6/1. *L. donovani* in East Africa affects adults and older children, with a reservoir in the grass rat (*Arvicanthis niloticus*), spiny mouse (*Acomys albigena*), serval (*Felis serval*), genet (*Genetta genetta*), jackal (*Canis.* sp.), squirrel, and gerbil. The principal vector is *Ph. papatasi. Ph. (Paraphlebotomus) alexandri* may also act as vector in China and Iraq; and *Ph. (Synphletobomus) martini* in Kenya.
- *L. chagasi* (currently considered synonymous with *L. infantum*) produces sporadic cases in Latin America, with a local reservoir in domestic dogs and foxes. The vector is *Lutzomyia longipalpis*; although, *Lu. ovalesi*

and *Lu. evansi* had been implicated in the past. Proven or suspected reservoirs include carnivores such as the cat (*Felis domesticus*), fox (*Cerdocyon thous*), *Lycalopex vetulus*, *Canis familiaris*; and opossums (*Didelphis albiventris* and *Di. marsupialis*). Asymptomatic human carriage has also been demonstrated.

- As of 2000, infection acquired through blood transfusion has been reported in Belgium, Brazil, France, and India.

- *Leishmania*/HIV co-infection has emerged in southwestern Europe as a result of the increasing overlap between visceral leishmaniasis (VL) and AIDS, which is due to the spread of the AIDS pandemic in rural areas and that of VL in suburban areas. Although cases of coinfection have so far been reported in 35 countries worldwide, most of the cases have been notified in southwestern Europe (1,911 cases in France, Italy, Portugal, and Spain as of 2001). The cases reported in these countries between January 1996 and June 1998 represented 49.8% of the total number of cases. AIDS increases the risk of VL by 100 to 1,000 times in endemic areas.

- As of June 1998, 1,663 cases of HIV-Leishmania coinfection were reported to WHO. Of southern European patients with visceral leishmaniasis, 25 to 70% are coinfected with AIDS, and 1.5 to 9% of AIDS patients in the area are coinfected with visceral leishmaniasis. Approximately 70% of coinfected patients are males, and 71.1% are drug abusers (1990 to 1998).

- Of the estimated 25 million dogs in southern Europe, 16.7% are infected. All breeds of dogs are equally affected, with peak rates at ages 3 and 8 years.

Clinical Presentation

Following an incubation period of 2 to 8 months, the patient develops chronic fever, abdominal pain (from an enlarged spleen) and swelling, weight loss, cough, and occasionally, diarrhea. The classical fever rises twice daily, without rigors; however, single spikes, irregular or undulant fevers are common. Caucasians may experience an abrupt onset of high fever, with rapid progression of illness, toxemia, weakness, dyspnea, and anemia.

Physical signs can be limited to splenomegaly, but chronically ill patients are typically pale and cachetic. Hyperpigmentation of face, extremities, and abdomen (kala-azar) could be present in advanced cases. The spleen is nontender, and it could be massively enlarged, reaching the left or even right iliac fossa. Moderate hepatomegaly is present in one third of cases. Generalized lymphadenopathy is found in 50% of African patients, and a smaller percentage of Indian and European cases. Jaundice, mucosal and retinal hemorrhage, and uveitis are occasionally encountered. A chronic rash (post kala-azar dermal leishmaniasis = PKDL) resembling leprosy and involving primarily the extremities and face often appears months to years following infection.

Laboratory studies reveal pancytopenia, hypoalbuminemia, hyperglobulinemia, and only mild hepatic dysfunction. Intercurrent infections are common, notably pneumococcal disease (otitis, pneumonia, or septicemia), tuberculosis, and measles. The case-fatality rate without treatment is 80 to 90%.

Further Reading

Alvar J. Leishmaniasis and AIDS co-infection: the Spanish example. *Parasitolol Today.* 1994;10:160-163.

Communicable Disease Surveillance and Response Web site. Available at: http://www.who.int/emc/diseases/leish/index.html. Accessed April 15, 2005.

Desjeux P. Leishmaniasis: current situation and new perspectives. *Comp Immunol Microbiol Infect Dis.* 2004;27:305-318.

Leishmania infection. Centers for Disease Control Web site. Available at: http://www.cdc.gov/ncidod/dpd/parasites/leishmania/default.htm. Accessed April 15, 2005.

Linguatula serrata

Halzoun, Marrara Syndrome

Agent
Pentastomid worm: *L. serrata*

Reservoir
Herbivore

Vector
None

Vehicle
Meat (liver or lymph nodes of sheep or goat)

Geographic Distribution
The parasite appears to have a worldwide distribution.

Incubation Period
Unknown

Diagnostic Tests
Identification of larvae in nasal discharge

Typical Therapy
No specific therapy available

Background

- *L. serrata* is found worldwide, and it lives in the nasal passages of dogs, foxes, and wolves.
- Eggs are discharged, and eaten by rodents, sheep, goats, and other domestic animals in which they hatch to invade visceral organs.
- Humans can develop either visceral infection (usually asymptomatic, with the exception of eye lesions) through ingestion of ova; or they can develop nasopharyngeal infection (halzoun in Greece, Marrara in Sudan) through migration of ingested larvae in foods such as semiraw sheep liver or lymph nodes. As of 1999, ocular infection had only been described in Israel, Ecuador, and the United States.

Clinical Presentation

Infestation is associated with pain and itching in the throat or ear, lacrimation, cough, hemoptysis, rhinorrhea, or hoarseness. Complications include respiratory obstruction, epistaxis, facial paralysis, or involvement of the eye.

Additional Reading

Ma KC, Qiu MH, Rong YL. Pathological differentiation of suspected cases of pentastomiasis in China. *Trop Med Int Health.* 2002;7:166-177.

Schacher JF, Saab S, Germanos R, Boustany N. The aetiology of halzoun in Lebanon: recovery of Linguatula serrata nymphs from two patients. *Trans R Soc Trop Med Hyg.* 1969;63:854-858.

Yagi H, el Bahari S, Mohamed HA, et al. The Marrara syndrome: a hypersensitivity reaction of the upper respiratory tract and buccopharyngeal mucosa to nymphs of Linguatula serrata. *Acta Trop.* 1996;62:127-134.

Malaria

Ague, Bilious Remittent Fever, Chagres Fever, Estiautumnal Fever, March Fever, Paludism, Paludismo

Agent
Protozoa. Sporozoa, Apicomplexa: *Plasmodium* spp.

Reservoir
Humans

Vector
Mosquitoes (*Anopheles* spp.)

Vehicle
Transfusion

Geographic Distribution
Malaria is endemic to 105 countries.
    Note: Chloroquine-resistant *P. falciparum* malaria is found in 78 countries (**in bold-face type**)

REGION II—CAm	CRI, BLZ, GTM, HND, MEX, NIC, **PAN**, SLV
REGION III—SAm	ARG, **BOL, BRA, COL, ECU, GUF, GUY, PER,** PRY, **SUR, VEN**
REGION IV—Carib	DOM, HTI
REGION V—NAfr	DZA, EGY, LBY, MAR
REGION VI—CAfr	**AGO, BDI, BEN, BFA, CAF, CIV, CMR, COD, COG, COM, CPV, DJI, ERI, ETH, GAB, GHA, GIN, GMB, GNB, GNQ, KEN, LBR, MDG, MLI, MOZ, MRT, MWI,** MUS, **NER,**

	NGA, RWA, SDN, SEN, SLE, SOM, STP, TCD, TGO, TZA, UGA, ZMB, ZWE
REGION VII—SAfr	**BWA, NAM, SWZ**
REGION VIII—Eur	GEO
REGION IX—MidEast	ARE, **IRN**, IRQ, **OMN, SAU,** SYR, TUR, **YEM**
REGION X—IndSub	**BDG, BTN, IND, LKA, NPL, PAK**
REGION XI—Asia	**AFG,** ARM, AZE, **CHN,** PRK, TKM, TJK, RUS, **UZB**
REGION XII—SEA	**IDN, KHM, LAO, MMR, MYS, PHL, THA, VNM**
REGION XIII—Poly	**PNG, SLB, VUT**

Incubation Period
12–30d. Note that disease can relapse after 7 (*P. ovale* and *P. vivax*) to 40 (*P. malariae*) years.

Diagnostic Tests
Examination of blood smear
Serology, antigen, and microscopic techniques
Nucleic acid amplification

Typical Adult Therapy
Chloroquine-resistant falciparum: quinine +
   (doxycycline or clindamycin)
Or mefloquine
Or atovaquone/proguanil
Or artemisinin
Other forms: chloroquine 1 g. Then, 500 mg at 6, 24, &
   48 hrs. If *P. ovale* or *vivax*, follow with primaquine.

Typical Pediatric Therapy

Chloroquine-resistant falciparum: quinine +
    (doxycycline or clindamycin)

Or atovaquone/proguanil

Or artemisinin

Other forms: chloroquine base 10 mg/kg, 5 mg/kg at 6,
    24, and 48 hrs. If *P. ovale* or *vivax*, follow with
    primaquine.

Background

- Malaria accounts for 2.3% of all disease globally, and
  9% in Africa. An estimated 200 to 500 million cases of
  malaria occur each year—50 to 90% of these in Africa.
  Two thirds of the remaining cases are reported from
  India, Brazil, Sri Lanka, Vietnam, Colombia and the
  Solomon Islands. Approximately 10,000 to 12,000
  cases are imported into Europe each year.
- Malaria was the eleventh most common cause of death
  worldwide in 1990. Worldwide mortality is estimated
  at 1.5 to 2.7 million per year, most among young
  children in sub-Saharan Africa. It is estimated that
  860,000 Africans die of the disease each year, and that
  one to two children die of malaria every minute.
  Malaria accounted for 6% of all deaths in Africa in
  1900, and 9% in 1997, compared to 8% of all deaths in
  the rest of the world in 1900, and 0.08% in 1997.
- As of 1994, 2.02 billion people lived in malarious
  areas, and an additional 1.62 billion lived in
  potentially malarious areas.
- *P. vivax* is the most common of four human malaria
  species, with a worldwide distribution within
  approximately 16 to 20°N and S of the summer
  isotherms.

- Chloroquine-resistant *P. falciparum* occurs in all endemic areas except Central America (north of Panama), the Caribbean, China (with some resistance in the southeast), the Middle East (except the Arabian/Gulf States), and Turkey. Resistance first appeared in Southeast Asia during the 1960s. Chloroquine-resistant strains first appeared in Africa in 1978 and had involved all countries on the continent by 1988.
- Resistance to sulfadoxine/pyrimethamine is widespread in Southeast Asia and South America and occurs sporadically in other parts of the world.
- Chloroquine-resistant *P. vivax* was first reported in Papua-New Guinea in 1989, and has been confirmed in Guatemala, India, Indonesia, Myanmar, Brazil, Colombia, Guyana, and Vanuatu. Possible chloroquine-resistant *P. malariae* has been reported in Indonesia.
- Africa accounts for 90% of the world's malaria cases.
- Transfusion-borne malaria was first described in 1911. More than 3,000 cases had been reported worldwide as of 1990.
- For reporting purposes, malaria is classified as (1) autochthonous—either indigenous or introduced (acquired by local mosquitoes and transmitted in an area where malaria does not occur regularly); (2) imported (acquired outside of the country or territory in question); (3) induced (acquired through blood products); (4) relapsing; or (5) cryptic (an isolated case that cannot be linked epidemiologically to secondary cases).
- During 1977 to 1999, 71 cases of airport malaria were reported in Europe—most cases were due to *P. falciparum*—and more than 33% cases were in France.

From 1969 to 1999, 12 European countries reported 87 cases of airport malaria.

Causal Agents

Blood parasites of the genus *Plasmodium*. There are approximately 156 named species of *Plasmodium* which infect various species of vertebrates. Four are known to infect humans: *P. falciparum*, *P. vivax*, *P. ovale* and *P. malariae*. In 2004, naturally-acquired *Plasmodium knowlesi* malaria was confirmed in a human in Thailand (CDC).

Life Cycle

The malaria parasite life cycle involves two hosts. During a blood meal, a malaria-infected female *Anopheles* mosquito inoculates sporozoites into the human host ❶ [Figure 4-38]. Sporozoites infect liver cells ❷ and mature into schizonts ❸, which rupture and release merozoites ❹. (Of note, in *P. vivax* and *P. ovale* a dormant stage [hypnozoites] can persist in the liver and cause relapses by invading the bloodstream weeks, or even years later.) After this initial replication in the liver (exo-erythrocytic schizogony Ⓐ), the parasites undergo asexual multiplication in the erythrocytes (erythrocytic schizogony Ⓑ). Merozoites infect red blood cells ❺. Ring stage trophozoites mature into schizonts, which rupture releasing merozoites ❻. Some parasites differentiate into sexual erythrocytic stages (gametocytes) ❼. Blood stage parasites are responsible for the clinical manifestations of the disease.

Male (microgametocytes) and female (macrogametocytes) gametocytes, are ingested by an *Anopheles* mos-

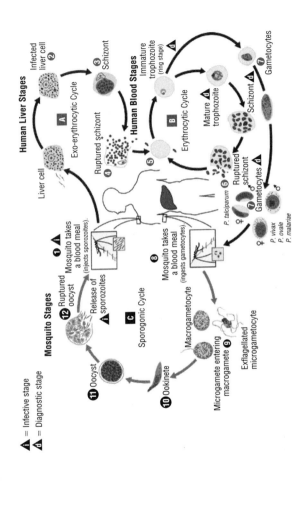

Figure 4-38   Life cycle of malaria.

301

quito during a blood meal ❽. The parasites' multiplication in the mosquito is known as "sporogony" 🅲. While in the mosquito's stomach, microgametes penetrate the macrogametes generating zygotes ❾. The zygotes in turn become motile and elongated (ookinetes) ❿ and invade the midgut wall of the mosquito, where they develop into oocysts ⓫. The oocysts grow, rupture, and release sporozoites ⓬, which make their way to the mosquito's salivary glands. Inoculation of the sporozoites into a new human host perpetuates the malaria life cycle ❶ (CDC).

Clinical Presentation

Malaria can be caused by any of four species of *Plasmodium*: *P. falciparum, P. vivax, P. malariae,* and *P. ovale.* Approximately 1% of cases involve coinfection by more than one species. Although signs and symptoms for any of these species are similar, *P. falciparum* infection is typified by relatively severe illness and even death.

Following acquisition of infection from a mosquito (genus *Anophles*) bite, parasites multiply in the patient's liver before entering the blood stream to infect erythrocytes. In infections caused by *P. vivax* and *P. ovale*, silent infection of the liver might persist, with one or more relapses following the initial infection—even after many years. *P. malariae* may circulate asymptomatically in the peripheral blood and relapse after several years.

Most cases of malaria present with nonspecific signs suggestive of sepsis, such as fever, headache, and myalgia. Clinical findings include the following: cough, fatigue, malaise, rigors, arthralgia, myalgia, headache, and diaphoresis. The classic paroxysm begins with rigors lasting 1 to 2 hours, followed by high fever. This is followed by marked diaphoresis and a fall in temperature.

Classical fever patterns are rarely helpful, and anemia and splenomegaly develop only after several attacks. Less common findings include anorexia, vomiting, diarrhea, and hypotension. Complications include pulmonary disease (acute respiratory distress syndrome—ARDS), encephalopathy, nephropathy, shock (algid malaria), massive diarrhea, myocarditis, and dysfunction of other organs.

Reference

Malaria. Centers for Disease Control Web site. Available at: http://www.dpd.cdc.gov/dpdx/HTML/Malaria.htm. Accessed June 30, 2005.

Further Reading

Clark IA, Alleva LM, Mills AC, Cowden WB. Pathogenesis of malaria and clinically similar conditions. *Clin Microbiol Rev.* 2004;17:509-539.

Hay SI, Guerra CA, Tatem AJ, Noor AM, Snow RW. The global distribution and population at risk of malaria: past, present, and future. *Lancet Infect Dis.* 2004;4:327-336.

Kremsner PG, Krishna S. Antimalarial combinations. *Lancet.* 2004;364:285-294.

Maitland K, Bejon P, Newton CR. Malaria. *Curr Opin Infect Dis.* 2003;16:389-395.

Malaria. Centers for Disease Control Web site. Available at: http://www.cdc.gov/malaria. Accessed April 15, 2005.

The Roll Back Malaria Partnership Web site. Available at: http://www.rbm.who.int. Accessed April 15, 2005.

Mammomonogamus (Syngamus) laryngeus

Syngamiasis, Gapeworm

Agent

Nematoda. Phasmidea: *M. (S.) laryngeus.*

Reservoir
Mammals

Vector
None

Vehicle
Uncooked vegetables, water

Geographic Distribution

REGION III—SAm	BRA, GUY, PER
REGION IV—Carib	DMA, GLP, LCA, MTQ, PRI, TTO
REGION XI—Asia	CHN
REGION XII—SEA	PHL

Incubation Period
6–11d

Diagnostic Tests
Identification of ova in feces or of adults from respiratory tract

Typical Therapy
Extraction or expulsion of parasite

Background

- Mammomonogamiasis is widely distributed in the tropics; however, most reports of human infection have originated from the Caribbean.
- Although the parasite is found in the respiratory tracts of cattle and other mammals, the life cycle is uncertain.

- Infected fowl exhibit spasms of dyspnea ("the gapes"), which can be fatal.

Clinical Presentation

Symptoms in the human suggest a foreign body in the upper respiratory tract, with cough, wheezing, and occasionally hemoptysis. The condition is usually diagnosed following expulsion of characteristic Y-shaped adult worms (male 5 mm and female 15 mm in length).

Further Reading

Kim HY, Lee SM, Joo JE, Na MJ, Ahn MH, Min DY. Human syngamosis: the first case in Korea. *Thorax.* 1998;53:717-718.

Mesocestoidiasis

Agent

Cestoda. Taenia: *Mesocestoides lineatus, M. variabilis.*

Reservoir

Insects

Vector

Small mammals

Vehicle

Ingestion of undercooked small mammals

Geographic Distribution

REGION I—NAm	USA
REGION XI—Asia	JPN, KOR

Background

- *Mesocestoides* species are cestodes similar to *Taenia.* The parasite is thought to enter the liver and peritoneal cavity of birds, snakes, lizards, amphibia, and rodents following ingestion of arthropods. Carnivores (skunks, opossums, raccoons, foxes, coyotes, dogs, and cats) serve as the definitive hosts and are infected through ingestion of these intermediates.

- A total of 22 human infections were documented as of 1991—including 14 Japanese (all adults over age 30), and 6 children in the United States. Additional cases have been reported from Korea and Africa, where 26 cases were reported to 2002—18 due to *M. lineatus* and 8 to *M. variabilis.*

- Human infection is characterized by abdominal pain and passage of motile proglottids. The presumed therapy is that of taeniasis.

Further Reading

Eom KS, Kim SH, Rim HJ. Second case of human infection with Mesocestoides lineatus in Korea. *Kisaengchunghak Chapchi.* 1992;30(2):147-150.

Fuentes MV, Galan-Puchades MT, Malone JB. Short report: a new case report of human Mesocestoides infection in the United States. *Am J Trop Med Hyg.* 2003;68:566-567.

Schultz LV, Roberto RR, Rutherford GW III, Hummert B, Lubell I. *Mesocestoides* (Cestoda) infection in a California child. *Pediatr Infect Dis J.* 1992;11:332-334.

Metagonimiasis

Agent

Platyhelminthes, Trematoda. Plagiorchiida, Heterophyidae: *Metagonimus yokogawai, M. takahashii, M. miyatai.*

Reservoir

Snails (*Cerithidea cingulata, Pirenella conica*), fish

Vector
None

Vehicle
Fish (mullet and tilapia [*Oreochromis nilo*])

Geographic Distribution
See: "*Heterophyid* Infections"

Incubation Period
7–14d

Diagnostic Tests
Identification of ova or adults in stool

Typical Therapy
Praziquantel 25 mg/kg t.i.d. × 3 doses

Background

- *M. yokogawai* is the smallest trematode found in humans; it infects cats, dogs, pigs, and fish-eating birds. The first intermediate hosts are molluscs (*Semisulcospira libertina, S. coreana,* and *Thiara granifera*). The principal fish host in Japan is ayu (*Plecoglossus altivelis*). Other hosts include golden carp (*Carassius auratus*), common carp (*Cyprinus carpio*), *Zacco temminckii, Photimus steindachneri, Acheilognathus lanceolata,* and *Pseudorasbora parva*.

Causal Agent

Metagonimus yokogawai, a minute intestinal trematode (and the smallest human fluke) (CDC).

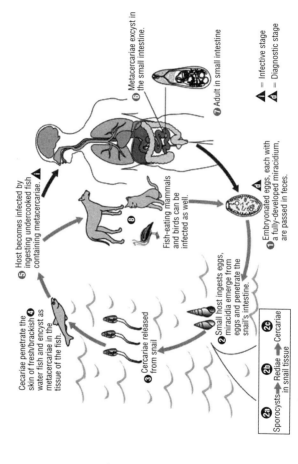

Cecariae penetrate the skin of fresh/brackish water fish and encyst as metacercariae in the tissue of the fish. ❹

❺ Host becomes infected by ingesting undercooked fish containing metacercariae. ▲

❻ Metacercariae excyst in the small intestine.

❼ Adult in small intestine

Fish-eating mammals and birds can be infected as well. ❽

❶ Embryonated eggs, each with a fully-developed miracidium, are passed in feces. ◭

▲ = Infective stage
◭ = Diagnostic stage

❸ Cercariae released from snail

❷ Small host ingests eggs, miracidia emerge from eggs and penetrate the snail's intestine.

❷ₐ Sporocysts → ❷ᵦ Rediae in snail tissue → ❷ᵧ Cercariae

Figure 4-39 Life cycle of metagonimiasis.

308

Life Cycle

Adults release embryonated eggs, each with a fully-developed miracidium, which are passed in the host's feces ❶ [Figure 4-39]. After ingestion by a suitable snail (first intermediate host), the eggs hatch and miracidia penetrate the snail's intestine ❷. Snails of the genus *Semisulcospira* are the most frequent intermediate host for *Metagonimus yokogawai*. Miracidia undergo several developmental stages in the snail, ie sporocysts ❷ₐ, rediae ❷ᵦ, and cercariae ❷꜀. Cercariae are released from the snail ❸ and encyst as metacercariae in the tissues of fresh/brackish water fish (second intermediate host) ❹. The definitive host becomes infected by ingesting contaminated undercooked or salted fish ❺. After ingestion, the metacercariae excyst, attach to the mucosa of the small intestine ❻ and mature into adults (1.0 mm to 2.5 mm by 0.4 mm to 0.75 mm) ❼. In addition to humans, fish-eating mammals (eg, cats and dogs) and birds can also be infected by *M. yokogawai* ❽ (CDC).

Reference

Metagonimiasis. Centers for Disease Control Web site. Available at: http://www.dpd.cdc.gov/dpdx/HTML/ Metagonimiasis.htm. Accessed June 30, 2005.

Further Reading

Also see "*Heterophyid* Infections" section.

Belizario VY, Bersabe MJ, de Leon WU, et al. Intestinal heterophyidiasis: an emerging food-borne parasitic zoonosis in southern Philippines. *Southeast Asian J Trop Med Public Health*. 2001;32(suppl 2):36-42.

Chai JY, Lee SH. Food-borne intestinal trematode infections in the Republic of Korea. *Parasitol Int*. 2002;51:129-154.

Hong SJ, Chung CK, Lee DH, Woo HC. One human case of natural infection by Heterophyopsis continua and three other species of intestinal trematodes. *Korean J Parasitol.* March 1996;34(1):87-89.

Metagonimiasis. Centers for Disease Control Web site. Available at: http://www.dpd.cdc.gov/dpdx/HTML/ Metagonimiasis.htm. Accessed June 30, 2005.

Waikagul J, Wongsaroj T, Radomyos P, Meesomboon V, Praewanich R, Jongsuksuntikul P. Human infection of Centrocestus caninus in Thailand. *Southeast Asian J Trop Med Public Health.* 1997;28:831-835.

Metorchiasis

North American Liver Fluke

Agent
Platyhelminthes, Trematoda. Plagiorchiida, Opisthorchiidae: *Metorchis conjunctus* and *M. orientalis.*

Reservoir
Snails (*Amnicola limosa limosa*), fish, cats, dogs, minks, foxes, raccoons, voles, wolves, bears, coyotes

Vector
None

Vehicle
Fish (white sucker = *Catostomus commersoni*; rarely brook trout and other species)

Geographic Distribution

REGION I—NAm	CAN, USA
REGION XI—Asia	CHN

Incubation Period
5–6d (range 1–15d)

Diagnostic Tests
Identification of ova in stool (appear after 10 days).
ELISA was used in the Canadian outbreak.

Typical Therapy
Praziquantel (anecdotal evidence)

Background

- The first human cases were described in 1993. To date, *Metorchis* has been identified in carnivores in the United States and Canada—from the Canadian Atlantic coast to the western prairies, and from South Carolina to the Northwest Territories.
- A focus of *M. orientalis* infection of humans, ducks, cats and dogs has been reported in China.
- *M. bilis* has been implicated in human infections in Siberia.

Clinical Presentation
Metorchiasis is characterized by abdominal pain, fever, headache and eosinophilia beginning 1 to 15 days after ingestion of raw fish (sashimi). Symptoms can persist for more than 4 weeks.

Further Reading
Behr MA, Gyorkos TW, Kokoskin E, Ward BJ, MacLean JD. North American liver fluke (Metorchis conjunctus) in a Canadian aboriginal population: a submerging human pathogen? *Can J Public Health.* 1998;89:258-259.

MacLean JD, Arthur JR, Ward BJ, Gyorkos TW, Curtis MA, Kokoskin E. Common-source outbreak of acute infection due to the North American liver fluke Metorchis conjunctus. *Lancet.* 1996;347:154-158.

Micronemiasis

Halicephalobus

Agent
Secernentea. Rhabditida. Cephalobina. Panagrolaimoidea. Panagrolaimidae. *Micronema deletrix. H. gingivalis.*

Reservoir
Soil, decaying vegetable matter

Vector
None

Vehicle
Direct contact with traumatized skin

Geographic Distribution
REGION I—NAm   CAN, USA

Incubation Period
Unknown

Diagnostic Tests
Identification of larvae in tissue. Culture in axenic: 1% pure agar or NA + 5 mg/ml cholesterol and *Escherichia coli.*

Typical Therapy
None

Background

- Normally free-living larvae in decaying organic material and soil could invade the body through abrasions and migrate to the central nervous system, kidneys, lungs, maxillae, and nasal cavity of equines.
- In its parasitic form, the nematode replicates parthenogenetically.
- At least three fatal infections by *H.* (*Micronema*) *deletrix* have been reported—all in North America and characterized by meningoencephalitis, with or without visceral involvement.

Clinical Presentation

Cases have followed lacerations contaminated with soil and manure. Clinical presentation is compatible with signs and symptoms of acute, multifocal meningoencephalitis, cerebral hemorrhage, and encephalomalacia.

Further Reading

Anderson RC, Linder KE, Peregrine AS. Halicephalobus gingivalis (Stefanski, 1954) from a fatal infection in a horse in Ontario, Canada with comments on the validity of H. deletrix and a review of the genus. *Parasite*. 1998;5:255-261.

Connor DH, Gibson DW, Ziefer A. Diagnostic features of three unusual infections: micronemiasis, pheomycotic cyst, and prototHecosis. *Monogr Pathol*. 1982;23:205-239.

Gardiner CH, Koh DS, Cardella TA. Micronema in man: third fatal infection. *Am J Trop Med Hyg*. 1981;30:586-589.

Stefanski W. Rhabditis gingivalis sp.n. parasite trouvé dans un granulome de la gencive chez un cheval. *Acta Parasitologica Polonica*. 1954;1:329-336.

Hoogstraten J, Young WG. Meningo-encephalomyelitis due to the saprophagous nematode, Micronema deletrix. *Can J Neurol Sci*. 1975;2:121-126.

Microsporidiosis

Agent
Protozoa. Microspora: *Enterocytozoon, Encephalitozoon* (*Septata*), *Vittaforma* (*Nosema*), *Pleistophora, Trachipleistophora, et al.*

Reservoir
Rabbits, rodents, carnivores, nonhuman primates, fish, dogs, birds

Vector
None

Vehicle
Fecal–oral contact

Geographic Distribution
Worldwide

Incubation Period
Unknown

Diagnostic Tests
Microscopy of duodenal aspirates.
Inform laboratory if this organism is suspected.
Nucleic acid amplification.

Typical Adult Therapy
Albendazole 400 mg PO b.i.d. × 3 weeks.
Encephalitozoon hellem might respond to fumagillin drops.
S. intestinalis might respond to albendazole.
Nitazoxanide has been used for *Enterocytozoon bieneusi.*
No proven therapy for *V. corneae* and *Pleistophora.*

Typical Pediatric Therapy

Albendazole 200 mg PO b.i.d. × 3 weeks.
E. hellem might respond to fumagillin drops.
S. intestinalis might respond to albendazole.
Nitazoxanide has been used for *E. bieneusi*.

Background

- Microsporidiosis accounts for 7 to 50% of chronic
  diarrhea among AIDS patients. Though associated
  with AIDS and other forms of immune suppression,
  these organisms are also found in normal individuals.
  For example, 8% of Dutch blood donors and 5% of
  pregnant French women are seropositive for
  Encephalitozoon.
- Intestinal disease is caused by *Enterocytozoon bieneusi*
  and *Encephalitozoon (Septata) intestinalis*.
- Recent data suggest that *E. bienusi* is a significant cause
  of diarrhea among non–immune-compromised
  elderly persons.
- Ocular microsporidiosis is caused by *E. hellem*,
  Microsporidium ceylonensis, *M. africanum*, *V. corneae*
  (Nosema corneum), *N. ocularum* and *Brachiola algerae*
  (N. algerae).
- Disseminated disease is caused by *E. hellum*, *E. cuniculi*,
  Trachipleistophora anthropophthera, *B. connori (N. con-
  nori)*, and *Pleistophora* sp.

Causal Agents

The term microsporidia is also used to denote obligate
intracellular protozoan parasites belonging to the phylum *Microsporidia*. To date, more than 1,200 species belonging to 143 genera have been described as parasites
infecting a wide range of vertebrate and invertebrate

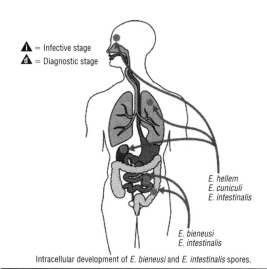

▲ = Infective stage
▲d = Diagnostic stage

E. hellem
E. cuniculi
E. intestinalis

E. bieneusi
E. intestinalis

Intracellular development of *E. bieneusi* and *E. intestinalis* spores.

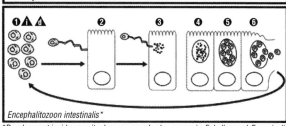

*Development inside parasitophorous vacuole also occurs in *E. hellem* and *E. cuniculi*.

Figure 4-40   Life cycle of microsporidiosis.

hosts. *Microsporidia* are characterized by the production of resistant spores that vary in size, depending on the species. They possess a unique organelle, the polar tubule or polar filament, which is coiled inside the spore as demonstrated by its ultrastructure. The microsporidia spores of species associated with human infection measure from 1 to 4 μm (a useful diagnostic feature). There are at least 14 microsporidian species that have been identified as human pathogens: *Enterocytozoon bieneusi*, *Encephalitozoon intestinalis*, *Encephalitozoon hellem*, *Encephalitozoon cuniculi*, *Pleistophora* sp., *Trachipleistophora hominis*, *T. anthropophthera*, *Nosema ocularum*, *N. algerae*, *Vittaforma corneae*, *Microsporidium ceylonensis*, *M. africanum*, *Brachiola vesicularum*, *B. connori*. *Encephalitozoon intestinalis* was previously named *Septata intestinalis*, but it was reclassified as *Encephalitozoon intestinalis* based on its similarity at the morphologic, antigenic, and molecular levels to other species of this genus. Based on recent data it is now known that some domestic and wild animals may be naturally infected with the following microsporidian species: *E. cuniculi*, *E. intestinalis*, *E. bieneusi* (CDC).

Life Cycle

The infective form of microsporidia is a resistant spore which can survive for long periods in the environment ❶ [Figure 4-40]. The spore extrudes its polar tubule and infects the host cell ❷ by injecting sporoplasm into the eukaryotic host cell ❸. Inside the cell, the sporoplasm undergoes extensive multiplication either by merogony (binary fission) or schizogony (multiple fission) ❹. This development can occur either in direct contact with the host cell cytoplasm (eg, *E. bieneusi*) or inside of a "parasitophorous vacuole" (eg, *E. intestinalis*). Once inside of either the cytoplasm or a parasitophorous vacuole, microsporidia develop by sporogony to mature spores ❺. During sporogony, a thick wall is formed around the spore, which provides resistance to adverse environmental conditions. When the spores increase in number and completely fill the host cell cytoplasm, the cell membrane is disrupted and spores are released into the surroundings ❻, from where they can infect new cells thus continuing the cycle (CDC).

Clinical Presentation

Immunocompetent patients can develop a self-limited diarrhea, traveler's diarrhea or asymptomatic carriage. Immunocompromised patients present with cholangitis, cholecystitis, sinusitis, or pneumonia. *E. hellum* has also been implicated in keratoconjunctivitis, sinusitis, pneumonia, nephritis, and prostatitis.

Pleistophora species have been implicated in myositis among immunocompromised patients. Myositis is caused by *T. hominis* and *B. vesicularum.*

Reference

Microsporidiosis. Centers for Disease Control Web site. Available at: http://www.dpd.cdc.gov/dpdx/HTML/Microsporidiosis.htm. Accessed April 15, 2005.

Further Reading

Coyle CM, Weiss LM, Rhodes LV, et al. Fatal myositis due to the microsporidian brachiola algerae, a mosquito pathogen. *NEJM.* July 2004;351:42-47.

Garcia LS. Laboratory identification of the microsporidia. *J Clin Microbiol.* 2002;40:1892-1901.

Gross U. Treatment of microsporidiosis including albendazole. *Parasitol Res.* 2003;90(supp 1):S14-S18.

Microsporidia infection. Centers for Disease Control Web site. Available at: http://www.cdc.gov/ncidod/dpd/parasites/microsporidia/default.htm. Accessed April 15, 2005.

Weiss LM. Microsporidia 2003: IWOP-8. *J Eukaryot Microbiol.* 2003;50(suppl):566-568.

Moniliformis moniliformis

Moniliform acanthocephalan

Agent
Archiacanthocephala (distinct phylum).
Moniformidae: *Moniliformis moniliformis.*

Reservoir
Rats

Vector
None

Vehicle
Insect (ingestion)

Geographic Distribution
The precise distribution of this disease is unknown.

REGION II—CAm	BLZ
REGION VI—CAfr	NGA, SDN
REGION VIII—Eur	ITA
REGION IX—MidEast	IRN, IRQ

Incubation Period
Unknown—presumed 15 to 40 days

Diagnostic Tests
Identification of worm in stool

Typical Therapy
There is no specific therapy; infection is self-limited.

Background

- *M. moniliformis* is an acanthocephalan helminth found in rats. The adult male is 4 to 5 cm in length; the female is 18 to 27 cm. Rats, and presumably humans, acquire infection through ingestion of the intermediate hosts, beetles and roaches. The worm attains maturity in the rat within 22 to 28 days; 15 to 40 days in humans.
- The precise distribution of the parasite is unknown; however, infected rats have been documented in Egypt, Malaysia, Nigeria, and Taiwan (Kaohsiung). Human infections have been reported in Italy, Nigeria, Sudan, Belize, Iran, and Iraq.
- A related acanthocephalan helminth, *Macracanthorhynchus hirudinaceus*, is a common parasite of pig, boar, and occasionally monkeys and dogs in many parts of the world. Human infection follows accidental ingestion of infested beetles and has been reported from Australia, Madagascar, Europe, Thailand, and Russia. Patients have presented with abdominal pain, intestinal obstruction, or perforation. *Macracanthorhynchus ingens*, a parasite of raccoons, has been recovered from the stool of a child in Texas.

Clinical Presentation
Most infections are characterized by asymptomatic passage of a worm; however, vague complaints such as periumbilical discomfort and giddiness have been described.

In one instance, a man developed marked abdominal pain following experimental self-infection.

Additional Reading

Anosike JC, Njoku AJ, Nwoke BE, et al. Human infections with Moniliformis moniliformis (Bremser 1811) Travassos 1915 in south-eastern Nigeria. *Ann Trop Med Parasitol.* 2000;94:837-838.

Bettiol S, Goldsmid JM. A case of probable imported Moniliformis moniliformis infection in Tasmania. *J Travel Med.* 2000;7:336-337.

Counselman K, Field C, Lea G, Nickol B, Neafie R. Moniliformis moniliformis from a child in Florida. *Am J Trop Med Hyg.* 1989;41:88-90.

Neafie RC, Marty AM. Unusual infections in humans. *Clin Microbiol Rev.* 1993;6:34-56.

Myiasis

Furuncular Myiasis, Maggot Infestation, Ophthalmomyiasis, Rectal Myiasis, Urinary Myiasis, Vaginal Myiasis

Agent
Insecta (Diptera) larvae

Reservoir
Mammals

Vector
Biting and nonbiting flies

Vehicle
Fly eggs deposited by biting arthropod

Geographic Distribution

Various forms of myiasis are found worldwide or in virtually every country.

Incubation Period

1w–3m

Diagnostic Tests

Identification of extracted maggot

Typical Therapy

Removal of maggot

Background

- Myiasis can be primary (active invasion) or secondary (colonization of wound).
- Secondary forms are caused by *Wohlfarthia magnifica* in southern Europe, Russia, Africa, Middle East; or by the Old World screw worm (*Chrysomyia bezziana*) in Asia and sub-Saharan Africa. Rare instances of secondary myiasis have been ascribed to *Calliphora vicina* and *Megaselia scalaris.*
- Primary furuncular myiasis is usually caused by the human botfly (*Dermatobia hominis*) in Latin America, and the Tumbu fly (*Cordylobia anthropophagia*) in Africa. Sporadic infestations by *Cordylobia rhodaini* (Lund's fly) and *C. ruandae* are also reported. Up to 1988, 55 cases of subcutaneous or ophthalmic myiasis due to rodent or rabbit botfly (*Cuterebra*) had been reported.
- Rare instances of creeping subdermal infection are caused by *Hypoderma lineatum* and *Gasterophilus intestinalis.*

- *Oestrus ovis, Cochliomyia macellaria, Co. hominivorax, Chrysomyia bezziana, W. magnifica, Dermatobia hominis, Oedemagena tarandia,* and *Hypoderma lineatum* can cause ophthalmomyiasis.
- Pharyngeal myiasis due to *Oestrus ovis* affects persons working with sheep and goats.
- *Psychoda, Musca, Calliphora,* and *Sarcophaga* cause urinary myiasis.
- *Lucilia sericata* causes infestation of the nares and vaginal myiasis.
- Five cases of tracheopulmonary myiasis had been reported to 2002: two caused by horse botfly (*Gasterophilus*), and four by rodent or rabbit botfly (*Cuterebra*).
- *Sarcophaga haemorrhoidalis* causes rectal myiasis. The larvae of *Musca, Fannia, Eristalis,* and *Sarcophaga* are occasionally recovered from stool.

Clinical Presentation
Myiasis is characterized by the appearance of one or more pruritic or painful draining nodules. Fever and eosinophilia may be present. Instances of brain, eye, middle ear, and other deep infestations are described. Signs and symptoms will vary somewhat depending on the anatomic location of the infestation.

Further Reading
Hall M, Wall R. Myiasis of humans and domestic animals. *Adv Parasitol.* 1995;35:257-334.

Jappe U. Unusual skin infections in military personnel. *Clin Dermatol.* 2002;20:425-434.

Jelinek T, Nothdurft HD, Rieder N, Loscher T. Cutaneous myiasis: review of 13 cases in travelers returning from tropical countries. *Int J Dermatol.* 1995;34:624-626.

Lucchina LC, Wilson ME, Drake LA. Dermatology and the recently returned traveler: infectious diseases with dermatologic manifestations. *Int J Dermatol.* 1997;36:167-181.

Mackey SL, Wagner KF. Dermatologic manifestations of parasitic diseases. *Infect Dis Clin North Am.* 1994;8:713-743.

Safdar N, Young DK, Andes D. Autochthonous furuncular myiasis in the United States: case report and literature review. *Clin Infect Dis.* 2003;36:e73-e80.

Veraldi S, Gorani A, Suss L, Tadini G. Cutaneous myiasis caused by Dermatobia hominis. *Pediatr Dermatol.* 1998;15:116-118.

Nanophyetus salmincola

Agent
Platyhelminthes, Trematoda. *N. (Troglotrema) salmincola* (symptoms possibly due to an associated bacterium (*Neorickettsia helminthoeca*).

Reservoir
Snails (*Semisulcospira*), fish

Vector
None

Vehicle
Fish (salmon)

Geographic Distribution
REGION I—NAm   CAN, USA
REGION XI—Asia   CHN

Incubation Period
7d

Diagnostic Tests
Identification of ova in stool

Typical Therapy
Praziquantel 25 mg/kg PO t.i.d. $\times$ 1 day

Background
- *N. salmincola* is a small trematode whose life cycle involves an intermediate snail host and a definitive host in raccoons and skunks.
- Human infection has been described in the United States and the former Soviet Union. Infection may also be acquired through importation of fish from endemic areas.
- Sporadic cases are encountered in the Pacific Northwest coastal region. This is the most common systemic trematode in North America.
- Humans are infected by ingestion of raw or undercooked fish (salmon, trout, steelhead, et al).

Clinical Presentation
Infection is usually asymptomatic or limited to mild diarrhea and abdominal discomfort.

Further Reading
Eastburn RL, Fritsche TR, Terhune CA Jr. Human intestinal infection with Nanophyetus salmincola from salmonid fishes. *Am J Trop Med Hyg.* 1987;36:586-591.

Harrell LW, Deardorff TL. Human nanophyetiasis: transmission by handling naturally infected coho salmon (Oncorhynchus kisutch). *J Infect Dis.* 1990;161:146-148.

Winward LD, Lattig GM. A new experimental second intermediate host of Nanophyetus salmincola with evidence of
transmission of Neorickettsia helminthoeca. *J Parasitol.*
1970;56:621-622.

Oesophagostomiasis

Dapaong Tumor

Agent
Nematoda. Phasmidea: *Oesophagostomum bifurcum* (*O. apiostomum, O. stephanostomum*).

Reservoir
Nonhuman primates, soil

Vector
None

Vehicle
Feces, water, soil

Geographic Distribution
REGION III—SAm	BRA, SUR
REGION VI—CAfr	AGO, BFA, CAF, CIV, CMR, COD, ERI, ETH, GAB, GHA, GMB, KEN, LBR, MLI, MOZ, MWI, NER, NGA, RWA, SDN, SEN, SLE, SOM, TGO, TZA, UGA, ZMB, ZWE
REGION XII—SEA	BRN, IDN, MYS

Incubation Period
2w–2m

Diagnostic Tests
Demonstration of parasite in tissue

Typical Therapy
Albendazole or pyrantel pamoate can be effective.
Excision as necessary.

Background
- Oesophagostomiasis is found in Africa, with sporadic cases from South America and Southeast Asia. It is estimated that 250,000 are infested and 1,000,000 at risk. The world's literature reported 116 cases to 1999; however, 156 cases were collected as of 2000 in a single series from Northern Ghana. Human-to-human transmission occurs during the rainy season, presumably by the oral route.
- Two species are encountered: *O. apiostomum* and *O. stephanostomum*. The latter is commonly identified in monkeys, with rare human infections in Brazil, French Guiana, and northern Nigeria.
- Ova of *O. bifurcum* are morphologically indistinguishable from those of *Necator americanus*. Coproculture and examination of third-stage larva or polymerase chain reaction (PCR) can be used to distinguish between the two.

Clinical Presentation
The disease is contracted through ingestion of soil-contaminated food or water and is characterized by development of an inflammatory mass in the ileum or colon. Approximately 15% of patients present with multinodular disease, characterized by abdominal pain, fever, vomiting, and mucous diarrhea. An intestinal mass

adherent to the overlying abdominal wall (Dapaong tumor) is present in 85% of cases, often associated with pain and fever.

Further Reading

Polderman AM, Anemana SD, Asigri V. Human oesophagostomiasis: a regional public health problem in Africa. *Parasitol Today.* 1999;15:129-130.

Storey PA, Faile G, Hewitt E, Yelifari L, Polderman AM, Magnussen P. Clinical epidemiology and classification of human oesophagostomiasis. *Trans R Soc Trop Med Hyg.* 2000;94:177-182.

Storey PA, Spannbrucker N, Yelifari L, et al. Ultrasonographic detection and assessment of preclinical oesophagostomum bifurcum-induced colonic pathology. *Clin Infect Dis.* 2001;33:166-170.

Storey PA, Steenhard NR, Van Lieshout L, Anemana S, Magnussen P, Polderman AM. Natural progression of Oesophagostomum bifurcum pathology and infection in a rural community of northern Ghana. *Trans R Soc Trop Med Hyg.* 2001;95:295-299.

Opisthorchiasis

Amphimeriasis, Cat Liver Fluke

Agent

Platyhelminthes, Trematoda. Plagiorchiida, Opisthorchiidae: *Opisthorchis felineus, O. guayaquilensis, O. viverrini.*

Reservoir

Cats, civet cats, dogs, other fish-eating mammals, snails (*Bythynia*)

Vector

None

Vehicle
Freshwater fish

Geographic Distribution
REGION VIII—Eur	BLR
REGION X—IndSub	IND
REGION XI—Asia	JPN, KAZ, KGZ, KOR, PRK, RUS, SGP
REGION XII—SEA	KHM, LAO, MYS, PHL, THA, VNM

Incubation Period
21–28d (range 7d–years)

Diagnostic Tests
Identification of ova in stool or duodenal aspirate

Typical Therapy
Praziquantel 25 mg/kg t.i.d. × 1d

Background
- *O. felineus* affects 1.5 million persons, predominantly in the central Russian Federation. *O. viverrini* infests 9 million, notably in northeastern Thailand, India, and Laos.
- The definitive hosts for *O. felineus* are humans and wild or domestic felines. The first intermediate (snail) host is *Bythnia leachi* (occasionally *B. tentaculata*). The most common second intermediate (fish) hosts are tench (*Tinca tinca*), ide (*Leucisus idus*), barbel (*Barbus barbus*) and roach (*Rutilus rutulus*).
- The definitive hosts for *O. viverrini* are the dog and civet cat. First intermediate (snail) hosts are *Bythnia*

funiculata, B. siamensis, B. goniomphales, and *B. laevis.*
Second intermediate (fish) hosts include *Cyclocheilich-thus siaja, Hampala dispar, Punctius orphoides, P. gonionotus, P. poctozyron, Labiabarbus lineatus* and *Osteochilus* sp.

- The relative risk of cholangiocarcinoma among infected patients is 5 to 15 times that for noninfected individuals.
- Rare instances of infection by *O. guayaquilensis* (*Amphimerus pseudofelineus*) have been reported in Ecuador.

Causal Agent

Trematodes (flukes) *Opisthorchis viverrini* (Southeast Asian liver fluke) and *O. felineus* (cat liver fluke) (CDC).

Life Cycle

The adult flukes deposit fully developed eggs, which are passed in the feces ❶ [Figure 4-41]. After ingestion by a suitable snail (first intermediate host) ❷, eggs release miracidia ❷ⓐ, which undergo several developmental stages (sporocysts ❷ⓑ, rediae ❷ⓒ, cercariae ❷ⓓ). Cercariae are released from the snail ❸ and penetrate freshwater fish (second intermediate host), encysting as metacercariae in the muscles or under the scales ❹. Mammalian definitive hosts (cats, dogs, and various fish-eating mammals including humans) become infected by ingesting under-cooked fish containing metacercariae. Metacercariae excyst in the duodenum ❺ and ascend through the ampulla of Vater into the biliary ducts, where they attach and develop into adults, which lay eggs after 3 to 4 weeks ❻. The adult

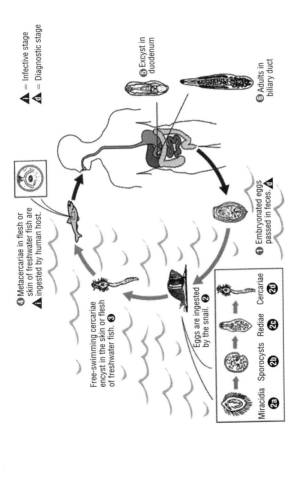

▲ = Infective stage
◆ = Diagnostic stage

⑤ Excyst in duodenum

⑥ Adults in biliary duct

④ Metacercariae in flesh or skin of freshwater fish are ▲ ingested by human host. ④

① Embryonated eggs passed in feces. ◆

Free-swimming cercariae encyst in the skin or flesh of freshwater fish. ③

Eggs are ingested by the snail. ②

Miracidia ②ⓐ Sporocysts ②ⓑ Rediae ②ⓒ Cercariae ②ⓓ

Figure 4-41 Life cycle of opisthorchiasis.

331

flukes (*O. viverrini*: 5 mm to 10 mm by 1 mm to 2 mm; *O. felineus*: 7 mm to 12 mm by 2 mm to 3 mm) reside in the biliary and pancreatic ducts of the mammalian host, where they attach to the mucosa (CDC).

Clinical Presentation

Most infections are asymptomatic. Some patients experience mild dyspepsia, abdominal pain, or diarrhea. Chronic infestations could be more clinically overt and associated with hepatomegaly or malnutrition. Rare instances of cholangitis, cholecystitis, and chlolangiocarcinoma are encountered. Infections due to *O. felineus* may present with an acute illness resembling the Katayama fever of schistosomiasis (fever, facial edema, lymphadenopathy, arthralgias, rash, and eosinophilia). Chronic forms of *O. felineus* may involve the pancreatic ducts in addition to the biliary tract.

Reference

Opisthorchiasis. Centers for Disease Control Web site. Available at: http://www.dpd.cdc.gov/dpdx/HTML/ opisthorchiasis.htm. Accessed April 15, 2005.

Further Reading

Harinasuta T, Pungpak S, Keystone JS. Trematode infections: opisthorchiasis, clonorchiasis, fascioliasis, and paragonimiasis. *Infect Dis Clin North Am.* 1993;7:699-716.

Haswell-Elkins MR, Satarug S, Elkins DB. Opisthorchis viverrini infection in northeast Thailand and its relationship to cholangiocarcinoma. *J Gastroenterol Hepatol.* 1992;7:538-548.

Liu LX, Harinasuta KT. Liver and intestinal flukes. *Gastroenterol Clin North Am.* 1996;25:627-636.

Opisthorchis infection. Centers for Disease Control Web site. Available at: http://www.cdc.gov/ncidod/dpd/parasites/ opisthorcis/default.htm. Accessed April 15, 2005.

Watanapa P, Watanapa WB. Liver fluke-associated cholangio-carcinoma. *Br J Surg.* 2002;89:962-970.

Paragonimiasis

Endemic Hemoptysis, Lung Fluke, Oriental Lung Fluke, Pulmonary Distomiasis

Agent
Platyhelminthes, Trematoda. *Paragonimus westermani, P. heterotemus, P. skrjabini, P. miyazakii, P. africanus, et al.*

Reservoir
Humans, dogs, cats, pigs, wild carnivores, snails (*Semisulcospira, Thiara,* etc.)

Vector
None

Vehicle
Freshwater crab (at least eight species) and crayfish (*Cambaroides*)

Incubation Period
6w–6m

Geographic Distribution

REGION I—NAm	USA
REGION II—CAm	CRI, HND, GTM, MEX, NIC, PAN, SLV
REGION III—SAm	BRA, COL, ECU, PER, PRY, VEN
REGION VI—CAfr	CMR, COD, COG, GAB, GIN, GMB, GNB, GNQ, LBR, NGA, SEN

REGION X—IndSub   BGD, IND, LKA, NPL, PAK
REGION XI—Asia   CHN, JPN, KOR, MAC,
                         PRK, RUS, TWN
REGION XII—SEA   IDN, LAO, MYS, PHL, THA
REGION XIII—Poly   ASM, PNG, SLB

Diagnostic Tests

Identification of ova in sputum or stool.
Serologic and skin tests are available.

Typical Therapy

Praziquantel 25 mg/kg t.i.d. $\times$ 2d
Or bithionol 40 mg/kg every other day $\times$ 10 doses
Or triclabendazole 10 mg/kg/d $\times$ 2

Background

- It is estimated that 22 million are infested by *Paragoni-mus* species worldwide, and 195 million live in areas of risk.
- *P. africanus* infects the mongoose (*Crossarchus obscurus, Atilax paludinosus*), dog, cat, and drill (*Mandrillus leucophaeus*) in Cameroon, Nigeria, and Democratic Congo (Zaire). The snail host is *Potadoma freethii.*
- The crab intermediates are *Sudanautes africanus, S. ambryi* and *Liberonautes latidactylus* (*S. pelii*).
- Disease is limited to mild pulmonary symptoms. Retroauricular cysts have also been described.
- *P. compactus* is found in India, with disease limited to pulmonary symptoms only.
- *P. hueitungensis* is found in China and India. The snail host is *Tricula cristella.* The crab hosts are *Sinopotamon denticalus, S. joshueiense, Isopotamon sinense,* and *I. papilonaceus.*

- Disease is largely limited to migratory subcutaneous swellings, without cerebral lesions. Pulmonary involvement is mild.
- *P. heterotremus* is found in Thailand, Cambodia, Laos, and southern China. The crab hosts are *Parathelphusa maculata* and *Potamon cognatus.*
- Pulmonary and cerebral involvement are described, and migratory subcutaneous swellings have been reported.
- *P. kelicotti* is found in North America.
- *P. mexicanus* (*peruvianus*) infects cats in Mexico, Guatemala, Panama, Colombia, Peru, Ecuador, Costa Rica, Honduras, Venezuela, El Salvador, Nicaragua, and Canada. The snail intermediates are *Pomiatopsis lapidaria* and *Aroapyrgus costarencis.* The crab intermediates are *Pseudothelphusa chilensis*, *Psychophallus tristani* and *Potamocarcinus magnus.* Disease is characterized by either pulmonary or cerebral inflammation.
- *P. miyazakii* infects crab-eating mammals (including boar and marten) in Japan. The crab host is *Geothelphusa dehaani.*
- *P. philippinensis* is found in the Philippines.
- *P. szechuanensis* (*skrjabini*) is found in the mountainous areas of China. The snail host is *Tricula humida.* The crab intermediate host is *Sinapotamon denticalus.* Infection is characterized by subcutaneous swellings and granulomata of the brain and liver.
- *P. tuanshenensis* is found in China. The snail host is *Oncomelania chiui.* The crab intermediate is *Sinopotamon denticulatus.* Disease is limited to pulmonary symptoms only.
- *P. uterobilateralis* infects civets (*Viverra civetta*) in Cameroon, Nigeria, Liberia, Congo, and Guinea. The crab intermediate is *Liberonautes latidactylus.* Disease is limited to pulmonary symptoms.

- *P. westermani* infects wild and domestic felines in China, Japan, Korea, Taiwan, India, Sri Lanka, Thailand, Laos, Indonesia, Philippines, Russia, the Solomon Islands, American Samoa, and Western Samoa.
- The optimum host crab (Japan) is *Eriocheir japonicus*; however, a variety of other crab and crayfish species could be involved. Pulmonary, dermal, and cerebral lesions are encountered.
- A related digenean trematode, *Poikilorchis* (*Achillurbania*) *congolensis*, has caused several cases of human soft tissue abscess in the region of the mastoid. The parasite is reported in Indonesia and Africa.

Causal Agent

More than 30 species of trematodes (flukes) of the genus *Paragonimus* have been reported which infect animals and humans. Among the more than 10 species reported to infect humans, the most common is *P. westermani*, the oriental lung fluke (CDC).

Life Cycle

The eggs are excreted unembryonated into the sputum, or alternately are swallowed and passed with stool [Figure 4-42] ❶. In the external environment, the eggs become embryonated ❷, and miracidia hatch and seek and penetrate the first intermediate host, a snail ❸. Miracidia go through several developmental stages inside the snail ❹: sporocysts ❹ⓐ, rediae ❹ⓑ, the latter giving rise to many cercariae ❹ⓒ, which emerge from the snail. Cercariae invade the second intermediate host, a crustacean such as a crab or crayfish, where they encyst and become metacercariae ❺. Human infection with *P. wes-*

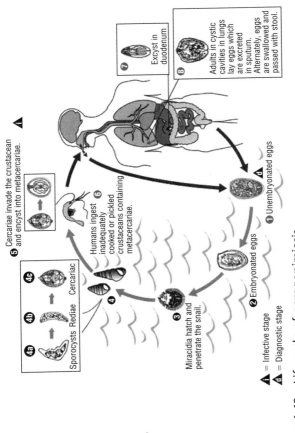

6 Cercariae invade the crustacean and encyst into metacercariae. ▲

5 Cercariae invade the crustacean and encyst into metacercariae.

Humans ingest inadequately cooked or pickled crustaceans containing metacercariae.

Sporocysts   Rediae   Cercariae

4a   **4b**   **4c**

4

Miracidia hatch and penetrate the snail.

3

2 Embryonated eggs

1 Unembryonated eggs ◢

▲ = Infective stage
◢ = Diagnostic stage

7 Excyst in duodenum

8 Adults in cystic cavities in lungs lay eggs which are excreted in sputum. Alternately, eggs are swallowed and passed with stool.

Figure 4-42   Life cycle of paragonimiasis.

337

termani occurs through ingestion of inadequately cooked or pickled crab or crayfish ❻. The metacercariae excyst in the duodenum ❼, penetrate through the intestinal wall into the peritoneal cavity, and then through the diaphragm into the lungs, where they become encapsulated and develop into adults ❽ (7.5 to 12 mm by 4 to 6 mm). The worms can also reach other organs and tissues, such as the brain and striated muscles. When this takes place completion of the life cycle is not achieved, since eggs laid in these sites cannot reach the environment. The time from infection to oviposition is 65 to 90 days.

Infections may persist for 20 years in humans. Animals such as pigs, dogs, and a variety of felines can also harbor *P. westermani* (CDC).

Clinical Presentation
The acute phase of parasitic invasion and migration is accompanied by diarrhea, abdominal pain, fever, urticaria, hepatosplenomegaly, wheezing, cough, pleuritic pain, and eosinophilia. Later, pulmonary manifestations include cough, expectoration of discolored sputum, hemoptysis, and chest roentgenographic abnormalities. Extrapulmonary infection could involve the brain (fewer than 1% of cases), subcutaneous tissues (most commonly the trunk and thighs), or other organs. Subcutaneous disease is found in 10% of patients with *P. westermani* infection and 20 to 60% of those with *P. skrjabini* (*P. szechuanensis*) infection.

Reference
Paragonimiasis. Centers for Disease Control Web site. Available at: http://www.cdc.gov/ncidod/dpd/parasites/paragonimus/default.htm. Accessed April 15, 2005.

Further Reading

Fain A, Vandepitte J. A new trematode, Poikilorchis congolensis, n.g., n.sp., living in subcutaneous retroauricular cysts in man from the Belgian Congo. *Nature.* 1957;179:740.

Lie KJ, Williams HI, Miyazaki I, Wong SK. A subcutaneous retro-auricular abscess in a Dyak boy in Sarawak, probably caused by a trematode of the genus Poikilorchis, Fain and Vandepitte, 1957. *Med J Malaya.* 1962;17:37-40.

Oyediran AB, Fajemisin AA, Abioye AA, Lagundoye SB, Olugbile AO. Infection of the mastoid bone with a Paragonimus-like trematode. *Am J Trop Med Hyg.* 1975;24:268-273.

Paragonimus infection. Centers for Disease Control Web site. Available at: http://www.cdc.gov/ncidod/dpd/parasites/paragonimus/default.htm. Accessed April 15, 2005.

Wong SK, Lie KJ. Another periauricular abscess from Sarawak, probably caused by a trematode of the genus Poikilorchis, Fain and Vandepitte. *Med J Malaya.* 1965;19:229-230.

Pediculosis (*humanus, capitis, corporis*)

Agent
Parasite—Insecta. Anoplura: *Pediculus humanus, Phthirus pubis.*

Reservoir
Humans

Vector
Louse

Vehicle
Contact

Causal Agent

Pediculus humanus capitis, the head louse, an insect of the order Anoplura, is an ectoparasite whose only hosts are humans. The louse feeds on blood several times daily and resides close to the scalp to maintain its body temperature (CDC).

Life Cycle

The life cycle of the head louse has three stages: egg, nymph, and adult.

Eggs: Nits are head lice eggs. They are difficult to see and are often mistaken for dandruff or hair spray droplets. Nits are laid by the adult female and are cemented at the base of the hair shaft nearest the scalp ❶ [Figure 4-43], and hatch after a period of 6 to 9 days. The eggs are 0.8 mm by 0.3 mm, oval, and yellow to white. Viable eggs are usually located within 6 mm of the scalp.

Nymphs: After hatching to release a nymph ❷, the nit shell becomes a dull yellow color, and remains attached to the hair shaft. The nymph resembles the adult louse, but is the size of a pinhead. Nymphs mature after three moults (❸, ❹) and become adults after 7 days.

Adults: The adult louse is the size of a sesame seed, has 6 legs (each with claws), and is tan to grayish-white ❺. In persons with dark hair, the adult louse will appear darker. Females are larger than males and can lay up to 8 nits per day. Adult lice live up to 30 days on the scalp. Adult lice require a blood meal several times daily (CDC).

Reference

Pediculosis. Centers for Disease Control Web site. Available at: http://www.dpd.cdc.gov/dpdx/HTML/HeadLice.htm. Accessed June 30, 2005.

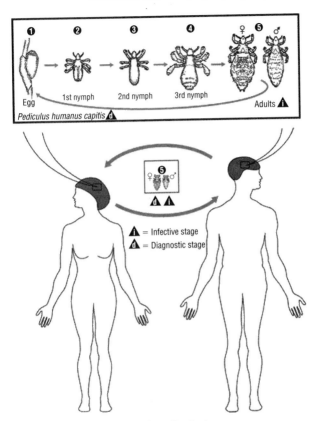

Figure 4-43   Life cycle of pediculosis.

Further Reading

Burkhart CG. Relationship of treatment-resistant head lice to the safety and efficacy of pediculicides. *Mayo Clin Proc.* 2004;79:661-666.

Heukelbach J, Feldmeier H. Ectoparasites—the underestimated realm. *Lancet.* 2004;363:889-891.

Pediculosis. Centers for Disease Control Web site. Available at:
    http://www.dpd.cdc.gov/dpdx/HTML/HeadLice.htm.
    Accessed June 30, 2005.

Steen CJ, Carbonaro PA, Schwartz RA. Arthropods in derma-
    tology. *J Am Acad Dermatol.* 2004;50:819-842.

Pelodera strongyloides and Related Species

Background

- *Strongyloides fulleborni* is found in Central Africa and
  eastern Africa, Zambia, and Papua New Guinea.
  S. fulleborni is found in primates, and has been implicated in cases of disseminated infection of humans.
- Three cases of human infection (dermatitis or larva
  migrans) by *Pelodera strongyloides* have been reported.
  P. strongyloides is a parasite of dogs, cattle, sheep,
  horses, lemmings, and murid rodents.
- *Turbatrix aceti* has been found in the vagina of a
  woman following use of vinegar douches.
- *Diploscapter coronata* is occasionally found in urine,
  and in the gastric contents of achlorhydric patients.

Further Reading

Jones CC, Rosen T, Greenberg C. Cutaneous larva migrans due
    to Pelodera strongyloides. *Cutis.* 1991;48:123-126.

Ginsburg B, Beaver PC, Wilson ER, Whitley RJ. Dermatitis due
    to larvae of a soil nematode, Pelodera strongyloides. *Pediatr
    Dermatol.* 1984;2:33-37.

Pasyk K. Dermatitis rhabditidosa in an 11-year-old girl: a new
    cutaneous parasitic disease of man. *Br J Dermatol.*
    1978;98:107-112.

Rallietiniasis

Raillietina celebensis, a tapeworm of rats, has been occasionally identified in children.

Geographic Distribution
REGION XIII—Poly   PYF

Further Reading
Rougier Y, Legros F, Durand JP, Cordoliani Y. Four cases of parasitic infection by Raillietina (R.) celebensis (Kanicki, 1902) in French Polynesia. *Trans R Soc Trop Med Hyg.* 1981;75:121.

Sarcocystosis

Isospora hominis infection, Sarcocystiasis, Sarcosporidiosis

Agent
Protozoa. Sporozoa, Apicomplexa: *Sarcocystis bovihominis* or *S. suihominis.*

Reservoir
Cattle, pigs

Vector
None

Vehicle
Meat, water

Geographic Distribution
The precise distribution of this disease is unknown.

Incubation Period
9–39d

Diagnostic Tests
Identification of cysts in stool

Typical Therapy
Supportive

Background

- More than 100 species of *Sarcocystis* occur worldwide in a wide range of domestic and wild animals, with prevalences of 10 to 100% among domestic livestock. Humans may serve as intermediate hosts for some *Sarcocystis* species and as definitive hosts for others.
- Most reports of human infection have originated from tropical and subtropical areas, primarily the Far East. Only 40 cases had been reported in the world literature to 1979; and 52 to 1998.
- The morphology and biology of *S. hominis* resemble those of *I. belli*; however, *Sarcocystis* requires alternating intermediate hosts such as cattle and pigs. In fact, some authorities describe two separate pathogens: *S. bovihominis* and *S. suihominis*.

Clinical Presentation
Human infection is limited to moderate diarrhea or asymptomatic infection of muscle (rare instances of myalgia with eosinophilia have also been reported).

Further Reading
Ackers JP. Gut Coccidia—Isospora, Cryptosporidium, Cyclospora and Sarcocystis. *Semin Gastrointest Dis.* 1997;8:33-44.

Arness MK, Brown JD, Dubey JP, Neafie RC, Granstrom DE. An outbreak of acute eosinophilic myositis attributed to human Sarcocystis parasitism. *Am J Trop Med Hyg.* 1999;61:548-553.

Beaver PC, Gadgil K, Morera P. Sarcocystis in man: a review and report of five cases. *Am J Trop Med Hyg.* 1979;28:819-844.

Mehrotra R, Bisht D, Singh PA, Gupta SC, Gupta RK. Diagnosis of human sarcocystis infection from biopsies of the skeletal muscle. *Pathology*. 1996;28:281-282.

Van den Enden E, Praet M, Joos R, Van Gompel A, Gigasse P. Eosinophilic myositis resulting from sarcocystosis. *J Trop Med Hyg*. 1995;98:273-276.

Wong KT, Pathmanathan R. High prevalence of human skeletal muscle sarcocystosis in south-east Asia. *Trans R Soc Trop Med Hyg*. 1992;86:631-632.

Scabies

Arachnid, Acarina (mite), Sarcoptiae: Sarcoptes (Acarus) scabiei, sarcoleptic mange

Reservoir
Humans

Vehicle
Contact, including sexual contact

Geographic Distribution
Worldwide

Incubation Period
3–42d

Diagnostic Tests
Identification of mites in skin scrapings

Typical Therapy
Permethrin 5%
Or lindane
Or crotamiton 10%
Or ivermectin 150 to 200 ug/kg PO as single dose
    (ivermectin may be used over the age of 5 years)

Background

- Scabies is found worldwide, with occasional reports of case clusters and epidemics. Nosocomial outbreaks have also been described.
- Sarcoptic mange (animal scabies) is acquired from animals and is not transmissible from person to person; it is usually self-limited.
- Mites do not survive for more than 48 hours away from the human host, and are acquired through close contact with patients or fomites, notably in the setting of poor hygiene and crowding. The entire life cycle takes place in the skin, with ova maturing to adults in approximately 14 days.
- Mites of the genus *Cheyletiella* commonly infest dogs, cats, and rabbits. Humans can acquire these arachnids through close animal contact and develop intensely pruritis macular, vesicular, or bullous eruptions. Unlike scabies, dermal burrows are not seen. At least three species have been described in human disease: *C. blakei*, *C. yasguri* and *C. parasitivorax*.

Causal Agent

Sarcoptes scabei, the human itch- or mange-mite, is an Arachnid, subclass Acari, family Sarcoptidae. The mites burrow into the skin but never below the stratum corneum. Burrows appear as raised serpentine lines up to several centimeters long. Other races of scabies may cause infestations in mammals such as domestic cats, dogs, pigs, and horses. Occasionally, races of mites found on other animals may establish infestations in humans. Although they cause temporary itching and dermatitis, they do not multiply on the human host (CDC).

Life Cycle

Sarcoptes scabei undergoes four stages in its life cycle; egg, larva, nymph and adult. Females deposit eggs at 2 to 3 day intervals as they burrow through the skin ❶ [Figure 4-44]. Eggs are oval and 0.1 to 0.15 mm in length ❷, and incubate for 3 to 8 days. After the eggs hatch, larvae migrate to the skin surface and burrow into the intact stratum corneum to construct almost invisible, short burrows called "molting pouches." The larva, which has only 3 pairs of legs ❸, exists for 2 to 3 days. After larvae molt, the resulting nymphs have 4 pairs of legs ❹. Nymphs molt once again into slightly larger nymphs, before developing into adults. Larvae and nymphs are often found in molting pouches or in hair follicles, and resemble small adults. Adults are round, sac-like eyeless mites. Females are 0.3 to 0.4 mm long and 0.25 to 0.35 mm wide, and males are slightly more than half that size. Mating occurs after the nomadic male penetrates the molting pouch of the adult female ❺. Impregnated females extend their molting pouches into the characteristic serpentine burrows, laying eggs in the process. The impregnated females burrow into the skin and spend the remaining 2 months of their lives in tunnels under the surface of the skin. Males are rarely seen, and produce a temporary gallery in the skin before mating. Transmission occurs by the transfer of ovigerous females during personal contact. Person to person contact is usually involved, but transmission may also occur via fomites (eg, bedding or clothing). Burrows are found predominantly between the fingers and on the wrists, where mites hold onto the skin using suckers attached to the two most anterior pairs of legs (CDC).

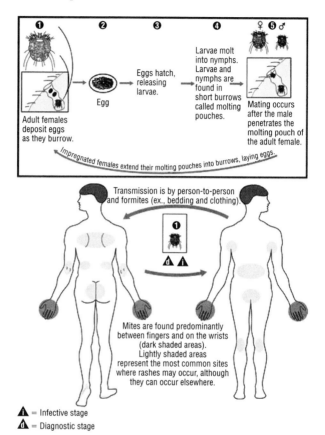

Figure 4-44   Life cycle of scabies.

Clinical Presentation

The lesions of scabies are usually symmetrical, and involve the interdigital webs, buttocks, penis, scrotum, breasts and nipples, axillae, and flexor surfaces of the wrists. Pruritis is often worse at night. Skin lesions consist of burrows, papules, or vesicles; however, exaggerated eczematous patches (crusted, or Norwegian scabies) may be encountered—notably in institutions for Down syndrome and leprosy. Lesions in children are atypical, are often vesicular, and tend to involve the buttocks and perineum. Complications include secondary infection and acute glomerulitis.

Cheyletiella dermatitis was reported in one community in 14 individuals over an 8-year period. All patients were females, aged 40 years or younger, who experienced pruritic papules during the winter months.

Reference

Scabies. Centers for Disease Control Web site. Available at: http://www.dpd.cdc.gov/dpdx/HTML/Scabies.htm. Accessed June 30, 2005.

Further Reading

Beck W. Farm animals as disease vectors of parasitic epizoonoses and zoophilic dermatophytes and their importance in dermatology. *Hautarzt.* 1999;50:621-628.

Dal Tio R, Taraglio S, Tomidei M, Vercelli A. Dermatitis caused by Cheyletiella: description of 8 cases and review of the literature. *G Ital Dermatol Venereol.* 1990;125:19-24.

Rivers JK, Martin J, Pukay B. Walking dandruff and Cheyletiella dermatitis. *J Am Acad Dermatol.* 1986;15:1130-1123.

Scabies. Centers for Disease Control Web site. Available at: http://www.dpd.cdc.gov/dpdx/HTML/Scabies.htm. Accessed June 30, 2005.

Steen CJ, Carbonaro PA, Schwartz RA. Arthropods in dermatology. *J Am Acad Dermatol.* 2004;50:819-842.

Tsianakas P, Polack B, Pinquier L, Levy Klotz B, Prost-Squarcioni C. Cheyletiella dermatitis: an uncommon cause of vesiculobullous eruption. *Ann Dermatol Venereol.* 2000;127:826-829.

Schistosoma haematobium

Urinary Bilharziasis, Egyptian Hematuria, Schistosomal Hematuria, Vesicle Bilharziasis

Agent
Platyhelminthes, Trematoda. Strigeida, Schistosomatidae: *S. haematobium*.

Reservoir
Snails (*Bulinus, Planobarius, Ferrissia*), rarely baboons or monkeys

Vector
None

Vehicle
Water (skin contact)

Geographic Distribution

REGION V—NAfr	DZA, EGY, LBY, MAR, TUN
REGION VI—CAfr	AGO, BDI, BEN, BWA, CAF, CIV, CMR, COD, COG, DJI, ERI, ETH, GAB, GHA, GIN, GMB, GNB, GNQ, KEN, LBR, MDG, MLI, MOZ, MRT, MUS, NER, NGA, RWA, SDN, SEN, SLE, SOM, STP, TCD, TGO, TZA, UGA, ZMB, ZWE
REGION VII—SAfr	NAM, SWZ, ZAF
REGION IX—MidEast	IRN, IRQ, JOR, LBN, OMN, SAU, SYR, TUR, YEM
REGION X—IndSub	IND

Incubation Period
2–6w

Diagnostic Tests
Identification of ova in urine or stool
Serological and antigen assay tests

Typical Therapy
Praziquantel 20 mg/kg PO q4h × 2 doses

Background

- *S. haematobium* infection is endemic to more than 50 countries in Africa, the eastern Mediterranean, including the Arabian peninsula, the Indian Ocean, and western Asia.
- It is estimated that 180 million are exposed and 90 million are infested worldwide; however, others estimate the prevalence in sub-Saharan Africa alone at 25.9% (131 million cases). Schistosomal hematuria afflicts 70 million persons, and 18 million people suffer from associated bladder wall pathology and 10 million from hydronephrosis.
- It is estimated that 150,000 die each year from resultant renal failure.
- During 1999 to 2001, 92 cases were identified through active surveillance among returning European travellers.
- The parasite is transmitted by approximately 30 species of *Bulinus* snails—notably *B. africanus* in Africa and the Sahara; the *B. forskalii* group in Africa, Arabia, and some Indian Ocean islands; the *B. truncatus/tropicus* complex in Africa and the Middle East (as far as Iran); and *B. reticulatus* in Ethiopia and the Arabian Peninsula.

Causal Agents

Schistosomiasis is caused by digenetic blood trematodes. The three main species infecting humans are *Schistosoma haematobium, S. japonicum,* and *S. mansoni.* Two additional species, more localized geographically, are *S. mekongi* and *S. intercalatum.* Other schistosome species, which parasitize birds and mammals, can cause cercarial dermatitis in humans (CDC).

Life Cycle

Eggs are eliminated with feces or urine ❶ [Figure 4-45]. Under optimal conditions the eggs hatch and release miracidia ❷, which swim and penetrate specific snail intermediate hosts ❸. The stages in the snail include 2 generations of sporocysts ❹ and the production of cercariae ❺. Upon release from the snail, the infective cercariae swim, penetrate the skin of the human host ❻, and shed their forked tail, becoming schistosomulae ❼. The schistosomulae migrate through several tissues and mature before establishing residence in the veins (❽, ❾). In humans, adults reside in the mesenteric venules ❿. *S. japonicum* is more frequently found in the superior mesenteric veins draining the small intestine 🄰, and *S. mansoni* occurs more often in the superior mesenteric veins draining the large intestine 🄱. Both species can occupy either location, and are capable of moving between sites. *S. haematobium* is most often found in the venous plexus of the urinary bladder 🄲 but can also be found in the rectal venules. Adult females (size 7 to 20 mm; males slightly smaller) deposit eggs in the small venules of the portal and perivesical systems. These eggs move progressively toward the lumen of the intestine (*S. mansoni* and

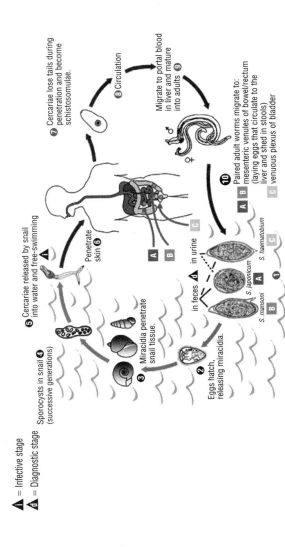

▲ = Infective stage
◮ = Diagnostic stage

① Cercariae lose tails during penetration and become schistosomulae.

⑧ Circulation

Migrate to portal blood in liver and mature into adults ⑨

⑥ Cercariae released by snail into water and free-swimming ▲

Penetrate skin ⑥

⑩ Paired adult worms migrate to: mesenteric venules of bowel/rectum (laying eggs that circulate to the liver and shed in stools) ᴬ ᴮ venous plexus of bladder ᶜ

A B

C in urine

④ Sporocysts in snail (successive generations)

Miracidia penetrate snail tissue. ③

in feces ◮

S. mansoni B   S. japonicum A   S. haematobium C ①

② Eggs hatch, releasing miracidia.

Figure 4-45   Life cycle of *Schistosoma haematobium*.

353

S. japonicum) and of the bladder and ureters (*S. haematobium*), and are eliminated with feces or urine, respectively ❶. The pathology of *S. mansoni* and *S. japonicum* infestation includes: Katayama fever, hepatic perisinusoidal egg granulomas, Symmers' pipe-stem periportal fibrosis, portal hypertension, and occasionally embolic egg granulomas in the brain or spinal cord. *S. haematobium* is associated with hematuria, scarring, calcification, squamous cell carcinoma, and occasional embolic egg granulomas in the brain or spinal cord. Various animals, such as dogs, cats, rodents, pigs, horses and goats, serve as reservoirs for *S. japonicum*, and dogs for *S. mekongi* (CDC).

Clinical Presentation

The clinical features caused by *Schistosoma* species infecting humans are similar and will be discussed together. Within 24 hours of penetration by cercariae, the patient develops a pruritic papular skin rash known as swimmer's itch. (The more overt form of cercarial dermatitis assocated with avian schistosomes is discussed elsewhere in this chapter.) One to two months after exposure, an overt systemic illness known as Katayama fever begins, heralded by acute onset of fever, chills, diaphoresis, sweating, headache, and cough. The liver, spleen, and lymph nodes are enlarged, and eosinophilia is present. Although deaths have been described at this point (notably in *S. japonicum* infection), these findings subside within a few weeks in most cases.

The likelihood of progression to chronic schistosomiasis is related to the extent of infestation. Chronic schistosomiasis caused by *S. mansoni*, *S. japonicum*, or *S. mekongi* is characterized by fatigue, abdominal pain, and intermittent diarrhea or dysentery. Blood loss from intestinal ulcerations may lead to moderate anemia. In *S. mansoni*,

S. japonicum, and *S. mekongi* infections, ova remain in the venous portal circulation and are carried to the liver where they produce granulomata and block portal blood flow. Portal hypertension and portosystemic collateral circulation result. Although liver function tests remain normal for a long time, hepatosplenomegaly and variceal hemorrhage develop. The spleen is firm and could reach massive size. Fatal hematemesis is unusual. Laboratory tests reveal moderate eosinophilia and anemia related to blood loss and hypersplenism. Eventually, hepatic function deteriorates, with late ascites and jaundice.

In *S. haematobium* infection, ova are located in the bladder and ureters, leading to granuloma formation, inflammation, hematuria, ureteral obstruction, secondary infection, and often carcinoma of the bladder. Terminal hematuria and dysuria are common symptoms.

S. intercalatum infection is characterized by abdominal pain and bloody diarrhea. *S. mekongi* is an important cause of hepatomegaly in endemic areas.

The following are some of the many complications described in chronic schistosomiasis. Pulmonary schistosomiasis is manifested by symptoms and signs of right ventricular congestion related to blockage of pulmonary capillaries by ova in the course of hepatosplenic schistosomiasis. Central nervous system schistosomiasis is manifested as a cerebral mass, generalized encephalopathy or focal epilepsy (notably in *S. japonicum* infection). Granulomata of *S. haematobium* and *S. mansoni* could involve the spinal cord, producing transverse myelitis. Although best known for damage to the urinary bladder and ureters, the female genitalia are involved in 50 to 70% of infected women—resulting in vaginal deformities and fistulae, hypogonadism, ectopic pregnancy, miscarriage, and malignancy.

Reference

Schistosomiasis. Centers for Disease Control Web site. Available at: http://www.dpd.cdc.gov/dpdx/HTML/ Schistosomiasis.htm. Accessed April 15, 2005.

Further Reading

Grobusch MP, Muhlberger N, Jelinek T, et al. Imported schistosomiasis in Europe: sentinel surveillance data from TropNetEurop. *J Travel Med.* 2003;10:164-169.

Kameh D, Smith A, Brock MS, Ndubisi B, Masood S. Female genital schistosomiasis: case report and review of the literature. *South Med J.* 2004;97:525-527.

Lengeler C, Utzinger J, Tanner M. Questionnaires for rapid screening of schistosomiasis in sub-Saharan Africa. *Bull World Health Organ.* 2002;80:235-242.

Savioli L, Albonico M, Engels D, Montresor A. Progress in the prevention and control of schistosomiasis and soil-transmitted helminthiasis. *Parasitol Int.* 2004;53:103-113.

Schistosomiasis. Centers for Disease Control Web site. Available at: http://www.cdc.gov/ncidod/dpd/parasites/ schistosomiasis/default.htm. Accessed April 15, 2005.

Schistosoma intercalatum

Agent
Platyhelminthes, Trematoda. Strigeida, Schistosomatidae: *S. intercalatum.*

Reservoir
Snail (*Bulinus forskalii* and *Bulinus africanus* group)

Vector
None

Vehicle
Water (skin contact)

Geographic Distribution

REGION VI—CAfr   AGO, BFA, CAF, CMR, COD, COG, GAB, GNQ, MLI, NGA, SEN, STP, TCD, UGA

Incubation Period

2–6w

Diagnostic Tests

Identification of ova in stool or biopsy specimens
Serology
Antigen detection

Typical Therapy

Praziquantel 20 mg/kg PO q4h $\times$ 3 doses

Background

- *S. intercalatum* infection was first reported in 1911 and is essentially confined to the forest areas of five countries in west and central Africa in addition to Sao Tome. Sporadic cases have been reported from Congo, Senegal, Mali, Burkina Faso, Nigeria, and Angola. The worldwide prevalence is estimated at 1.73 million.
- The Lower Guinea strain (reservoir *B. forskalii*) is found in Gabon, Cameroon, Nigeria, Equatorial Guinea, and Sao Tome (with possible sporadic foci in Mali, Central African Republic, Chad, Angola, Burkina Faso, Congo, Uganda, and Senegal).
- The Zaire strain (reservoir *B. africanus*) is confined to the Democratic Republic of Congo (Zaire).
- During 1999 to 2001, four cases were identified through active surveillance among returning European travelers.

Life Cycle

See the representative schema in the "*Schistosoma haematobium*" section.

Clinical Presentation

S. intercalatum infection is characterized by abdominal pain, bloody diarrhea, eosinophilia and hepatomegaly. Unlike the disease associated with *S. mansoni*, portal hypertension or overt and severe disease of the liver or lungs is unusual.

Further Reading

Corachan M, Escosa R, Mas J, Ruiz L, Campo E. Clinical presentation of Schistosoma intercalatum infestation. *Lancet.* 1987;1:1139-1140.

Cosgrove CL, Southgate VR. Interactions between Schistosoma intercalatum (Zaire strain) and *S. mansoni. J Helminthol.* 2003;77:209-218.

Jourdane J, Southgate VR, Pages JR, Durand P, Tchuem Tchuente LA. Recent studies on Schistosoma intercalatum: taxonomic status, puzzling distribution and transmission foci revisited. *Mem Inst Oswaldo Cruz.* 2001;96(suppl):45-48.

Tchuem Tchuente LA, Southgate VR, Njiokou F, Njine T, Kouemeni LE, Jourdane J. Competitive exclusion in human schistosomes: the restricted distribution of Schistosoma intercalatum. *Parasitology.* 1996;113(pt 2):129-136.

Schistosoma japonicum

Kabure Itch, Oriental Blood Fluke, Oriental Schistosomiasis

Agent

Platyhelminthes, Trematoda. Strigeida, Schistosomatidae: *S. japonicum.*

Reservoir
Snails (*Oncomelania*), water buffaloes, dogs, cats, rats, pigs, horses, goats

Vector
None

Vehicle
Water (skin contact)

Geographic Distribution
REGION XI—Asia	CHN, JPN
REGION XII—SEA	IDN, KHM, LAO, MYS, PHL, THA, VNM

Incubation Period
2–6w

Diagnostic Tests
Identification of ova in stool or biopsy specimens
Serology
Antigen detection

Typical Therapy
Praziquantel 20 mg/kg PO q4h $\times$ 3 doses

Background

- *S. japonicum* infection of humans is found in mainland China, Indonesia, and the Philippines. Other countries listed in the Geographic Distribution section appear for historic interest, as transmission is rare or no longer occurs.
- It is estimated that 95 million are infested by *S. japonicum*, and 120,000 die of the disease each year.

- The parasites thrive in fresh water having a mean temperature of 20 to 30°C, between the latitudes 36°N and 34°S.
- *S. japonicum* is transmitted by amphibious snails belonging to six species: *Oncomelania hupensis hupensis* in mainland China; *O.h lindoensis* in Sulawesi, Indonesia; *O.h. quadrasi* in the Philippines; *O.h. nosophora* in Japan; *O.h. formosana* and *O.h. chiui* in Taiwan.
- *S. japonicum* infection has been identified in approximately 31 species of wild mammals and 13 domestic mammals in China.

Life Cycle
See the life cycle schema in the "*Schistosoma haematobium*" section.

Clinical Presentation
See "*Schistosoma haematobium*," earlier in this chapter.

Further Reading
Blas BL, Rosales MI, Lipayon IL, Yasuraoka K, Matsuda H, Hayashi M. The schistosomiasis problem in the Philippines: a review. *Parasitol Int.* 2004;53:127-134.

Cioli D, Liberti P. Schistosoma japonicum: modern tools for an ancient disease. *Lancet.* 2004;363:180-181.

Ross AG, Li YS, Sleigh AC, McManus DP. Schistosomiasis control in the People's Republic of China. *Parasitol Today.* 1997;13:152-155.

Schistosoma mansoni

Intestinal Bilharziasis

Agent
Platyhelminthes, Trematoda. Strigeida, Schistosomatidae: *S. mansoni*

Reservoir
Snails (*Biomphalaria*), dogs, cats, pigs, cattle, rodents, horses, nonhuman primates

Vector
None

Vehicle
Water (skin contact)

Geographic Distribution

REGION III—SAm	BRA, SUR, VEN
REGION IV—Carib	ATG, DOM, ES-CN, GLP, MTQ, LCA, PRI, ZO
REGION V—NAf	EGY, LBY
REGION VI—CAfr	AGO, BDI, BEN, BFA, CAF, CIV, CMR, COD, COG, DJI, ERI, ETH, GAB, GHA, GIN, GMB, GNB, KEN, LBR, MDG, MLI, MRT, MWI, MOZ, NGA, NER, RWA, SEN, SDN, SLE, SOM, STP, TCD, TGO, TZA, UGA, ZMB, ZWE
REGION VII—SAfr	BWA, NAM, ZAF
REGION IX—MidEast	LBN, OMN, SAU, YEM

Incubation Period
2–6w

Diagnostic Tests
Identification of ova in stool or biopsy specimens
Serology
Antigen detection

Typical Therapy
Praziquantel 20 mg/kg PO q 4h $\times$ 2 doses

Background

- It is estimated that 65 million are infested by
  S. mansoni; however, the prevalence in sub-Saharan
  Africa is estimated at 18.3% (98 million cases). Each
  year, 130,000 die of the disease.
- The parasites thrive in fresh water having a mean
  temperature of 20 to 30°C, between the latitudes
  36°N to 34°S.
- Snail intermediates of the genus *Biomphalaria* are
  widely distributed in the Old World, Africa, the Nile
  Valley, the Arabian Peninsula, the southern United
  States, the Caribbean, Brazil, Suriname, and Venezuela.
  B. pfeifferi is most important in the Old World, with a
  lesser role for the *B. choanomphala* group and *B.
  alexandrina* group. *B. glabrata*, *B. straminea,* and *B.
  tenagophila* are naturally infected in the New World.
- Although *S. mansoni* infection has been identified in a
  wide range of primates, insectovora, arteriodactyla,
  marsupials, rodents, carnivores, and edentes, evidence
  for a role in human disease is lacking. The only
  exceptions are baboons (Tanzania) and rats
  (Guadeloupe and Brazil).
- During 1999 to 2001, 130 cases were identified through
  active surveillance among returning European travellers.

Life Cycle
See the representative life cycle schema in the "*Schistosoma haematobium*" section.

Clinical Presentation
See "*Schistosoma haematobium*," earlier in this chapter.

Further Reading

Garba A, Labbo R, Tohon Z, Sidiki A, Djibrilla A. Emergence of Schistosoma mansoni in the Niger River valley, Niger. *Trans R Soc Trop Med Hyg.* 2004;98:296-298.

Grobusch MP, Muhlberger N, Jelinek T, et al. Imported schistosomiasis in Europe: sentinel surveillance data from TropNetEurop. *J Travel Med.* 2003;10:164-169.

Malone JB, Abdel-Rahman MS, El-Bahy MM, Huh OK, Shafik M, Bavia M. Geographic information systems and the distribution of Schistosoma mansoni in the Nile delta. *Parasitol Today.* 1997;13:112-119.

Nozais JP. The origin and dispersion of human parasitic diseases in the Old World (Africa, Europe and Madagascar). *Mem Inst Oswaldo Cruz.* 2003;98(suppl 1):13-19.

Schistosoma mattheei

Agent
Platyhelminthes, Trematoda. Strigeida, Schistosomatidae: *S. mattheei.*

Reservoir
Snails (*Bulinus globosus*), sheep, goats, cattle, horses, zebras, antelope, baboons

Vector
None

Vehicle
Water (skin contact)

Geographic Distribution
REGION VI—CAfr   COG, ZMB, ZWE

Incubation Period
2–6w

Diagnostic Tests
Identification of ova in stool or biopsy specimens
Serology
Antigen detection

Typical Therapy
Praziquantel 20 mg/kg PO q4h $\times$ 3 doses

Background

- *S. mattheei* infection is not discussed in most standard parasitology texts. Clinical information appears to be based on a small number of clinical reports. Similarly, *S. bovis*, a parasite of cattle, sheep, goats, horses, and monkeys, has been described as a rare cause of hematuria in humans. *S. bovis* is found in South Africa, Sudan, Egypt, Iran, Iraq, and southern Europe.

Life Cycle
See the representative life cycle schema in the "*Schistosoma haematobium*" section.

Clinical Presentation
S. mattheei infection is characterized by abdominal pain, bloody diarrhea, eosinophilia, and hepatomegaly. Unlike the disease associated with *S. mansoni*, portal hypertension or overt and severe disease of the liver or lungs is unusual.

Further Reading
Berry A. First recorded finding of ova of the cattle parasite Schistosoma mattheei in human cervical smears. *Trans R Soc Trop Med Hyg.* 1974;68:263-264.

Kruger FJ, Evans AC. Do all human urinary infections with
Schistosoma mattheei represent hybridization between
S. haematobium and S. mattheei? *J Helminthol.* 1990;64:
330-332.

Van Wyk JA. The importance of animals in human schistosomiasis in South Africa. *S Afr Med J.* 1983;63:201-203.

Schistosoma mekongi

Agent
Platyhelminthes, Trematoda. Strigeida, Schistosomatidae:
S. mekongi.

Reservoir
Snails (*Tricula aperta*), dogs

Vector
None

Vehicle
Water

Geographic Distribution
REGION XII—SEA   KHM, LAO, THA, VNM

Incubation Period
2–6w

Diagnostic Tests
Identification of ova in stool or biopsy specimens
Serology
Antigen detection

Typical Therapy
Praziquantel 20 mg/kg PO q4h $\times$ 2 doses

Background

- *S. mekongi* infection was first described in 1957 and is endemic to Laos (Khong Island) and areas of Cambodia. The worldwide prevalence is estimated at 910,000.
- An estimated 80,000 Cambodians and 60,000 Laotians were at risk as of 2000.
- The parasite is transmitted by aquatic snails (*Tricula aperta*) and has been found to infect dogs as well as humans.

Life Cycle

See representative schema in the "*Schistosoma haematobium*" section.

Clinical Presentation

Within 24 hours of penetration by cercariae, the patient develops a pruritic papular skin rash known as swimmer's itch. One to two months after exposure, an overt systemic illness known as Katayama fever begins, heralded by acute onset of fever, chills, diaphoresis, sweating, headache, and cough. The liver, spleen, and lymph nodes are enlarged, and eosinophilia is present.

The likelihood of progression to chronic schistosomiasis is related to the extent of infestation. Chronic schistosomiasis is characterized by fatigue, abdominal pain and intermittent diarrhea or dysentery. Blood loss from intestinal ulcerations could lead to moderate anemia. Ova remain in the venous portal circulation and are carried to the liver, where they produce granulomata and block portal blood flow. Portal hypertension and portosystemic collateral circulation result. Although liver function tests remain normal for a long time, hepatosplenomegaly and variceal hemorrhage develop. The spleen is firm and could reach massive size. Fatal hematemesis is unusual. Laboratory tests reveal moderate eosinophilia and anemia related to blood loss and hypersplenism.

Eventually, hepatic function deteriorates, with late ascites and jaundice. *S. mekongi* is an important cause of hepatomegaly in endemic areas. Clinical features of *S. mekongi* infection are similar to those of *S. japonicum* infection; however, the disease is somewhat milder in *S. mekongi*, and cerebral and cardiopulmonary complications are not reported. The clinical presentation may be complicated by the fact that patients in endemic areas are often coinfected by *Opisthorchis* spp.

Further Reading

Attwood SW. Schistosomiasis in the Mekong region: epidemiology and phylogeography. *Adv Parasitol.* 2001;50:87-152.

Attwood SW, Upatham ES, Meng XH, Qiu DC, Southgate VR. The phylogeography of Asian Schistosoma (Trematoda: Schistosomatidae). *Parasitology.* 2002;125(pt 2):99-112.

Schistosomiasis. Centers for Disease Control Web site. Available at: http://www.cdc.gov/ncidod/dpd/parasites/schistosomiasis/default.htm. Accessed April 15, 2005.

Urbani C, Sinoun M, Socheat D, et al. Epidemiology and control of mekongi schistosomiasis. *Acta Trop.* 2002;82:157-168.

Woodruff DS, Merenlender AM, Upatham ES, Viyanant V. Genetic variation and differentiation of three Schistosoma species from the Philippines, Laos, and Peninsular Malaysia. *Am J Trop Med Hyg.* 1987;36:345-354.

Sparganosis

Agent
Platyhelminthes, Cestoda. Pseudophyllidea, Diphyllobothriidae: *Spirometra* spp.

Reservoir
Copepod—ingested by birds, amphibians, or reptiles

Vector
None

Vehicle
Water, undercooked reptile, amphibian, bird, or mammal meat

Geographic Distribution

REGION I—NAm	CAN, USA
REGION II—CAm	BLZ
REGION III—SAm	ARG, COL, ECU, GUY, URY, VEN
REGION IV—Carib	PRI
REGION VI—CAfr	BDI, ERI, ETH, KEN, MDG, MOZ, RWA, SOM, UGA
REGION VIII—Eur	NLD
REGION X—IndSub	IND, LKA
REGION XI—Asia	CHN, JPN, KOR, PRK, SGP, TWN
REGION XII—SEA	IDN, KHM, LAO, MYS, PHL, THA, VNM
REGION XIII—Poly	AUS

Incubation Period
20d–3y

Diagnostic Tests
Identification of parasite in tissue

Typical Therapy
Excision

Background

- Human sparganosis is attributed to pseudophyllidean tapeworms of the species *Spirometra mansoni* and *S. mansonoides* (*S. theileri* in Africa). Infection follows ingestion of *Cyclops* or uncooked meat (amphibian, reptile, bird, mammal), which are infected with procercoid larvae.
- The larva then penetrate the intestinal wall and migrate to subcutaneous tissue, muscle, the central nervous tissue, and other sites where they develop into second-stage plerocercoids. Application of raw amphibian flesh to the eye may result in direct inoculation. In rare cases, massive numbers of larvae were found to proliferate in the subcutaneous tissue of humans (sparganum proliferum).
- The disease is widely distributed in the tropics and subtropics, with highest rates in Southeast Asia and eastern Africa.
- Autochthonous cases are reported from North America and Central America.
- Seven cases of sparganonsis were reported in Europe to 2002—five in Italy and two in France.

Clinical Presentation

The worm usually lodges in subcutaneous tissue or muscle in the chest, abdominal wall, extremities, or scrotum. Infection typically presents as a nodular mass, swelling, and painful edema. Orbital sparganosis is also common. Less common sites have included the urinary tract, pleura, pericardium, brain, spinal canal, and abdominal viscera. The patient may notice lumps which appear and then spontaneously disappear over a period of weeks to months. The overlying skin is red and pruritic, and local bleeding or necrosis might occur.

Further Reading

Beaver PC, Rolon FA. Proliferating larval cestode in a man in Paraguay. A case report and review. *Am J Trop Med Hyg*. 1981;30:625-637.

Holodniy M, Almenoff J, Loutit J, Steinberg GK. Cerebral sparganosis: case report and review. *Rev Infect Dis*. 1991;13:155-159.

Mueller JF. The biology of Spirometra. *J Parasitol*. 1974;60:3-14.

Nakamura T, Hara M, Matsuoka M, Kawabata M, Tsuji M. Human proliferative sparganosis: a new Japanese case. *Am J Clin Pathol*. 1990;94:224-228.

Strongyloides stercoralis

Cochin China Gastroenteritis, Threadworm

Agent
Nematoda. Phasmidea: *S. stercoralis*.

Reservoir
Humans, possibly dogs

Vector
None

Vehicle
Skin contact, soil, feces, autoinfection, sexual contact (rare)

Geographic Distribution
Worldwide

Incubation Period
14–30d

Diagnostic Tests

Identification of larvae (or ova, for *Strongyloides fülleborni*) in stool or duodenal aspirate

Typical Adult Therapy

Ivermectin 200 μg/kg/d PO daily × 2d
Or thiabendazole 25 mg/kg b.i.d. (max 3g) × 2d
Or albendazole 400 mg/d × 3d

Typical Pediatric Therapy

Ivermectin 200 μg/kg/d PO daily × 2d
Or thiabendazole 25 mg/kg b.i.d. (max 3g) × 2d
Or albendazole 200 mg/d × 3d

Background

- The global prevalence of strongyloidiasis was estimated at 39 million in 1947, and 100 million in 1996.
- *S. stercoralis* is encountered in virtually all countries.
- Prevalence ranges from 1.4 to 40% in mental institutions, and 0.5 to 37% among World War II veterans who served in endemic areas.

Causal Agent

The nematode (roundworm) *Strongyloides stercoralis*. Other *Strongyloides* include *S. fülleborni*, which infects chimpanzees and baboons and may produce limited infections in humans (CDC).

Life Cycle

The *Strongyloides* life cycle [Figure 4-46] is more complex than that of most nematodes with its alternation between free-living and parasitic cycles, and its potential for autoinfection and multiplication within the host. Two types of cycles exist:

Free-living cycle: Rhabditiform larvae passed in the stool ❶ (see "Parasitic cycle" below) can either molt twice to become infective filariform larvae (direct development), ❻ or moult four times to become free living adult males and females ❷ that mate and produce eggs ❸ from which rhabditiform larvae hatch ❹. The latter in turn can either develop ❺ into a new generation of free-living adults ❷, or into infective filariform larvae ❻. Filariform larvae penetrate the human host skin to initiate the parasitic cycle (see below) ❻.

Parasitic cycle: Filariform larvae in soil enter human skin ❻, and are transported to the lungs where they penetrate the alveolar spaces; they are carried through the bronchial tree to the pharynx, swallowed, and reach the small intestine ❼. Here, they molt twice to become adult female worms ❽. Females live threaded in the epithelium of the small intestine and, by parthenogenesis, produce eggs ❾ which yield rhabditiform larvae. Rhabditiform larvae can either be passed in the stool ❶ (see "Free-living cycle" above), or cause autoinfection ❿. In autoinfection, rhabditiform larvae become infective filariform larvae, which penetrate either the intestinal mucosa (internal autoinfection) or the perianal skin (external autoinfection). In either case, the filariform larvae may follow the previously described route, being carried successively to the lungs, the bronchial tree, the pharynx, and the small intestine where they mature into adults; or they may disseminate widely in the body. To date, occurrence of autoinfection in humans is recognized only in *Strongyloides stercoralis* and *Capillaria*

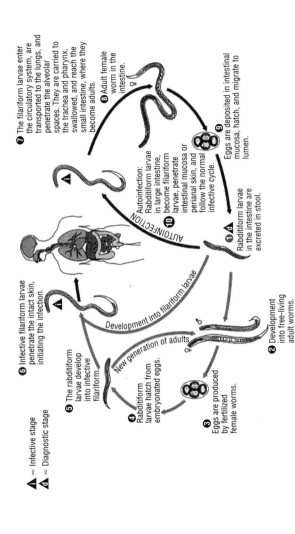

▲ = Infective stage

△ = Diagnostic stage

❶ Rabditiform larvae in the intestine are excreted in stool. △

❷ Development into free-living adult worms.

❸ Eggs are produced by fertilized female worms.

❹ Rabditiform larvae hatch from embryonated eggs.

New generation of adults

Development into filariform larvae

❺ The rabditiform larvae develop into infective filariform.

❻ Infective filariform larvae penetrate the intact skin, initiating the infection. ▲

❼ The filariform larvae enter the circulatory system, are transported to the lungs, and penetrate the alveolar spaces. They are carried to the trachea and pharynx, swallowed, and reach the small intestine, where they become adults.

❽ Adult female worm in the intestine. ♀

❾ Eggs are deposited in intestinal mucosa, hatch, and migrate to lumen.

AUTOINFECTION

❿ Autoinfection: Rabditiform larvae in large intestine become filariform larvae, penetrate intestinal mucosa or perianal skin, and follow the normal infective cycle.

Figure 4-46 Life cycle of *Strongyloides stercoralis*.

373

philippinensis infections. In the case of *Strongyloides*, autoinfection may explain the possibility of persistent infections for many years in persons who have not been in an endemic area and of hyperinfections in immunodepressed individuals (CDC).

Clinical Presentation

The symptoms of strongyloidiasis reflect invasion of the skin, larval migration of larvae intestinal penetration. Approximately one third of patients are asymptomatic. Dermal and pulmonary symptoms resemble those of hookworm, pruritic papular rash and a Loeffler-like syndrome.

Intestinal penetration is characterized by abdominal pain, mucous diarrhea, and eosinophilia. Vomiting, weight loss, and protein-losing enteropathy are occasionally encountered. Some patients develop a generalized or localized urticarial rash beginning in the anal region and extending to the buttocks, abdomen, and thighs; this occurs in 5 to 22% of patients.

Autoinfection is characterized by massive larval invasion of the lungs and other organs. Massive systemic strongyloidiasis occurs in patients with lymphoma, leukemia, and AIDS; and during high-dose therapy with corticosteroids. Findings include generalized abdominal pain, bilateral diffuse pulmonary infiltrates, ileus, and concurrent gram-negative bacillary septicemia. Eosinophilia may be absent at this stage.

Reference

Strongyloidiasis. Centers for Disease Control Web site. Available at: http://www.dpd.cdc.gov/dpdx/HTML/ Strongyloidiasis.htm. Accessed April 15, 2005.

Further Reading

Fincham JE, Markus MB, Adams VJ. Could control of soil-transmitted helminthic infection influence the HIV/AIDS pandemic? *Acta Trop.* 2003;86:315-333.

Jorgensen T, Montresor A, Savioli L. Effectively controlling strongyloidiasis. *Parasitol Today.* 1996;12:164.

Keiser PB, Nutman TB. Strongyloides stercoralis in the immunocompromised population. *Clin Microbiol Rev.* 2004;17:208-217.

Safdar A, Malathum K, Rodriguez SJ, Husni R, Rolston KV. Strongyloidiasis in patients at a comprehensive cancer center in the United States. *Cancer.* 2004;100:1531-1536.

Strongyloides infection. Centers for Disease Control Web site. Available at: http://www.cdc.gov/ncidod/dpd/parasites/strongyloides/default.htm. Accessed April 15, 2005.

Taeniasis

Beef Tapeworm, Pork Tapeworm

Agent
Platyhelminthes, Cestoda. Cyclophyllidea, Taeniidae: *Taenia solium* and *Taenia saginata*.

Reservoir
Cattle, pigs

Vector
None

Vehicle
Meat

Geographic Distribution
Worldwide

Incubation Period
6–14w

Diagnostic Tests
Identification of ova or proglottids in feces

Typical Therapy
Praziquantel 10 mg/kg (T. solium) or 20 mg/kg (*T. saginata*) PO as single dose

Background

- It is estimated that 70 million are infested with *T. saginata* and 5 million with *T. solium* worldwide.
- Prevalence rates vary from > 10% in parts of central and east Africa, the Near East and southern part of the former Soviet Union to 1 to 5% in parts of western Europe, Southeast Asia and Latin America; to < 0.1%, in North America and Australia.
- A recently described species (*Asian Taenia* = *T. saginata asiatica*) is discussed separately later in the text. See "Taeniasis—Other."

Causal Agents

The cestodes (tapeworms) *Taenia saginata* (beef tapeworm) and *T. solium* (pork tapeworm). *Taenia solium* can also cause cysticercosis (CDC).

Life Cycle

Humans are the only definitive hosts for *Taenia saginata* and *Taenia solium*. Eggs or gravid proglottids are passed with feces ❶ [Figure 4-47], and can survive for days to

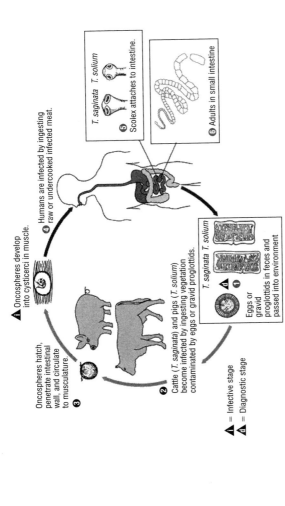

T. saginata   T. solium

❺ Scolex attaches to intestine.

❻ Adults in small intestine

❹ Humans are infected by ingesting raw or undercooked infected meat.

▲ Oncospheres develop into cysticerci in muscle.

Oncospheres hatch, penetrate intestinal wall, and circulate to musculature.
❸

T. saginata T. solium

Eggs or gravid proglottids in feces and passed into environment
❶

Cattle (*T. saginata*) and pigs (*T. solium*) become infected by ingesting vegetation contaminated by eggs or gravid proglottids.
❷

▲ = Infective stage
◬ = Diagnostic stage

Figure 4-47   Life cycle of taeniasis.

377

months in the environment. Cattle (*T. saginata*) and pigs (*T. solium*) become infected by ingesting vegetation contaminated with eggs or gravid proglottids ❷. Ingested oncospheres hatch ❸, invade the intestinal wall, and migrate to striated muscles, where they develop into cysticerci. A cysticercus can survive for several years in the animal. Humans become infected by ingesting raw or undercooked meat ❹. In the human intestine, the cysticercus develops over 2 months into an adult tapeworm, which can survive for years. The tapeworm attaches to the small intestine using its scolex ❺ and resides in the lumen ❻. Adult worms attain lengths of 5 m or less (*T. saginata*) to 7 m (*T. solium*). Proglottids mature, become gravid, detach from the tapeworm, and migrate to the anus or are passed in the stool (approximately 6 per day). *T. saginata* adults usually have 1,000 to 2,000 proglottids, while *T. solium* adults have an average of 1,000 proglottids. The eggs contained in the gravid proglottids are released after the proglottids are passed with the feces. *T. saginata* may produce up to 100,000 and *T. solium* may produce 50,000 eggs per proglottid respectively (CDC).

Clinical Presentation

Most infestations are subclinical. Symptomatic taeniasis may be associated with nausea, vomiting, epigastric fullness, weight loss or diarrhea. *T. saginata* often becomes apparent when motile proglottids are passed through the anus; however, this is uncommon with *T. solium* infestations. Eosinophilia is not a prominent finding. Rare complications include appendicitis, cholangitis, pancreatitis, or intestinal obstruction. The best known complication of *T. solium* infection, cysticercosis, is discussed in the "Cystercercosis" section.

Reference

Taeniasis. Centers for Disease Control Web site. Available at: http://www.dpd.cdc.gov/dpdx/HTML/Taeniasis.htm. Accessed April 15, 2005.

Further Reading

Hoberg EP. Taenia tapeworms: their biology, evolution and socioeconomic significance. *Microbes Infect.* 2002;4:859-866.

Ito A, Wandra T, Yamasaki H, et al. Cysticercosis/taeniasis in Asia and the pacific. *Vector Borne Zoonotic Dis.* 2004;4:95-107.

Roberts T, Murrell KD, Marks S. Economic losses caused by foodborne parasitic diseases. *Parasitol Today.* 1994;10:419-423.

Song EK, Kim IH, Lee SO. Unusual manifestations of Taenia solium infestation. *J Gastroenterol.* 2004;39:288-291.

Taenia infection. Centers for Disease Control Web site. Available at: http://www.cdc.gov/ncidod/dpd/parasites/taenia/default.htm. Accessed April 15, 2005.

Taeniasis—Other

Taenia asiatica

A recently described species (Asian *Taenia* = *T. saginata asiatica*) is acquired from pork and pig viscera, though clinically and morphologically similar to *T. saginata.* Humans are the only definitive host of this parasite, while the domestic pig (Taiwan and Korea) and wild boar (Taiwan) are intermediate hosts. *T. saginata asiatica* has been detected in Indonesia, Korea, Myanmar, the Philippines, Taiwan, and Thailand.

Taenia serialis

T. serialis, a parasite of rabbits and squirrels, is occasionally recovered from humans.

380 Chapter 4: Parasites

Taenia taeniaformis

Accidental human infection by a cat tapeworm. *T. taeniaformis* has been reported from Argentina, Japan, and Sri Lanka.

Taenia crassiceps

Rare instances of *T. crassiceps* (a fox-rodent parasite) cysticercosis have been reported in humans, and characterized by mass lesions in brain, eyes or subcutaneous tissues.

Geographical Distribution

REGION III—SAm	ARG
REGION X—IndSub	LKA
REGION XI—Asia	JPN, KOR, PRK, TWN
REGION XII—SEA	IDN, MMR, THA

Further Reading

Bueno EC, Snege M, Vaz AJ, Leser PG. Serodiagnosis of human cysticercosis by using antigens from vesicular fluid of Taenia crassiceps cysticerci. *Clin Diagn Lab Immunol.* 2001;8:1140-1144.

Ito A, Nakao M, Wandra T. Human taeniasis and cysticercosis in Asia. *Lancet.* 2003;362:1918-1920.

Peralta RH, Vaz AJ, Pardini A, et al. Evaluation of an antigen from Taenia crassiceps cysticercus for the serodiagnosis of neurocysticercosis. *Acta Trop.* August 2002;83(2):159-168.

Ternidensiasis

Geographic Distribution

REGION VI—CAfr	ZMB, ZWE

Background

- *Ternidens diminutus* is carried by monkeys in Africa, India, and Indonesia.

- Human disease is usually asymptomatic or characterized by colonic nodules and ulcers.

Further Reading

Bradley M. Rate of expulsion of Necator americanus and the false hookworm Ternidens deminutus Railliet and Henry 1909 (Nematoda) from humans following albendazole treatment. *Trans R Soc Trop Med Hyg.* 1990;84:720.

Lyons NF, Goldsmid JM. Abnormal Ternidens deminutus Railliet and Henry, 1909 (Nematoda) from man in Rhodesia. *J Parasitol.* 1973;59:219-220.

Thelaziasis

Conjunctival Spirurosis, Oriental Eye Worm

Agent
Nematoda. Phasmidea: *Thelazia callipaeda* (rarely *T. californiensis) Ructularia* spp.

Reservoir
Dogs, rabbits, deer, cats

Vector
Flies (presumably *Musca* and *Fannia* spp.)

Vehicle
None

Geographic Distribution
The precise distribution of this disease is unknown.

Incubation Period
Not known

Diagnostic Tests
Identification of parasite

Typical Therapy
Extraction of parasite

Background

- Thelaziasis has been reported in Africa, Asia, Europe, and North America.
- *T. callipaeda* is found in India, Thailand, China, and Japan. The intermediate host is a fly, *Amiota variegata.*
- Although the vector is uncertain, flies of the genera *Musca* and *Fannia* have been implicated.
- The threadlike adult worms reach a length of 4 to 6 mm and are identified in the conjunctival sac.

Clinical Presentation
Infestation is characterized by conjunctivitis and lacrimation associated with the sensation of an ocular foreign body. *Rictularia* spp., a similar nematode found in the intestines of several mammal species, has been identified in the human appendix.

Additional Reading

Kenney M, Eveland LK, Yermakov V, Kassouny DY. A case of Rictularia infection of man in New York. *Am J Trop Med Hyg.* 1975;24:596-599.

Koyama Y, Ohira A, Kono T, Yoneyama T, Shiwaku K. Five cases of thelaziasis. *Br J Ophthalmol.* 2000;84:441.

Mahanta J, Alger J, Bordoloi P. Eye infestation with Thelazia species. *Indian J Ophthalmol.* 1996;44:99-101.

Teekhasaenee C, Ritch R, Kanchanaranya C. Ocular parasitic infection in Thailand. *Rev Infect Dis.* 1986;8:350-356.

Toxocariasis

Visceral Larva Migrans

Agent
Nematoda. Phasmidea: *Toxocara cati* and *T. canis.*

Reservoir
Cats, dogs, mice

Vector
None

Vehicle
Soil ingestion

Geographic Distribution
Worldwide
Incubation Period
1w–2y

Diagnostic Tests
Identification of larvae in tissue
Serology

Typical Therapy
Albendazole 400 mg b.i.d. × 5d
Or mebendazole 100 to 200 mg PO b.i.d. × 5d

Background

- *T. canis* infection of dogs is found worldwide, with rates varying from 2 to 90%. Infected dogs are usually healthy; however, young animals may have diarrhea, intussusception or intestinal obstruction. Transplacental infection is common in both dogs and cats. Foxes may also serve as a host and source for infection.

- Human infection by *Toxocara* spp. was first reported in 1950. Most cases of human visceral larva migrans are reported from the southern and eastern United States, eastern and western Europe, the Caribbean, Mexico, Hawaii, Australia, the Philippines, and South Africa.
- Humans usually acquire infection through ingestion of fertilized ova shed by puppies (which are infected in-utero). Ova become infective 2 to 3 weeks after passing in feces, and can survive in soil for 1 to 3 years, depending on environmental conditions.
- Children, particularly those who ingest foreign material (pica), are at highest risk. Thus other ingested agents such as lead-containing paint, *Ascaris* and *Trichuris,* are often evident.
- Human infection by *T. cati* is rarely reported. The first case was reported in 1824, in Ireland, and a total of approximately 24 cases had appeared in the world's literature to 2002.

Causal Agents

Toxocariasis is caused by larvae of *Toxocara canis* (dog roundworm) and less frequently of *T. cati* (cat roundworm), two nematode parasites of animals (CDC).

Life Cycle

Toxocara canis accomplishes its life cycle [Figure 4-48] in dogs, with humans acquiring the infection as accidental hosts. Following ingestion of infective eggs by dogs, larvae penetrate the gut wall and migrate to various tissues,

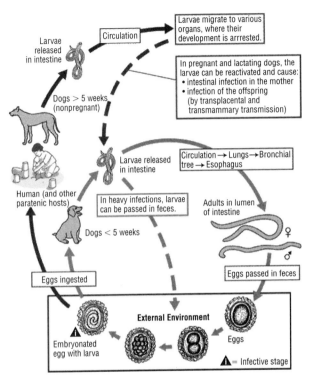

Figure 4-48 Life cycle of toxocariasis.

where they encyst. In dogs below the age of five weeks, the larvae migrate through the lungs, bronchial tree, and esophagus; and adult worms develop and oviposit in the small intestine. In older dogs, the encysted stages are reactivated during pregnancy, and infect puppies via the transplacental and transmammary routes. Thus, infective eggs are excreted both by puppies and lactating adults. Humans are accidentally infected by ingesting infective eggs in contaminated soil. After ingestion, the eggs hatch and larvae penetrate the intestinal wall and are carried by the circulation to various organs (liver, heart, lungs, brain, muscle, eyes). While the larvae do not develop further in these sites, they can cause severe local reactions that are the basis of visceral larva migrans (VLM) and ocular larva migrans (OLM)* (CDC).

Clinical Presentation

Most infections present in children under the age of 5 years, and are asymptomatic or mild. Overt disease is characterized by fever, cough, wheezing, eosinophilia, myalgia, tender hepatomegaly, and abdominal pain. A tender nodular rash might be present on the trunk and legs. Myocarditis, pulmonary infiltrates, seizures, nephritis, encephalopathy, transverse myelitis and renal dysfunction have been described in heavy infections. Ocular toxocariasis usually presents in children ages 5 to 10 years, and is characterized by formation of a retinal granuloma at or near the macula, resulting in strabismus, iridocyclitis, glaucoma, papillitis, or visual loss.

Reference

Toxocariasis. Centers for Disease Control Web site. Available at: http://www.dpd.cdc.gov/dpdx/HTML/Toxocariasis.htm. Accessed April 15, 2005.

Further Reading

Despommier D. Toxocariasis: clinical aspects, epidemiology, medical ecology, and molecular aspects. *Clin Microbiol Rev.* 2003;16:265-272.

Fisher M. Toxocara cati: an underestimated zoonotic agent. *Trends Parasitol.* 2003;19:167-170.

Baylisascaris procyonis, a roundworm of raccoons, has been reported to cause similar VLM and OLM syndromes in humans.

Kaplan M, Kalkan A, Hosoglu S, et al. The frequency of
   Toxocara infection in mental retarded children. *Mem Inst
   Oswaldo Cruz.* 2004;99:121-125.

Taylor MR. The epidemiology of ocular toxocariasis.
   J Helminthol. 2001;75:109-118.

Toxocara infection. Centers for Disease Control Web site.
   Available at: http://www.cdc.gov/ncidod/dpd/parasites/
   toxocara/default.htm. Accessed April 15, 2005.

Toxoplasma gondii

Agent
Protozoa. Sporozoa, Apicomplexa: *T. gondii.*

Reservoir
Rodents, pigs, cattle, sheep, chickens, birds, cats, marsupials (kangaroos)

Vector
None

Vehicle
Transplacental, meat ingestion, soil ingestion, water or milk (rare), flies

Geographic Distribution
Worldwide

Incubation Period
1–3w (range 5–21d)

Diagnostic Tests
Serology
Cultivation or identification of organisms per specialized
   laboratories
Nucleic acid amplification

Typical Adult Therapy

Pyrimethamine 25 mg/d + sulfadiazine 100 mg/kg (max
   6g)/d $\times$ 4w—give with folinic acid.
Alternatives: clindamycin, azithromycin, dapsone.
Spiramycin (in pregnancy) 4 g/d $\times$ 4w.

Typical Pediatric Therapy

Pyrimethamine 2 mg/kg/d $\times$ 3d, then 1 mg/kg/d + sulfadiazine 100 mg/kg/d $\times$ 4w—give with folinic acid.
Alternatives: clindamycin, azithromycin, dapsone.

Background

- The first cases of human toxoplasmosis were reported
  in 1923 in Czechoslovakia.
- Toxoplasmosis occurs worldwide, with up to 30% of
  the human population infected.
- Approximately 50% of European adults are infected.
  Congenital toxoplasmosis affects 10 to 100/100,000
  European newborns, with resulting learning abilities
  in 1 to 2%, and eye disease in 4 to 27%.
- Seropositivity rates increase with age, and both sexes
  are equally affected. The disease incidence is lower in
  cold climates and arid or elevated regions.
- Most infections are acquired through ingestion (lamb,
  pork—rarely beef). Undercooked pork, lamb, and beef
  account for 30 to 60% of infection among pregnant
  women in Europe.
- Meat accounts for 5 to 10 times more infections than
  does soil ingestion.
- Tachyzoites of *T. gondii* have been found in the milk of
  sheep, goats, cows, cats, and mice; and human
  infection has resulted from ingestion of raw goat milk.
- Felines are the only animals which act as definitive
  hosts and excrete oocysts. The oocyst becomes

infective in soil after 2 to 4 days and can remain viable for as long as 12 to 18 months. Cats suffer a transitory, self-limited disease, but can pass millions of oocysts. The relative importance of cats in transmission of human infection varies between countries.

Causal Agent

Toxoplasma gondii is a protozoan parasite that infects most species of warm blooded animals, including humans, causing the disease toxoplasmosis (CDC).

Life Cycle

Members of the cat family (Felidae) are the only known definitive hosts for the sexual stages of *T. gondii*, and thus are the main reservoirs of infection. Cats become infected with *T. gondii* by carnivorism ❶ [Figure 4-49]. After tissue cysts or oocysts are ingested by the cat, viable organisms invade epithelial cells of the small intestine where they undergo first asexual, and then sexual development to form oocysts, which are excreted. The oocyst sporulates (becomes infective) 1 to 5 days after excretion. Cats shed large numbers of oocysts for 1 to 2 weeks. Oocysts survive in the environment for several months and are remarkably resistant to disinfectants, freezing, and drying, but are killed by heating to 70°C for 10 minutes.

Human infection may be acquired in several ways: A) ingestion of undercooked meat containing *Toxoplasma* cysts ❷; B) ingestion of oocysts from fecally contaminated hands or food ❸; C) organ transplantation or blood transfusion; D) transplacental transmission; E) accidental inoculation of tachyzoites. The parasites form tissue cysts, most commonly in skeletal muscle, myocardium, and brain. Cysts may remain viable throughout the life of the host (CDC).

Clinical Presentation

The clinical features of acquired toxoplasmosis can range from subclinical infection to lymphadenopathy (the most common presentation) to fatal, fulminant disease. In

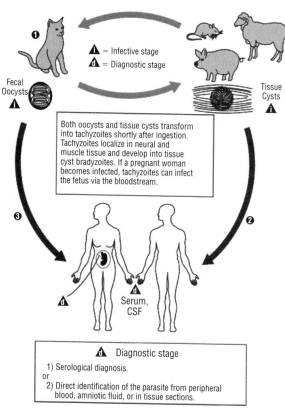

Figure 4-49   Life cycle of *Toxoplasma gondii*.

healthy adults, infection is usually subclinical or mimics infectious mononucleosis; however, pharyngitis and posterior cervical lymphadenopathy are unusual in toxoplasmosis. In immunocompromised hosts, toxoplasmosis may mimic other opportunistic infections, such as tuberculosis or infection with *P. jiroveci* (formerly *P. carinii*). In patients with AIDS, central nervous system (CNS) involvement is the most common manifestation, followed by pulmonary disease.

Ocular toxoplasmosis occurs from reactivation of cysts in the retina. Focal necrotizing retinitis is characteristic lesion, and approximately 35% of all cases of retinochoroiditis can be attributed to toxoplasmosis.

The manifestations of CNS toxoplasmosis in the immunocompromised patient range from an insidious process evolving over several weeks to acute onset of a confusional state. Signs may be focal or symmetrical. *T. gondii* has a predilection to localize in the basal ganglia and brain stem, producing extrapyramidal symptoms resembling those of Parkinson's disease. Nonfocal evidence of neurologic dysfunction can include generalized weakness, headache, confusion, lethargy, alteration of mental status, personality changes, and coma. Infection in transplant recipients is often diffuse and disseminated. In patients with underlying malignancy (eg, Hodgkin's disease), the presentation is evenly distributed between focal and nonfocal forms of encephalitis.

Patients with AIDS tend to present subacutely with nonspecific symptoms such as neuropsychiatric complaints, headache, fever, weight loss, disorientation, confusion, and lethargy evolving over 2 to 8 weeks. Later findings include evidence of focal CNS mass lesions, ataxia, aphasia, hemiparesis, visual field loss, vomiting, confusion, dementia, stupor and seizures.

Reference

Toxoplasmosis. Centers for Disease Control Web site. Available at: http://www.dpd.cdc.gov/dpdx/HTML/ Toxoplasmosis.htm. Accessed April 15, 2005.

Further Reading

Bhopale GM. Pathogenesis of toxoplasmosis. *Comp Immunol Microbiol Infect Dis.* 2003;26:213-222.

Jones JL, Lopez A, Wilson M, Schulkin J, Gibbs R. Congenital toxoplasmosis: a review. *Obstet Gynecol Surv.* 2001;56:296-305.

Rothova A. Ocular manifestations of toxoplasmosis. *Curr Opin Ophthalmol.* 2003;14:384-388.

Tenter AM, Heckeroth AR, Weiss LM. Toxoplasma gondii: from animals to humans. *Int J Parasitol.* 2000;30:1217-1258.

Toxoplasmosis. Centers for Disease Control Web site. Available at: http://www.cdc.gov/ncidod/dpd/parasites/ toxoplasmosis/default.htm. Accessed April 15, 2005.

Trichinosis

Trichinellosis

Agent

Nematoda. Aphasmidia: *Trichinella spiralis* (occasionally *T. nativa, T. britovi, T. pseudospiralis, T. nelsoni, et al*).

Reservoir

Wild carnivores, omnivores, marine mammals

Vector

None

Vehicle

Meat ingestion

Geographic Distribution
Worldwide

Incubation Period
10–20d (range 1–10w)

Diagnostic Tests
Identification of larvae in tissue or serology

Typical Adult Therapy
Albendazole 400 mg PO b.i.d. × 14d.
Or mebendazole 200 to 400 mg PO t.i.d. × 3 days, then
    400 to 500 mg PO t.i.d. × 10d.
Give with prednisone 50 mg PO daily × 3 to 5 days
    (then taper dosage).

Typical Pediatric Therapy
Thiabendazole 22 mg/kg b.i.d. × 7d with prednisone

Background

- It is estimated that 11 million are infested by
  Trichinella species worldwide. Most infections are due
  to *T. spiralis* (T1). Trichinosis accounted for 1.5% of all
  food-related outbreaks in Europe during 1991 to 1992.
- In most parts of Europe, the specific reservoir is the
  red fox (*Vulpes vulpes*), living at elevations above 400
  to 500 meters; however, the raccoon dog (*Nyctereutes
  procyonoides*) serves as an additional reservoir in
  Finland.
- More than 3,000 cases of human trichinosis were
  acquired from horse meat in Italy and France from
  1975 to 2000.

- European countries investigated 745 outbreaks (total 1,975 cases) during 1993 to 1998—accounting for 3.2% of all food-related outbreaks.
- During January 1995 to June 1997, 10,030 cases were officially reported, including 3,092 in Romania and 1,806 in Yugoslavia.
- *T. nativa* (T2) is found in arctic regions (including Canada, Finland, and central to northern Sweden), and transmitted by horse, bear, and walrus. Unlike *T. spiralis*, *T. nativa* is resistant to freezing at −10 to −20°C for up to 4 years. *T. britovi* can also survive freezing for long periods of time. The highest concentration of trichinella in walrus is found in the tongue.
- *T. britovi* (T3) occurs in temperate zones and is acquired from horses and boar.
- *T. pseudospiralis* (T4) occurs in the Nearctic and Oceania and is found in birds and omnivores. This is the only *Trichinella* species that infects both mammals and birds and was first reported to infect humans in 1995 (New Zealand). It is detected in sylvatic animals (raccoon dogs, corsac foxes, tiger cats, tawny eagles, and rooks) in remote regions (Caucasus, Kazakhstan, and Tasmania); and in wildlife in the United States, in domestic and synanthropic animals and humans in Russia (including an outbreak of approximately 30 cases in Kamchatka), and in humans in Thailand (an outbreak of 59 cases, 1 fatal). Additional identifications include a raccoon dog (*Nyctereutes procyonoides*) in the Krasnodar region of Caucasus; night birds of prey in central Italy; raccoon dogs, wild boars, and the brown rat in Finland; and domestic pigs and brown rats in Kamchatka.
- *Trichinella murrelli* (T5) is found in temperate areas of the Nearctic region. It is not resistant to freezing; it is

characterized by a long incubation period and moderate to severe pathogenicity for humans.

- *T. nelsoni* (T7) is found in the tropics and is acquired from wart hogs.
- *Trichinella papuae* (T10) is found in wild and domestic pigs in Papua New Guinea and is suspected to be the pathogen of human disease as well.

Causal Agents

Trichinellosis (trichinosis) is caused by nematodes (roundworms) of the genus *Trichinella*. In addition to *Trichinella spiralis* (found worldwide in many carnivorous and omnivorous animals), nine other species of *Trichinella* are now recognized (CDC).

Life Cycle

Trichinellosis is acquired by ingesting meat containing cysts (encysted larvae) ❶ [Figure 4-50] of *Trichinella*. After exposure to gastric acid and pepsin, the larvae are released ❷ from the cysts and invade the small bowel mucosa, where they develop into adult worms ❸ (female 2.2 mm in length, males 1.2 mm; life span in the small bowel: 4 weeks). After 1 week, the females release larvae ❹ that migrate to the striated muscles, where they encyst ❺. *Trichinella pseudospiralis*, however, does not encyst. Encystment is completed in 4 to 5 weeks, and encysted larvae may remain viable for several years. Carnivorous/omnivorous animals, such as pigs or bears, feed on infected rodents or meat from other animals. Various animal hosts are implicated in the life cycle of the different species of *Trichinella*. Humans are accidentally infected when eating improperly processed meat of these carniv-

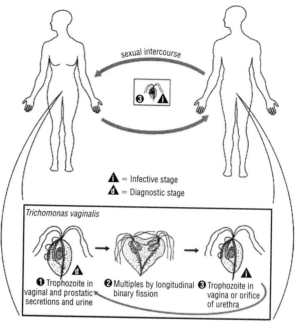

Figure 4-50   Life cycle of trichinosis.

orous animals (or eating food contaminated with such meat) (CDC).

Clinical Presentation

The majority of infections are subclinical, and development of symptoms depends on the number of larvae ingested. During the first week of illness, the patient may experience diarrhea, abdominal pain, and vomiting. Symptoms associated with larval invasion appear during the second week and include fever, periorbital edema, subconjunctival hemorrhages and chemosis. Myositis is also common and often appears in the extraocular muscles, progressing to involve the masseters, neck muscles, and limb and lumbar muscles.

Additional symptoms can include headache, cough, dyspnea, hoarseness, and dysphagia. Occasionally, a macular or petechial rash or retinal or subungual splinter hemorrhages are seen. Laboratory studies could reveal marked eosinophilia, hypoalbuminemia, and decreased erythrocyte sedimentation rate.

Systemic symptoms usually peak 2 to 3 weeks after infection and then slowly subside; however, weakness may persist for weeks. Deaths are ascribed to myocarditis, encephalitis, or pneumonia.

Reference

Trichinellosis. Centers for Disease Control Web site. Available at: http://www.dpd.cdc.gov/dpdx/HTML/Trichinosis.htm. Accessed April 15, 2005.

Further Reading

Bruschi F, Murrell KD. New aspects of human trichinellosis: the impact of new Trichinella species. *Postgrad Med J.* 2002;78:15-22.

International Commission on Trichinellosis Web site. Available at: http://www.med.unipi.it/ict/welcome.htm. Accessed April 15, 2005.

Murrell KD, Pozio E. Trichinellosis: the zoonosis that won't go quietly. *Int J Parasitol.* 2000;30:1339-1349.

Roy SL, Lopez AS, Schantz PM. Trichinellosis surveillance—United States, 1997–2001. *MMWR Surveill Summ.* 2003;52:1-8.

Trichinellosis. Centers for Disease Control Web site. Available at: http://www.cdc.gov/ncidod/dpd/parasites/trichinosis/default.htm. Accessed April 15, 2005.

Trichomonas vaginalis

Agent
Protozoa. Archezoa, Parabasalia, Trichomonadea. Flagellate: *T. vaginalis*.

Reservoir
Humans

Vector
None

Vehicle
Sexual contact

Geographic Distribution
Worldwide

Incubation Period
4–28d

Diagnostic Tests
Microscopy of vaginal discharge.
ELISA and other antigen detection tests are available.
Nucleic acid amplification.

Typical Adult Therapy
Metronidazole or tinidazole 2g PO as single dose to both sexual partners

Typical Pediatric Therapy
Metronidazole 5 mg/kg PO t.i.d. × 7d
Or tinidazole 50 mg/kg PO × 1 (maximum 2 grams)

Background

- The World Health Organization estimated 170 million cases of trichomoniasis in the age group 15 to 49 years for the year 1995 (male/female = 1.02/1)—75.43 million in south Asia and Southeast Asia and 30.42 million in sub-Saharan Africa. In 1996, 17,722,000 persons were infected in Latin America—with an incidence among adolescents of 7,085/100,000 per year.

- Trichomoniasis accounts for as many as 56% of visits to sexually transmitted disease (STD) clinics. One third of asymptomatic carriers can be expected to develop vaginitis within 6 months. Infected women are symptomatic in 25 to 50% of cases.

- Trichomoniasis is implicated in as many as 11% of nongonococcal urethritis cases in males. Infection is most common in the age group 20 to 45 years; with lower rates among users of oral contraceptives.

Causal Agent

Trichomonas vaginalis, a flagellate, is the most common pathogenic protozoan of humans in industrialized countries (CDC).

Life Cycle

Trichomonas vaginalis resides in the female lower genital tract and the male urethra and prostate ❶ [Figure 4-51], where it replicates by binary fission ❷. The parasite does not appear to have a cyst form, and does not survive well in the external environment. *Trichomonas vaginalis* is transmitted among humans, the only known host, primarily by sexual intercourse ❸ (CDC).

Clinical Presentation

Infections are asymptomatic in 10 to 50% of cases. Symptoms often begin or worsen during the menstrual period. Infection is usually characterized by vaginal discharge and vulvovaginal irritation. Dysuria may be present, and dyspareunia is common. As many as two thirds of infected women complain of a disagreeable odor. Abdominal discomfort is present in 5 to 12% of infected women. Examination reveals a copious, loose discharge that pools in the posterior vaginal fornix. The discharge is yellow or green in 5 to 40% of cases, and bubbles are observed in the discharge in 10 to 33%. The material has a

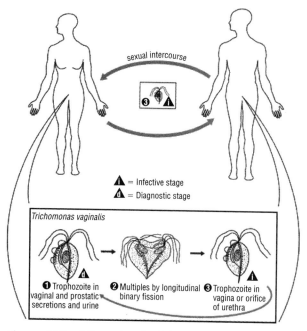

Figure 4-51   Life cycle of *Trichomonas vaginalis*.

pH above 4.5 in 66 to 91% of cases. Endocervical disease is not caused by *T. vaginalis*. Punctate hemorrhages (colpitis macularis or strawberry cervix) are seen colposcopically in 45% of infected women, but in only 2% by visual inspection alone. Parasites can be recovered from the urethra and paraurethral glands in more than 95% of the women, and this could explain the association of the infection with urinary frequency and dysuria.

Complications of trichomonal vaginitis include *vaginitis emphysematosa*—the presence of gas-filled blebs in the vaginal wall. Gestational trichomoniasis can be associated with premature labor and low birth weight, postabortal infection or premature rupture of the membranes. Spread of trichomonads beyond the lower urogenital tract is extremely rare.

Most men carrying trichomonads are asymptomatic; however, the organism is implicated in 5 to 15% of nongonococcal urethritis cases. The discharge from trichomonal urethritis is usually milder than that seen with other infections. Epididymitis, superficial penile ulcerations (often beneath the prepuce) and prostatitis are also described.

Reference
Trichomoniasis. Centers for Disease Control Web site. Available at: http://www.dpd.cdc.gov/dpdx/HTML/Trichomoniasis.htm. Accessed April 15, 2005.

Further Reading
Anderson MR, Klink K, Cohrssen A. Evaluation of vaginal complaints. *JAMA*. 2004;291:1368-1379.

Communicable Disease Surveillance and Response. World Health Organization Web site. Available at: http://www.who.int/emc/diseases/hiv/index.html. Accessed April 15, 2005.

Landers DV, Wiesenfeld HC, Heine RP, Krohn MA, Hillier SL. Predictive value of the clinical diagnosis of lower genital tract infection in women. *Am J Obstet Gynecol.* 2004;190:1004-1010.

Soper D. Trichomoniasis: under control or undercontrolled? *Am J Obstet Gynecol.* 2004;190:281-290.

Trichomonas Infection. Centers for Disease Control Web site. Available at: http://www.cdc.gov/ncidod/dpd/parasites/trichomonas/default.htm. Accessed April 15, 2005.

Trichostrongyliasis

Agent
Nematoda. Phasmidea: *Trichostrongylus colubriformis, T. orientalis, T. probolurus.*

Reservoir
Herbivores

Vector
None

Vehicle
Water, food, vegetation

Geographic Distribution

REGION I—NAm	USA
REGION III—SAm	BRA, CHL, PER
REGION V—NAfr	EGY
REGION VI—CAfr	AGO, CAF, COG, GMB, MLI, MWI, NER, NGA
REGION VIII—Eur	FRA, GRC
REGION IX—MidEast	IRN, IRQ, ISR, JOR, TUR
REGION X—IndSub	IND
REGION XI—Asia	CHN, JPN, KOR, PRK, RUS, TWN

REGION XII—SEA   IDN
REGION XIII—Poly   AUS, FJI

Incubation Period
21d

Diagnostic Tests
Identification of ova in stool or duodenal aspirate

Typical Therapy
Albendazole 400 mg PO × 1
Or pyrantel pamoate 11 mg/kg (max 1g) PO once
Or mebendazole 100 mg PO b.i.d. × 7d

Background

- *Trichostrongylus* spp. are normally found in the proximal small intestine of sheep and goats.
- Human infection by *T. colubriformis* is common among persons raising sheep and goats, and may infest 70% in some areas.
- *T. orientalis* is common among persons who work with donkeys and goats—particularly when human excreta are used as fertilizer.
- *T. probolurus* is found in camels and gazelles and rarely infects humans.
- *T. axei* infection has been reported in humans in the Caribbean region and Italy.
- *T. capricola* infection has been reported in humans in Iran and Italy.
- *T. vitrinus* infections have been reported in humans in Italy and Morocco.
- *T. lerouxi* infections have been reported in humans in Iran.

- *T. brevis* has been reported in humans (details not available).
- Related parasites found in humans include *Haemonchus contortus*, *Ostertagia ostertagi* and *Marshallagia marshalli* (all reported in Iran).

Clinical Presentation

Most infections are asymptomatic or characterized by mild, nonspecific abdominal symptoms. Heavy infections may result in episodic diarrhea, abdominal pain, and weight loss. Rare instances of cholecystitis are reported.

Further Reading

Boreham RE, McCowan MJ, Ryan AE, Allworth AM, Robson JM. Human trichostrongyliasis in Queensland. *Pathology.* 1995;27:182-185.

Bundy DA, Terry SI, Murphy CP, Harris EA. First record of Trichostrongylus axei infection of man in the Caribbean region. *Trans R Soc Trop Med Hyg.* 1985;79:562-563.

Cancrini G, Boemi G, Iori A, Corselli A. Human infestations by Trichostrongylus axei, T. capricola and T. vitrinus: 1st report in Italy. *Parassitologia.* 1982;24:145-149.

Ghadirian E, Arfaa F. First report of human infection with Haemonchus contortus, Ostertagia ostertagi, and Marshallagia marshalli (family Trichostrongylidae) in Iran. *J Parasitol.* 1973;59:1144-1145.

Ghadirian E, Arfaa F, Sadighian A. Human infection with Trichostrongylus capricola in Iran. *Am J Trop Med Hyg.* 1974;23:1002-1003.

Ghadirian E. Human infection with Trichostrongylus lerouxi (Biocca, Chabaud, and Ghadirian, 1974) in Iran. *Am J Trop Med Hyg.* 1977;26(6, pt 1):1212-1213.

Magambo JK, Zeyhle E, Wachira TM. Prevalence of intestinal parasites among children in southern Sudan. *East Afr Med J.* 1998; 75:288-290.

Massoud J, Arfaa F, Jalali H, Keyvan S. Prevalence of intestinal helminths in Khuzestan, southwest Iran, 1977. *Am J Trop Med Hyg*. 1980;29:389-392.

Ostoru M .Trichostrongylus brevis sp. nov. from man (Nematoda: Trichostrongylidae). *Acta Med Biol (Niigata)*. 1962;9:273-278.

Poirriez J, Dei-Cas E, Guevart E, Abdellatifi M, Giard P, Vernes A. Human infestation by Trichostrongylus vitrinus in Morocco. *Ann Parasitol Hum Comp*. 1984;59:636-638.

Trichuris trichiura

Trichocephaliasis, Whipworm

Agent
Nematoda. Aphasmidia: *T. trichiura.*

Reservoir
Humans

Vector
None

Vehicle
Soil ingestion, sexual contact (rare), flies

Geographic Distribution
Worldwide

Incubation Period
2m–2y

Diagnostic Tests
Stool microscopy or visualization of adult worms (adults are approximately 3 cm long)

Typical Adult Therapy

Mebendazole 100 mg PO b.i.d. × 3d

Or albendazole 400 mg PO × 1

Typical Pediatric Therapy

Mebendazole 100 mg PO b.i.d. × 3d (> age 2)

Or albendazole 400 mg PO × 1

Background

- Infection is common in areas of high rainfall and humidity and is most often associated with poor hygiene, ingestion of raw produce, and the pediatric age group.
- It is estimated that 902 million are infested (as compared to 355 million in 1947). The prevalence in sub-Saharan Africa is estimated at 20.9% (100 million cases).
- In 1998, 5,000 fatal cases were estimated; 2000 in 1999.
- Adult worms live in the cecum and appendix, attaining a length of 3.0 to 4.5 cm. Embryonation of ova takes at least 21 days. Ova are resistant to cold, but not to drying.
- *T. vulpis* has been recovered from a dog owner. The parasite is twice as large as *T. trichiura*.

Causal Agent

The nematode (roundworm) *Trichuris trichiura*, also called the human whipworm (CDC).

Life Cycle

Unembryonated eggs are passed with the stool ❶ [Figure 4-52]. In the soil, eggs develop into a 2-cell stage ❷, an advanced cleavage stage ❸, and mature embryos ❹. Eggs become infective in 15 to 30 days. After ingestion (soil-

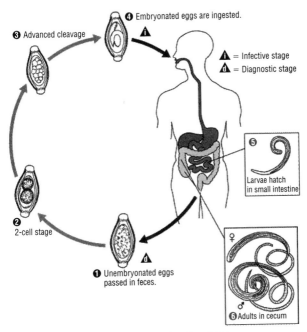

❹ Embryonated eggs are ingested.

❸ Advanced cleavage

ⓘ = Infective stage
ⓓ = Diagnostic stage

❺ Larvae hatch in small intestine

❷ 2-cell stage

❶ Unembryonated eggs passed in feces.

♀
♂
❻ Adults in cecum

Figure 4-52   Life cycle of *Trichuris trichiura*.

contaminated hands or food), the eggs release larvae ❺ that mature and establish themselves in the cecum and ascending colon ❻. Adults (approximately 4 cm in length) are fixed, with their anterior portions threaded into the mucosa. Females begin to oviposit 60 to 70 days after infection. Female worms in the cecum shed between 3,000 and 20,000 eggs per day. The life span of the adults is 1 year (CDC).

Clinical Presentation

The vast majority of infections are asymptomatic. Symptoms are aggravated by concurrent shigellosis, balantidiasis, or amebiasis. Heavy infestations are characterized by dysentery or rectal prolapse. Infants could develop hypoproteinemia, anemia, mental retardation, and digital clubbing.

Reference
Trichuriasis. Centers for Disease Control Web site. Available at: http://www.dpd.cdc.gov/dpdx/HTML/Trichuriasis.htm. Accessed April 15, 2005.

Further Reading
Bennett A, Guyatt H. Reducing intestinal nematode infection: efficacy of albendazole and mebendazole. *Parasitol Today*. 2000;16:71-74.

de Silva NR. Impact of mass chemotherapy on the morbidity due to soil-transmitted nematodes. *Acta Trop*. 2003;86: 197-214.

Fincham JE, Markus MB. Human immune response to Trichuris trichiura. *Trends Parasitol*. 2001;17:121.

Partners for parasite control (PPC). World Health Organization Web site. Available at: http://www.who.int/ctd/ intpara/. Accessed April 15, 2005.

Pedersen S, Murrell KD. Whipworm-nutrition interaction. *Trends Parasitol*. 2001;17:470.

Whipworm infection. Centers for Disease Control Web site. Available at: http://www.cdc.gov/ncidod/dpd/parasites/ whipworm/default.htm. Accessed April 15, 2005.

Trypanosomiasis—African

African Sleeping Sickness, Gambian Fever
Agent
Protozoa. Neozoa, Euglenozoa, Kenetoplastea. Flagellate: *Trypanosoma (Trypanozoon) brucei gambiense* and *Trypanosoma brucei rhodesiense*.

Reservoir
Humans, deer, wild carnivore, cattle

Vector
Flies (*Glossina* = tsetse fly)

Vehicle
None

Geographic Distribution

REGION VI—CAfr	AGO, BDI, BEN, BFA, CAF, CIV, CMR, COD, COG, ERI, ETH, GAB, GHA, GIN, GMB, GNB, GNQ, KEN, LBR, MLI, MOZ, MWI, NER, NGA, RWA, SDN, SEN, SLE, TCD, TGO, TZA, UGA, ZMB, ZWE
REGION VII—SAfr	NAM

Incubation Period
3–21d (acute illness)

Diagnostic Tests
Identification of protozoa in CSF, blood, lymph node
   aspirate
Serology
Nucleic acid amplification

Typical Adult Therapy
Early: pentamidine 4 mg/kg IM. qod × 10 doses
Or suramin 1 g i.v. days 1, 3, 7, 14, 21 (after test dose 100
   mg)

Or elfornithine (gambiense only) 100 mg q6h i.v. × 14
d; then 75 mg/kg PO × 21–30d

Late + CNS disease: melarsoprol

Typical Pediatric Therapy

Early: pentamidine 4 mg/kg IM qod × 10 doses

Or suramin 20 mg/kg i.v. days 1, 3, 7, 14, 21 (after test,
dose 20 mg)

Late + CNS: melarsoprol

Background

- *T. brucei* is transmitted by the bite of the tsetse fly
  (*Glossina* spp.). The disease is found over vast areas of
  tropical Africa and exists in two main forms. The east
  African form (caused by *T. b. rhodesiense*) runs a rapid
  course, while in the west and central African form
  (*T. b. gambiense*), the disease runs a much longer
  course, over several years, before death occurs.
  Without appropriate treatment both forms are fatal.
  Early diagnosis of *T. b. gambiense* infection is difficult
  because specific clinical signs are absent. Only
  serological tests can be used in population surveys.
- Human African trypanosomiasis is rural and focal,
  with humans as the principal reservoir of infection of
  T. b. gambiense and domestic cattle and wild animals
  as important reservoirs of *T. b. rhodesiense*. By the
  1960s, the disease had been brought under control, but
  since 1970 the situation has deteriorated, with major
  flare-ups in countries which have not maintained
  surveillance activities. Four main levels of endemicity
  have been identified: epidemic, high endemnicity, low
  endemnicity, and status uncertain.
- In Angola, Democratic Republic of Congo, Sudan, and
  Uganda the disease is considered epidemic due to a
  high prevalence and an important transmission level.

- Cameroon, Central African Republic, Chad, Congo, Côte d'Ivoire, Guinea, and Tanzania have been classified as countries of high endemicity where prevalence is increasing.
- Benin, Burkina Faso, Equatorial Guinea, Gabon, Ghana, Guinea, Kenya, Mali, Mozambique, Nigeria, Togo, and Zambia are considered of low endemicity although the epidemiological situation is poorly known in foci in some countries.
- Countries where the present epidemiological status is poorly known or not known include Burundi, Botswana, Ethiopia, Liberia, Namibia, Rwanda, Senegal, and Sierra Leone.
- It is estimated that 250,000 humans in sub-Saharan Africa carry the parasite and 55 million are at risk. Approximately 45 million cattle and 100 million sheep are considered at risk for the disease. In countries such as Angola, Democratic Republic of Congo, and Sudan, the operational capacity to respond to the epidemic situation is largely surpassed. In certain foci, the observed prevalence is more than 20%, and in many villages it is even greater than 50%. In some provinces, sleeping sickness has become the principal cause of mortality. To date, the Democratic Republic of Congo has estimated the number of deaths due to human trypanosomiasis as equal to or greater than that due to AIDS.
- In 2001, 10 cases were reported among western tourists returning from Tanzania.
- In 1998, 40,000 fatal cases were estimated; 66,000 in 1999—181 deaths each day.
- Animal reservoirs are thought to be more important in the transmission of *T.b. rhodesiense* to humans than in the transmission of *T.b. gambiense*. Nagana (the cattle disease) has occurred over as much as one quarter of

the African continent. The disease is fatal to horses, mules, camels, and dogs—resulting in an estimated 3 million livestock deaths per year in Africa. Cattle, sheep, and goats usually survive. Many of the wild ungulates native to Africa show no evidence of disease.

- Tsetse flies inhabit 10 million square kilometers of sub-Saharan Africa.

Causal Agents

Protozoan hemoflagellates belonging to the complex *Trypanosoma brucei*. Two subspecies that are morphologically indistinguishable cause distinct disease patterns in humans: *T. b. gambiense* causes West African sleeping sickness and *T. b. rhodesiense* causes East African sleeping sickness. (A third member of the complex, *T. b. brucei*, under normal conditions, does not infect humans.) (CDC)

Life Cycle

During a blood meal on the mammalian host, the infected tsetse fly (genus *Glossina*) injects metacyclic trypomastigotes into skin tissue. The parasites enter the lymphatic system and pass into the bloodstream ❶ [Figure 4-53], where they transform into trypomastigotes ❷. These are carried to other sites throughout the body, and continue the replication by binary fission ❸. The entire life cycle of African Trypanosomes is represented by extracellular stages. The tsetse fly becomes infected with bloodstream trypomastigotes when taking a blood meal on an infected mammalian host (❹, ❺). In the fly's midgut, parasites transform into procyclic trypomastigotes, multiply by binary fission ❻, leave the midgut, and transform into epimastigotes ❼. The epimastigotes reach the fly's salivary glands and continue to multiply by binary fission ❽. The cycle in the fly takes approximately 3 weeks. Humans are the main reservoir for *Trypanosoma brucei gambiense*, but this species can also be found in animals. Wild game animals are the main reservoir of *T. b. rhodesiense* (CDC).

Clinical Presentation

The initial sign of trypanosomiasis is a chancre which develops at the site of inoculation, 1 to 2 weeks following the bite of a tsetse fly. The chancre can reach a diameter of several centimeters and be associated with regional adenopathy, but resolves over several weeks. In most cases, the chancre is noted by neither the patient nor the clinician. Fever appears weeks to months following inoculation and is characteristically intermittent.

Lymphadenopathy is a fairly constant feature of west African trypanosomiasis. The nodes are discrete, movable, rubbery, and nontender. Supraclavicular and cervical nodes are often visibly discernible, and enlargement of the nodes of the posterior cervical triangle (Winterbottom's sign) is common in the west African form. Additional findings at this point may include hepatosplenomegaly; edema of the face, hands and feet; pruritis; an irregular circinate, 5 to 10 cm rash on the trunk, shoulders, buttocks, and thighs; headache, asthenia, weight loss, arthralgias, and tachycardia.

In the west African form, the meningoencephalitic stage could develop months or even years after the initial infection. Findings include irritability, personality changes, indifference, apathy, daytime somnolence (often with insomnia at night), slurred speech, choreiform movements of the trunk, neck, and extremities, tremors of the tongue

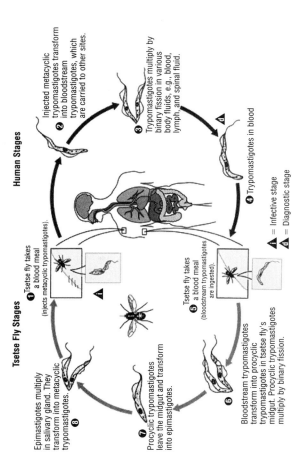

Tsetse Fly Stages

Human Stages

❶ Tsetse fly takes a blood meal (injects metacyclic trypomastigotes).

❷ Injected metacyclic trypomastigotes transform into bloodstream trypomastigotes, which are carried to other sites.

❸ Trypomastigotes multiply by binary fission in various body fluids, e.g., blood, lymph, and spinal fluid.

❹ Trypomastigotes in blood

▲ = Infective stage

▲ = Diagnostic stage

❺ Tsetse fly takes a blood meal (bloodstream trypomastigotes are ingested).

❻ Bloodstream trypomastigotes transform into procyclic trypomastigotes in tsetse fly's midgut. Procyclic trypomastigotes multiply by binary fission.

❼ Procyclic trypomastigotes leave the midgut and transform into epimastigotes.

❽ Epimastigotes multiply in salivary gland. They transform into metacyclic trypomastigotes.

Figure 4-53   Life cycle of trypanosomiasis—African.

414

and fingers, ataxia, and muscular fasciculations. The final phase of the CNS disease is progression to coma and death.

The east African form tends to follow a more acute course, with an incubation of a few weeks to several weeks. Intermittent fever, headache, myalgia, and rash develop early, while lymphadenitis is not a prominent feature. Persistent tachycardia is common, and some patients die of arrhythmias, congestive heart failure, or pericarditis before the onset of neurological disease. If untreated, the east African form is fatal within weeks to months.

Reference

Trypanosomiasis, African. Centers for Disease Control Web site. Available at: http://www.dpd.cdc.gov/dpdx/HTML/TrypanosomiasisAfrican.htm. Accessed April 15, 2005.

Further Reading

African trypanosomiasis (sleeping sickness). Communicable Disease Surveillance and Response Web page. Available at: http://www.who.int/emc/diseases/tryp/index.html. Accessed April 15, 2005.

African trypanosomiasis. Centers for Disease Control Web site. Available at: http://www.cdc.gov/ncidod/dpd/parasites/trypanosomiasis/default.htm. Accessed April 15, 2005.

Barrett MP, Burchmore RJ, Stich A, et al. The trypanosomiases. *Lancet.* 2003;362:1469-1480.

Cox FE. History of sleeping sickness (African trypanosomiasis). *Infect Dis Clin North Am.* 2004;18:231-245.

Fairlamb AH. Chemotherapy of human African trypanosomiasis: current and future prospects. *Trends Parasitol.* 2003;19:488-494.

Kennedy PG. Human African trypanosomiasis of the CNS: current issues and challenges. *J Clin Invest.* 2004;113:496-504.

Lejon V, Boelaert M, Jannin J, Moore A, Buscher P. The challenge of Trypanosoma brucei gambiense sleeping sickness diagnosis outside Africa. *Lancet Infect Dis.* 2003;3: 804-808.

Trypanosomiasis—American

Chagas' Disease

Agent
Protozoa. Neozoa, Euglenozoa, Kenetoplastea. Flagellate: *Trypanosoma cruzi.*

Reservoir
Humans, dogs, cats, pigs, guinea pigs, armadillos, rats, foxes, opossum, raccoons, bats, mice, monkeys

Vector
Bugs (Triatome or kissing bug = *Panstrongylus, Rhodnius* and *Triatoma* spp.)

Vehicle
Blood

Geographic Distribution

REGION II—CAm	BLZ, CRI, GTM, HND, MEX, NIC, PAN, SLV
REGION III—SAm	ARG, BOL, BRA, CHL, COL, ECU, GUF, GUY, PER, PRY, URY, VEN

Incubation Period
5–14d (acute illness)

Diagnostic Tests
Identification of protozoa in blood or tissue or serology
Xenodiagnosis
Nucleic acid amplification

Typical Adult Therapy
Nifurtimox 2 mg/kg PO q.i.d. × 3m
Or benznidazole 7 mg/kg/d × 30 to 120d

Typical Pediatric Therapy
Nifurtimox:
Age 1 to 10 years: 5 mg/kg PO q.i.d. × 3m
Age 11 to 16 years: 3.5 mg/kg PO q.i.d. × 3m (age 11 to 16y)
Or benznidazole 3.75 mg/kg PO b.i.d. × 2m

Background

- Chagas disease represents the third largest tropical disease burden worldwide, after malaria and schistosomiasis. Infections are limited to Latin America, between 42°N and 40°S latitudes. In those countries, 121 million persons (25% of the population) are at risk.
- During the early 1990s, 16 to 18 million were estimated to have the disease, of whom 2 to 3 million are in the chronic stages. As of 2000, 11 million infections were estimated.
- Each year, there are approximately 1 million new cases.
- In 1990, 72,677 new cases were estimated for Mexico and Central America and 86,237 for the Andean Pact region.
- In 1990, 23,000 deaths were estimated; 43,000 in 1995; 17,000 in 1998; 21,000 in 1999.

- The ecological unit of American trypanosomiasis is constituted by an ecotype composed of sylvatic or peridomestic mammals and sylvatic triatome bugs, both infested with *T. cruzi*.

Causal Agent

The protozoan parasite, *Trypanosoma cruzi*, causes Chagas disease, a zoonotic disease that can be transmitted to humans by blood-sucking triatomine bugs (CDC).

Life Cycle

An infected triatomine vector ("kissing" bug) takes a blood meal and releases trypomastigotes in its feces near the site of the bite wound. Trypomastigotes enter the host through the wound or through intact mucosal membranes, such as the conjunctiva ❶ [Figure 4-54]. Inside the host, the trypomastigotes invade cells, where they differentiate into intracellular amastigotes ❷. Amastigotes multiply by binary fission ❸ and differentiate into trypomastigotes, which are released into the bloodstream as trypomastigotes ❹. Trypomastigotes infect a variety of tissues and transform into intracellular amastigotes at new infection sites. Bloodstream trypomastigotes do not replicate (unlike African trypanosomes). Replication resumes only when the parasites enter another cell or are ingested by another vector. The "kissing" bug becomes infected by feeding on human or animal blood that contains circulating parasites ❺. Ingested trypomastigotes transform into epimastigotes in the vector's midgut ❻. The parasites differentiate in the midgut ❼ into infective metacyclic trypomastigotes in the hindgut ❽.

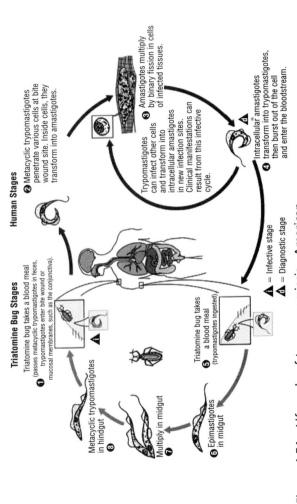

Triatomine Bug Stages

Human Stages

❶ Triatomine bug takes a blood meal (passes metacyclic trypomastigotes in feces, trypomastigotes enter bite wound or mucosal membranes, such as the conjunctiva).

❷ Metacyclic trypomastigotes penetrate various cells at bite wound site. Inside cells, they transform into amastigotes.

❸ Amastigotes multiply by binary fission in cells of infected tissues.

Trypomastigotes can infect other cells and transform into intracellular amastigotes in new infection sites. Clinical manifestations can result from this infective cycle.

❹ Intracellular amastigotes transform into trypomastigotes, then burst out of the cell and enter the bloodstream.

▲ = Infective stage
◆ = Diagnostic stage

❺ Triatomine bug takes a blood meal (trypomastigotes ingested).

❻ Epimastigotes in midgut

❼ Multiply in midgut

❽ Metacyclic trypomastigotes in hindgut

Figure 4-54   Life cycle of trypanosomiasis—American.

Trypanosoma cruzi can also be transmitted through blood transfusion, organ transplantation, transplacentally, and in laboratory accidents (CDC).

Clinical Presentation

The clinical features of acute and chronic infection are distinct. Acute infection can occur at any age, but is usually an illness of children in endemic areas. The first signs of illness occur one week or more following inoculation and consist of a chagoma, indurated area of erythema, and swelling with local lymph node involvement. Romana's sign consists of painless edema of the eyelids and periocular tissues which follows conjunctival inoculation. Later, the patient develops fever, malaise, anorexia, and edema of the face and legs. Generalized lymphadenopathy and mild hepatosplenomegaly also might appear.

Overt central nervous system signs are uncommon; however, the occurrence of meningoencephalitis at this stage is associated with a very poor prognosis. Severe myocarditis with arrhythmias and hearing failure can also develop during the acute disease and accounts for most deaths at this stage. Symptoms resolve gradually over a period of weeks to months in untreated patients; however, periocular swelling, lymphadenopathy, and splenomegaly can persist.

Chronic Chagas' disease presents years or decades after the initial infection. Acute infections will progress to chronic disease in 10 to 30% of cases. The heart is most often involved, with signs of arrhythmia, congestive heart failure, and thromboembolism. These arrhythmias may present as episodes of vertigo, syncope, or seizures. The cardiomyopathy primarily affects the right ventricle. Once congestive heart failure develops, death occurs in a matter of months.

The signs and symptoms of megaesophagus are similar to those of idiopathic achalasia, consisting of dysphagia, odynophagia, chest pain, cough, and regurgitation. Aspiration may occur during sleep, and recurrent pneumonia is common. An increased incidence of cancer of the esophagus is reported in patients with chagasic esophageal disease. Megacolon is characterized by chronic constipation and abdominal pain, occasionally complicated by volvulus or perforation.

Reference
Trypanosomiasis, American. Centers for Disease Control Web site. Available at: http://www.dpd.cdc.gov/dpdx/HTML/TrypanosomiasisAmerican.htm. Accessed April 15, 2005.

Further Reading
Barrett MP, Burchmore RJ, Stich A, et al. The trypanosomiases. *Lancet.* 2003;362:1469-1480.

Chagas Disease. Centers for Disease Control Web site. Available at: http://www.cdc.gov/ncidod/dpd/parasites/chagasdisease/default.htm. Accessed April 15, 2005.

Miles MA. The discovery of Chagas disease: progress and prejudice. *Infect Dis Clin North Am.* 2004;18:247-260.

Urbina JA, Docampo R. Specific chemotherapy of Chagas disease: controversies and advances. *Trends Parasitol.* 2003;19:495-501.

Tunga penetrans

Bicho de pe, Chica, Chigger, Chigoe Flea, Jigger, Nigua, Puce-chique, Tu

Agent
Insecta. Siphonaptera (flea), Tungidae: *Tunga penetrans* (sand fleas); *Tunga trimamillata.*

Reservoir
Pigs, dogs, various other mammals

Vector
None

Vehicle
Contact

Geographic Distribution

REGION I—NAm	BMU
REGION II—CAm	BLZ, CRI, GTM, HND, MEX, NIC, PAN, SLV
REGION III—SAm	ARG, BOL, BRA, CHL, COL, ECU, GUY, GUF, PER, PRY, SUR, URY, VEN
REGION IV—Carib	ABW, AIA, ANT, ATG, BHS, BRB, CUB, CYM, DMA, DOM, GLP, GRD, HTI, JAM, KNA, LCA, MSR, MTQ, PRI, TCA, TTO, VCT, VGB, VIR
REGION V—NAfr	MAR
REGION VI—CAfr	BDI, BEN, BFA, CAF, COD, COG, CIV, CMR, COM, ERI, ETH, GAB, GHA, GIN, GMB, GNB, GNQ, KEN, LBR, MDG, MLI, MOZ, MRT, MWI, NER, NGA, RWA, SDN, SEN, SLE, SOM, SYC, TCD, TGO, TZA, UGA, ZMB, ZWE

REGION VII—SAfr   ZAF
REGION X—IndSub   IND, PAK

Incubation Period
8–12d

Diagnostic Tests
Identification of parasite

Typical Therapy
Extraction of parasite

Background

- Tungiasis appears to have originated in Latin America and was inadvertently introduced into Africa by ships during the 1800s. Currently, tungiasis is endemic to Latin America (Mexico to northern Argentina and Chile), the Caribbean and sub-Saharan Africa (Sierra Leone, Ivory Coast, Nigeria, and Ethiopia to South Africa; Zanzibar and Madagascar); however, sporadic cases are also reported in Asia and Oceania. In Mexico and Colombia, the parasite has been encountered at elevations above 2000 m.
- Highest rates are reported among children ages 5 to 10 years, with a male predominance. Acquisition appears to be most common during the dry season.
- The female *T. penetrans* measures 1 mm in length and is adapted for permanent intracutaneous attachment to humans, pigs, cats, dogs, poultry, and other animals. Infection has also been reported in cattle, sheep, goats, horses, rats, mice, birds, elephants, and monkeys. The fertilized female can penetrate any portion of the body (most commonly does so to the feet) and subsequently

swells to resemble a small, white pea—only the posterior spiracles are exposed to air.

- Larvae live freely in dusty or sandy soil. After penetration into the host, the flea undergoes hypertrophy, expels hundreds of eggs over a period of less than 3 weeks, and then dies. Within 10 days of infection, the flea increases its volume by a factor of 2000. Its hindquarters serve for breathing, defecation, and expulsing eggs. The associated skin lesion measures 0.24 to 0.5 mm and serves as an entry point for pathogenic microorganisms.

- A second Tunga species, *Tunga triamillata*, has been described in humans, goats, sheep, cattle, and pigs in Ecuador.

Clinical Presentation

Virtually all infestations are limited to the feet, notably the interdigital and periungual regions. Ectopic infections are occasionally noted on the hands, elbows, thighs, or gluteal region. Irritation begins 8 to 12 days following infection and is manifested as a small pit which evolved into a circular ulcer associated with pain, edema, erythema, and pruritis. Secondary bacterial infection, thrombophlebitis, or even tetanus may follow. Most infestations are characterized by 2 to 3 fleas, although hundreds could be present. Severe disease may be characterized by deep ulcerations, necrosis leading to denudation of underlying bone, and autoamputation of digits. Ectopic infection (hands, elbows, neck, anus, and genitals) is encountered in small children.

Further Reading

http://www.cdfound.to.it/HTML/tunga.htm

Chapter 5: International Organization for Standardization (ISO) Country Codes*

AFG	Afghanistan	BVT	Bouvet Island
ALB	Albania	BRA	Brazil
DZA	Algeria	BRN	Brunei Darussalam
ASM	American Samoa		
AND	Andorra	BGR	Bulgaria
AGO	Angola	BFA	Burkina Faso
AIA	Anguilla	BDI	Burundi
ATG	Antigua and Barbuda	KHM	Cambodia
		CMR	Cameroon
ARG	Argentina	CAN	Canada
ARM	Armenia	ES-CN	Canary Islands
ABW	Aruba	CPV	Cape Verde
AUS	Australia	CYM	Cayman Islands
AUT	Austria	CAF	Central African Republic
AZE	Azerbaijan		
ZO	Azores	TCD	Chad
BHS	Bahamas	CHL	Chile
BHR	Bahrain	CHN	China
BGD	Bangladesh	CXR	Christmas Islands
BRB	Barbados	CCK	Cocos Islands
BLR	Belarus	COL	Colombia
BEL	Belgium	COM	Comoros
BLZ	Belize	COG	Congo
BEN	Benin	COK	Cook Islands
BMU	Bermuda	CRI	Costa Rica
BTN	Bhutan	CIV	Côte d'Ivoire
BOL	Bolivia	HRV	Croatia
BIH	Bosnia and Herzegovena	CUB	Cuba
		CYP	Cyprus
BWA	Botswana	CZE	Czech Republic

---

*For corresponding regions listed in text.

COD	Democratic Republic of the Congo	GUY	Guyana
		HTI	Haiti
		HND	Honduras
DNK	Denmark	HKG	Hong Kong
DJI	Djibouti	HUN	Hungary
DMA	Dominica	ISL	Iceland
DOM	Dominican Republic	IND	India
		IDN	Indonesia
TMP	East Timor	IRN	Iran
ECU	Ecuador	IRQ	Iraq
EGY	Egypt	IRL	Ireland
SLV	El Salvador	IMY	Isle of Man
GNQ	Equatorial Guinea	ISR	Israel
ERI	Eritrea	ITA	Italy
EST	Estonia	JAM	Jamaica
ETH	Ethiopia	JPN	Japan
FLK	Falkland Islands	JOR	Jordan
FRO	Faroe Islands	KAZ	Kazakhstan
FJI	Fiji	KEN	Kenya
FIN	Finland	KIR	Kiribati
FRA	France	PRK	Korea, Democratic People's Republic of
GUF	French Guiana		
PYF	French Polynesia	KOR	Korea, Republic of
GAB	Gabon	KWT	Kuwait
GMB	Gambia	KGZ	Kyrgyzstan
GEO	Georgia	LAO	Lao People's Democratic Republic
DEU	Germany		
GHA	Ghana		
GIB	Gibraltar	LVA	Latvia
GRC	Greece	LBN	Lebanon
GRL	Greenland	LSO	Lesotho
GRD	Grenada	LBR	Liberia
GLP	Guadeloupe	LBY	Libya
GUM	Guam	LIE	Liechtenstein
GTM	Guatemala	LTU	Lithuania
GIN	Guinea	LUX	Luxembourg
GNB	Guinea-Bissau	MAC	Macau

MKD	Macedonia	OMN	Oman
MDG	Madagascar	PAK	Pakistan
MWI	Malawi	PLW	Palau
MYS	Malaysia	PAN	Panama
MDV	Maldives	PNG	Papua New Guinea
MLI	Mali	PRY	Paraguay
MLT	Malta	PER	Peru
MYT	Mamoutzou	PHL	Philippines
MHL	Marshall Islands	PCN	Pitcairn
MTQ	Martinique	POL	Poland
MRT	Mauritania	PRT	Portugal
MUS	Mauritius	PRI	Puerto Rico
MEX	Mexico	QAT	Qatar
FSM	Micronesia, Federated States of	REU	Réunion
		ROM	Romania
MDA	Moldova	RUS	Russian Federation
MCO	Monaco	RWA	Rwanda
MNG	Mongolia	SHN	Saint Helena
MSR	Montserrat	KNA	Saint Kitts-Nevis
MAR	Morocco	LCA	Saint Lucia
MOZ	Mozambique	VCT	Saint Vincent and the Grenadines
MMR	Myanmar		
NAM	Namibia	WSM	Samoa
NRU	Nauru	SMR	San Marino
NPL	Nepal	STP	São Tomé Príncipe
NLD	Netherlands	SAU	Saudi Arabia
ANT	Netherlands Antilles	SCG	Serbia and Montenegro
NCL	New Caledonia		
NZL	New Zealand	SEN	Senegal
NIC	Nicaragua	SYC	Seychelles
NER	Niger	SLE	Sierra Leone
NGA	Nigeria	SGP	Singapore
NIU	Niue	SVK	Slovakia
NFK	Norfolk Island	SVN	Slovenia
MNP	Northern Mariana Islands	SLB	Solomon Islands
		SOM	Somalia
NOR	Norway	ZAF	South Africa

ESP	Spain	TUV	Tuvalu
LKA	Sri Lanka	UGA	Uganda
SDN	Sudan	UKR	Ukraine
SUR	Suriname	ARE	United Arab Emirates
SJM	Svalbard and Jan Mayen		
		GBR	United Kingdom
SWZ	Swaziland	USA	United States
SWE	Sweden	URY	Uruguay
CHE	Switzerland	UZB	Uzbekistan
SYR	Syria	VUT	Vanuatu
TWN	Taiwan	VEN	Venezuela
TJK	Tajikistan	VNM	Vietnam
TZA	Tanzania	VGB	Virgin Islands, British
THA	Thailand		
TGO	Togo	VIR	Virgin Islands, United States
TKL	Tokelau		
TON	Tonga	WLF	Wallis and Futuna Islands
TTO	Trinidad and Tobago		
		ESH	Western Sahara
TUN	Tunisia	YEM	Yemen
TUR	Turkey	YUG	Yugoslavia
TKM	Turkmenistan	ZMB	Zambia
TCA	Turks and Caicos	ZWE	Zimbabwe

All ISO Country Codes by Region

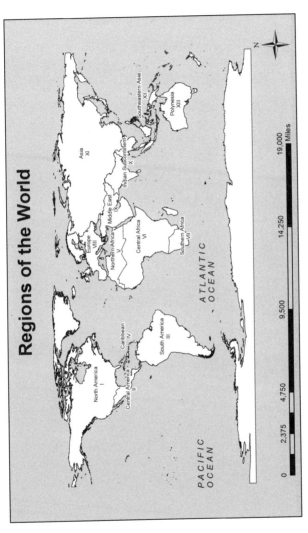

I—NAm   BMU, CAN, USA

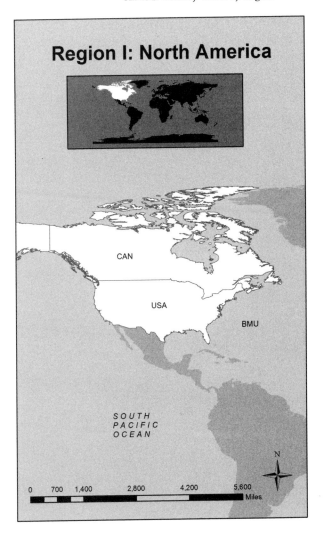

II—CAm   BLZ, CRI, GTM, HND, MEX, NIC, PAN,
          SLV

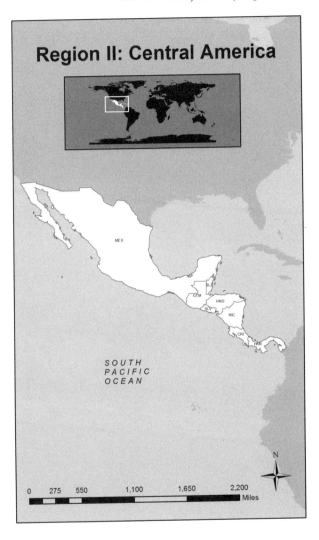

Region II: Central America

III—SAm   ARG, BOL, BRA, CHL, COL, ECU, FLK,
           GUF, GUY, PER, PRY, SUR, URY, VEN

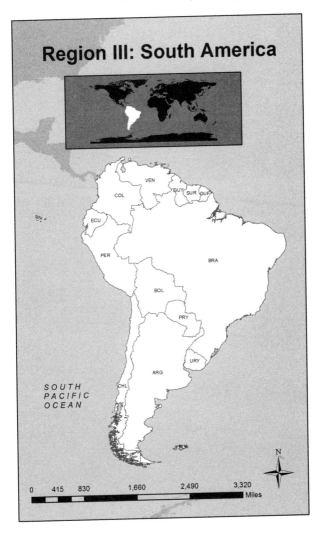

Region III: South America

IV—Carib   ABW, AIA, ANT, ATG, BHS, BRB, CUB,
            CYM, DMA, DOM, GLP, GRD, HTI, JAM,
            KNA, LCA, MSR, MTQ, PRI, TCA, TTO,
            VCT, VGB, VIR

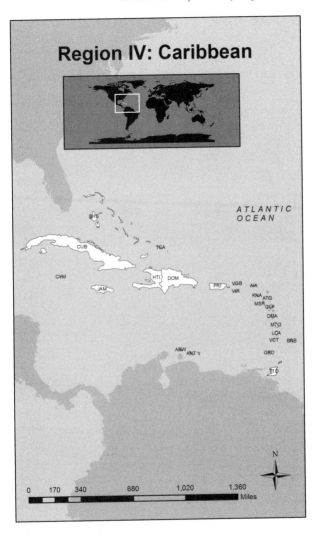

V—NAfr   DZA, EGY, ESH, LBY, MAR, TUN

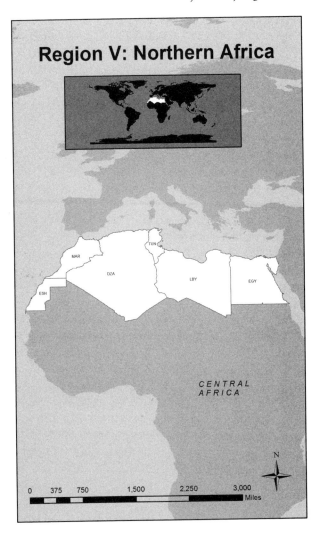

VI—CAfr   AGO, BDI, BEN, BFA, CAF, CIV, CMR,
            COD, COG, COM, CPV, DJI, ERI, ES-CN,
            ETH, GAB, GHA, GIN, GMB, GNB, GNQ,
            KEN, LBR, MDG, MLI, MOZ, MRT, MUS,
            MWI, MYT, NER, NGA, REU, RWA, SDN,
            SEN, SHN, SLE, SOM, STP, SYC, TCD, TGO,
            TZA, UGA, ZMB, ZWE

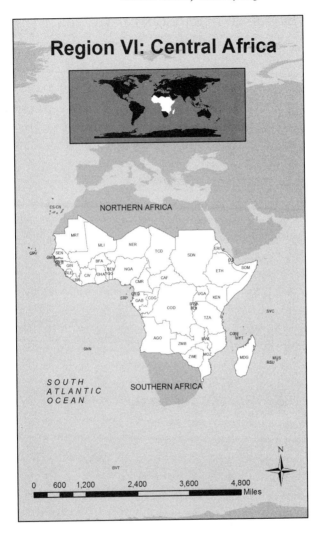

Region VI: Central Africa

VII—SAfr   BVT, BWA, LSO, NAM, SWZ, ZAF

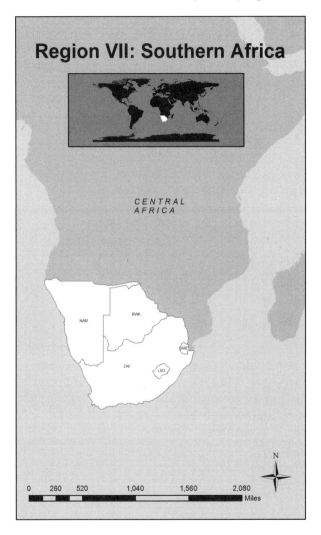

Region VII: Southern Africa

CENTRAL
AFRICA

NAM

BWA

SWZ

ZAF

LSO

N

| 0 | 260 | 520 | 1,040 | 1,560 | 2,080 |
Miles

VIII—Eur   ALB, AND, AUT, BEL, BGR, BIH, BLR,
            CHE, CYP, CZE, DEU, DNK, ESP, EST, FIN,
            FRA, FRO, GBR, GEO, GIB, GRC, GRL,
            HRV, HUN, IMY, IRL, ISL, ITA, LIE, LTU,
            LUX, LVA, MCO, MDA, MKD, MLT, NLD,
            NOR, POL, PRT, ROM, SCG, SJM, SMR,
            SVK, SVN, SWE, UKR, YUG

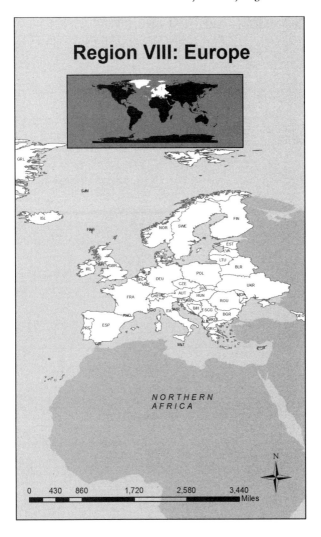

Region VIII: Europe

IX—MidEast   ARE, ARM, BHR, IRN, IRQ, ISR, JOR,
              KWT, LBN, OMN, QAT, SAU, SYR, TUR,
              YEM

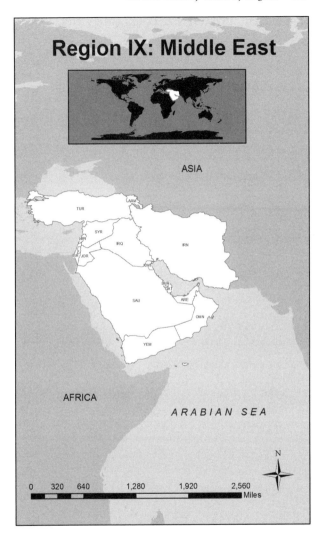

X—IndSub   BGD, BTN, IND, LKA, MDV, NPL, PAK

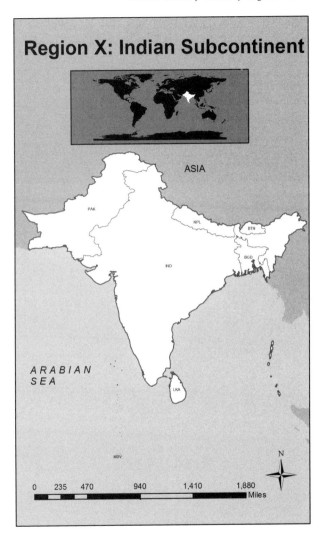

XI—Asia   AFG, AZE, CHN, HKG, JPN, KAZ, KGZ,
KOR, MAC, MNG, PRK, RUS, TJK, TKM,
TWN, UZB

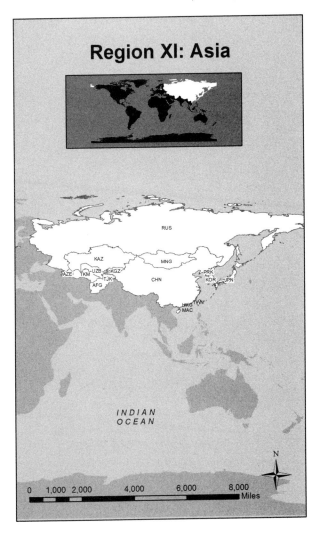

XII—SEA   BRN, CCK, CXR, IDN, KHM, LAO, MMR,
MYS, PHL, PLW, SGP, THA, VNM

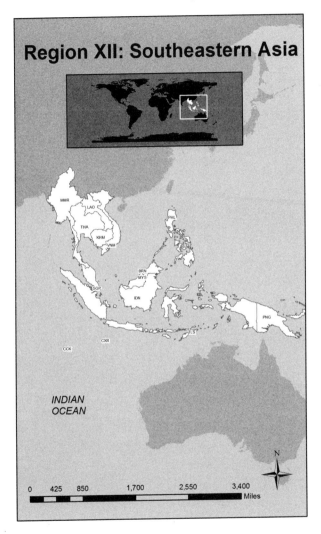

Region XII: Southeastern Asia

XIII—Poly   ASM, AUS, COK, FJI, FSM, GUM, KIR,
             MHL, MNP, NCL, NFK, NIU, NRU, NZL,
             PCN, PNG, PYF, SLB, TKL, TMP, TON,
             TUV, VUT, WLF, WSM

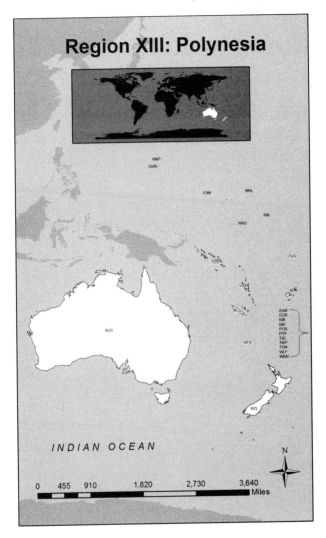

Region XIII: Polynesia

MWP
GUM

FSM   MHL

KIR

NRU

TUV

ASM
COK
KIR
NIU
PCN
PYF
TKL
TMP
TON
WLF
WSM

AUS

NCL

NFK

NZL

INDIAN OCEAN

N

0   455   910   1,820   2,730   3,640
                                              Miles

Chapter 6: Drugs Used in the Treatment of Parasitic Disease

As of 2005, more than 55 generic drugs are marketed for the treatment of parasitic disease. These agents vary widely in therapeutic spectrum, dosage, toxicity, and effectiveness. The reader should note that many of the diseases in this text are self-limited, and few are directly contagious from one human to another. Thus, the need for treatment will often depend on the clinical features of parasitism in the individual patient. In some diseases (eg, echinococcosis, anisakiasis), drug therapy might be supplemented by surgical intervention. As when using any drug, the clinician must be aware of ongoing diseases, allergies, concurrent medications, cost, and potential side effects. In the following lists, an asterisk (*) denotes that a given agent is drug of choice. Lists of trade names are not intended to endorse any given product, and do not include drugs marketed in combination.

Albendazole

Mechanism of Action
A benzimidazole
Binds to free beta tubulin and inhibits tubulin
    polymerization—resultant inhibition of glucose uptake

Typical Adult Dosage
Intestinal nematodes: 400 mg PO single dose
Echinococcosis: 5 to 7 mg/kg PO b.i.d. × 30d

Typical Pediatric Dosage
Intestinal nematodes: 200 mg PO single dose
Echinococcosis: 5 to 7 mg/kg PO b.i.d. × 30d

457

Potential Side Effects

Allergy

Alopecia

Anemia

Constipation

Diarrhea

Headache

Hepatic
   dysfunction/hepatitis

Leukopenia/neutropenia

Nausea/vomiting

Pregnancy—
   contraindicated

Pseudomembranous
   colitis

Vertigo or dizziness

Interactions

- Carbamazapine and phenytoin interact with albendazole (details not given)

- The activity of cimetidine is decreased by albendazole

- Grapefruit juice and praziquantel increase levels of albendazole

Spectrum

Ascaris lumbricoides

Brugia malayi

Brugia timori

Capillaria philippinensis

Clonorchis sinensis

Cutaneous larva migrans

Cysticercosis

Echinococcus granulosus*

Echinococcus
   multilocularis*

Enterobius vermicularis

Fasciolopsis buski

Giardia intestinalis
   (lamblia)

Gnathostoma spinigerum

Hookworm

Opisthorchis

Strongyloides

Taenia saginata

Toxocara

Trichinella spiralis*

Trichostrongylus*

Trichuris trichiura*

Wuchereria bancrofti

Trade Names

Abentel	Adazol	Albatel
ABZ	Alba-3	Alben

Albenda
Albendy
Albenza
Albenzol
Albezole
Alda
Alfazol
Alfuca
Alib
Alin
Alminth
Alzental
Alzol
Amplozol
Anthel
Bendapar
Bendex
Bendex-400
Bentiamin
Bradelmin
Ciclopar
Dabenzol
Dazocan
Dazol
Dazolin
Digezanol
Emanthal
Entoplus
Eskazol
Euralben
Fintel
Gascop
Gendazel
Helben
Helmindazol
Helmintal
Helminzol
Helmisons
Kontil
Labenda
Leo-400
Loveral
Lurdex
Masaworm
Mebenix
Monozol
Mycotel
Nemozole
Paranthil
Parasin
Plus
Rotopar
Tenibex
Thelban
Valbazen
Vemizol
Veranzol
Vericlase
Vermilan
Vermin
Vermisen
Vermital
Vermixide
Zeben
Zelfin
Zenaxin
Zentel
Zenzera
Zoben
Zolben
Zozolex

Amodiaquine
Note: This drug has been largely replaced by chloroquine because of concerns over toxicity.

Mechanism of Action
A 4-aminoquinoline
Interferes with acidification of vacuoles

Typical Adult Dosage
600 mg (base) PO, then 300 mg at 6, 24, and 48h

Typical Pediatric Dosage
10 mg/kg (base) PO, then 5 mg/kg at 24 and 48h

Potential Side Effects

Alopecia

Altered skin or nail color

Cardiac toxicity/conduction disturbance

Diarrhea

Headache

Hearing loss

Hypoglycemia

Leukopenia/neutropenia

Nausea/vomiting

Photosensitivity

Pruritis

Psoriasis—exacerbation reported

Psychosis

Rash

Retinopathy

Thrombocytopenia

Tinnitus

Visual disturbance

Interaction
Quinacrine enhances the toxicity of amodiaquine.

Trade Names
Basoquin
Camoquine
Flavoquine

Spectrum
Plasmodium falciparum (chloroquine-sensitive)
Plasmodium malariae
Plasmodium ovale
Plasmodium vivax

Artemisinin (Qinghaosu)

Mechanism of Action
An endoperoxide sesquiterpene (extracted from *Artimesia annua*).
Acts through free radicals

Alkalates heme-derived or parasite macromolecules
Bonds (covalent) with parasite proteins
Inhibits hematin polymerization

Typical Adult Dosage
Artesunate (po/iv/im); artemether (po/im); artemisinin (po/suppos); artemether (im)—4 mg/kg day 1, 2 mg/kg day 2–3, and 1 mg/kg day 4–7

Typical Pediatric Dosage
3.2 mg/kg i.m., then 1.6 mg/kg i.m. daily—switch when possible to PO and complete 7d therapy

Potential Side Effects
Abdominal pain

Nausea/vomiting

Cardiac arrhythmia

Rash

Diarrhea

Vertigo or dizziness

Fever

Interactions

- Aurothioglucose increases the risk for hematotoxicity from artemisinin (qinghaosu).

- Pyrimethamine levels are increased by artemisinin (qinghaosu).

Spectrum
Plasmodium (all species)

Trade Names
Alaxin

Arteether

Artesunate

Arinate

Artemether

B-Artemether

Arteannuin

Artemotil

Coartem

Artecef

Artenam

E Mal	Gsunate	Larither
(Artemotil)	Gvither	Paluther
Falcigo	Huanghuahaosu	Plasmotrim

Atovaquone

Mechanism of Action
A hydroxynaphthoquinone
Interferes with cytochrome electron transport
(dihydroorotate dehydrogenase) and mitochondrial
membrane potential

Typical Adult Dosage
750 mg PO t.i.d. × 21d

Typical Pediatric Dosage
Weight > 40 kg: as for adult

Potential Side Effects
Abdominal pain
Anemia
Candidiasis
Conjunctivitis
Constipation
Diarrhea
Erythema multiforme
Fever
Headache
Hepatic dysfunction/
  hepatitis
Hypoglycemia
Hyponatremia
Insomnia
Keratopathy
Leukopenia/neutropenia
Nausea/vomiting
Pruritis
Rash
Rhinitis
Vertigo or dizziness

Interactions

- Erythromycin can cause rhabdomyolysis with
  atovaquone.

- Fluconazole, indinavir, itraconazole, and ketoconazole interact with atovaquone (details not given).

- Metoclopramide, rifabutin, rifampin, and ritonavir decrease levels of atovaquone.

- Levels of sulfonamides, trimethoprim, and zidovudine are decreased by atovaquone.

Spectrum
Babesia (in combination)
Plasmodium spp. (in combination)

Trade Names

Acuvel	Metrone
Mepron	Wellvone

Note: Atovaquone is also marketed in fixed combination with proguanil (qv) under the trade names Malarone and Promal. This combination is extremely effective in the treatment and prevention of malaria, including disease caused by drug-resistant strains of *P. falciparum*. The usual adult dosage for prevention is one tablet daily, to be continued for one week after leaving endemic areas. The therapeutic dosage for adults is four tablets daily for 3 days. Toxicity and interactions as per individual components.

Benznidazole

Mechanism of Action
A 2-nitroimidazole (mechanism unknown)

Typical Adult Dosage
5 mg/kg/d PO × 30–60d

Typical Pediatric Dosage
3.75 to 5.0 mg/kg PO b.i.d. × 30–60d

Potential Side Effects

Abdominal pain	Rash
Nausea/vomiting	Seizures
Neuropathy	Somnolence
Photosensitivity	
Pregnancy—contraindicated	

Interactions
None reported

Spectrum
Trypanosoma cruzi (also effective against a variety of anaerobic bacteria)

Trade Names
Radinil
Ragonil
Rochagan

Bephenium Hydroxynaphthoate
Note: This drug has been largely replaced by other drugs.

Mechanism of Action
Unknown

Typical Adult Dosage
2.5 g PO × 1 dose

Typical Pediatric Dosage
2.5 g PO × 1 dose (1.25 g if < age 2y)

Potential Side Effects

Abdominal pain	Headache
Diarrhea	Vertigo

Interactions
None reported

Spectrum
Ascaris lumbricoides
Hookworm
Trichostrongylus

Trade Names
Alcopar
Alcopara
Debefenium

Bithionol

Mechanism of Action
A chlorinated bisphenol
Mechanism unknown
Use (in fascioliasis) has been superceded by
  triclabendazole

Typical Dosage
30 to 50 mg/kg PO alternate days × 10 doses

Potential Side Effects
Abdominal pain	Hepatic	Rash
Diarrhea	dysfunction/	Salivation
Headache	hepatitis	Vertigo or
	Photosensitivity	dizziness

Interactions
None reported

Trade Names
Actamer
Bitin
Lorothidol

Spectrum
Fasciola hepatica
Paragonimus

Chloroquine

Mechanism of Action
A 4-amino quinoline
Competes for degradation of ferriprotoporphyrin IX by
    glutathione—resulting substance possibly interferes
    with vacuole acidification

Typical Adult Dosage
600 mg (base) PO, then 300 mg at 6, 24, and 48h
Prophylaxis = 500 mg/w

Typical Pediatric Dosage
10 mg/kg (base) PO, then 5 mg/kg at 6, 24, and 48h
Prophylaxis = 8.3 mg/kg weekly

Potential Side Effects

Allergy
Alopecia
Altered skin or nail color
Amnesia
Ataxia
Cardiac toxicity/conduction
    disturbance
Confusion
Methemoglobinemia
Myasthenia gravis—
    exacerbation
Nausea/vomiting
Neuropathy
Nystagmus
Photosensitivity
Porphyria—exacerbation

Delusions
Depression
Diarrhea
G6PD-related hemolysis
Hallucinations
Headache
Hearing loss
Hyperpigmentation
Hypoglycemia
Hypopigmentation
Leukopenia/neutropenia
Mania
Pruritis
Psoriasis—exacerbation reported
Rash
Retinopathy
Stevens-Johnson syndrome
Thrombocytopenia
Tinnitus
Toxic epidermal necrolysis
Visual disturbance

Interactions

- Ampicillin absorption is decreased by chloroquine.

- Antacids, famotidine, kaolin preparations, ranitidine, and roxatidine reduce absorption of chloroquine.

- Aurothioglucose increases the risk for hematotoxicity from chloroquine.

- Botulinum toxin A (Botox) and levothyroxine activities are decreased by chloroquine.

- Cholestyramine decreases levels of chloroquine.

- Cimetidine increases levels of chloroquine.

- Cyclosporine, penicillamine, and praziquantel levels are increased by chloroquine.

- Digoxin and fluoxetine increase the risk for arrhythmias with chloroquine.

- Diltiazem interacts with chloroquine (details not available).

- Mefloquine and quinacrine enhance the toxicity of chloroquine.

- Methotrexate levels are decreased by chloroquine.

- Neuromuscular blockers increase the risk for neurotoxicity from chloroquine.

Spectrum

Clonorchis sinensis
Entamoeba histolytica
Giardia intestinalis (lamblia)
Paragonimus
Plasmodium falciparum,
  chloroquine sensitive*
Plasmodium malariae*
Plasmodium ovale*
Plasmodium vivax*

Trade Names

Anoclor	Diroquine	Novo-
Aralen	Emquin	Chloroquine
Arthrabas	Genocin	Paluken
Avloclor	Heliopar	Palux
Cadiquin	Klorokin	Pharmaquine
Chlorochin	Klorokinfosfat	Plasmoquine
Chlorofoz	Lagaquin	Promal
Chloroquini	Lariago	P-Roquine
Diphosphas	Malaquin	Quinalen
Chlorquin	Malarex	Repal
Cidanchin	Malaviron	Reso
Clo-Kit Junior	Maquine	Resochin
Daramal	Melubrin	Resochina
Delagil	Mexaquin	Resochine
Dichinalex	Mirquin	Syncoquin
Difosquin	Nivaquine	Weimerquin
Dilex		

Dehydroemetine and Emetine

Note: These drugs are rarely used because of concerns over cardiac toxicity.

Mechanism of Action
An alkaloid derived from ipecacuanha
Possible effect on nucleus and endoplasmic reticulum

Typical Adult Dosage
1 to 1.5 mg/kg i.m. daily × 5d

Typical Pediatric Dosage
0.5 to 0.75 mg/kg i.m. q12h × 5d

Potential Side Effects

Cardiac toxicity	Myocarditis	Rash
Diarrhea	Nausea/	Vertigo or
Headache	vomiting	dizziness
Myalgia or	Neuropathy	
myopathy		

Interactions
None reported

Spectrum

Balantidium coli	*Entamoeba*	*Fasciola hepatica*
Blastocystis	*histolytica*	*Paragonimus*
hominis		

Trade Names
Supplied as generic drugs

Diethylcarbamazine Citrate

Mechanism of Action
A piperazine derivative
Paralysis and membrane damage
Unmasks worm antigens to host immunity
Kills adults (lymphatic parasites)
Immobilizes microfilariae (nonlymphatic species)

Typical Adult Dosage
50 mg PO on day 1, 50 mg PO t.i.d. on day 2, 100 mg PO t.i.d. on day 3, 6 mg/kg PO t.i.d. on days 4–21

Typical Pediatric Dosage
1 mg/kg PO on day 1, 1 mg/kg PO t.i.d. on day 2, 1 to 2 mg/kg PO t.i.d. on day 3, 3 mg/kg PO t.i.d. on days 4–21

Potential Side Effects
Allergy
Arthralgia or
  arthritis
Fever
Headache
Lymph-
  adenopathy

Myalgia or
  myopathy
Nausea/
  vomiting
Optic neuritis or
  atrophy
Proteinuria

Somnolence
Vertigo or
  dizziness

Interactions
None described

Spectrum
Balantidium coli
Brugia malayi
Brugia timori
*Loa loa**

*Mansonella
  perstans*
*Mansonella
  streptocerca**

*Onchocerca
  volvulus*
Toxocara
*Wuchereria
  bancrofti*

Trade Names

Banocide	Helmazan (with	Pec-Dec
Diethizine	Piperazine)	Unicarbazam
Filarcidan	Hetrazan	
Filardidin	Notezine	

Diiodohydroxyquin

Mechanism of Action
A halogenated hydroxyquinoline
Chelates ferrous ions essential for metabolism

Typical Adult Dosage
650 mg PO t.i.d. × 20d

Typical Pediatric Dosage
10 mg/kg PO t.i.d. × 20d

Potential Side Effects

Abdominal pain	Nausea/vomiting	Paresthesia
Allergy	Neuropathy	Rash
Diarrhea	Optic neuritis or	
Headache	atrophy	

Interactions
Zalcitabine (ddC) increases the risk for neurotoxicity from diiodohydroxyquin.

Spectrum

Balantidium coli	*Entamoeba histolytica*
Blastocystis hominis	*Giardia intestinalis (lamblia)*
*Dientamoeba fragilis**	

Trade Names

Amabagyl
Antidifar
Carsuquin
Collila
Depofin
Diameb
Diodolina
Diodoquin
Direxiode
Diyomex

Diyosul
Diyowil
Drioquilen
Dysetrin
Entero-Diyod
Entodiba
Facetin-D
Farmeban
Flanoquin
Floraquin

Iodoquinol
Ovoquinol
Sebaquin
Threchop
   (Furazolidone)
Vytone
Yodoxin
Yopin

Diloxanide Furoate

Mechanism of Action
A dichloroacetamide derivative
Possibly inhibits protein synthesis

Typical Adult Dosage
500 mg PO t.i.d. × 10d

Typical Pediatric Dosage
7 mg/kg PO t.i.d. × 10d (maximum daily dose: 1.5 grams)

Potential Side Effects
Abdominal pain
Breast-feeding—
   contraindication
Diarrhea

Nausea/vomiting
Pruritis
Rash

Interactions
None reported

Spectrum
Entamoeba histolytica
Entamoeba polecki

Trade Names
Furamid
Furamide

Eflornithine

Mechanism of Action
Alpha difluoromethylornithine HCL
Inhibits polyamine synthesis (ornithine decarboxylase)
    and cell differentiation.

Typical Adult Dosage
100 mg/kg PO or i.v. q.i.d. $\times$ 10d

Typical Pediatric Dosage
Not established

Potential Side Effects

Alopecia	Hepatic	Thrombo-
Anemia	dysfunction	cytopenia
Diarrhea	Neutropenia	
Headache	Seizures	

Interactions
None reported

Spectrum
This drug is also used against Pneumocystis jerovici (a
    fungus).
Trypanosoma brucei gambiense

Trade Names
DFMO
Ornidyl
Vaniqa

Flubendazole

Mechanism of Action
A benzimidazole
Inhibits glucose uptake and possibly affects microtubule
   formation

Typical Dosage
100 mg PO $\times$ 1 to 3 doses

Potential Side Effects

Abdominal pain	Leukopenia/	Vertigo or
Allergy	neutropenia	dizziness
Alopecia	Nausea/vomiting	
Anemia	Pregnancy—	
Diarrhea	contra-	
Headache	indicated	

Interactions

- Amiodarone, astemizole, cisapride, phenothiazines, and procainamide increase the risk for arrhythmias with flubendazole.

- Carbamazapine increases metabolism/clearance of flubendazole.

- Cyclosporine could be more toxic when combined with flubendazole.

- Phenytoin interacts with flubendazole (details not given).

Spectrum

Ascaris lumbricoides	*Enterobius vermicularis*	*Trichuris trichiura*
Cysticercosis	Hookworm	
Echinococcus granulosus	*Onchocerca volvulus*	

Trade Names

Flicum
Fluvermal
Teniverme

Furazolidone

Note: Furazolidone's use is limited to treatment of giardiasis and bacterial diarrhea.

Mechanism of Action

A nitrofuran (mechanism unknown)

Typical Adult Dosage

100 mg PO q.i.d. × 10d

Typical Pediatric Dosage

Age > 1 month: 1.25 mg/kg PO q.i.d. × 10d

Potential Side Effects

Allergy	G6PD-related hemolysis	Serum sickness
Breast-feeding—contraindication	Hypoglycemia	Somnolence
Erythema multiforme	Pulmonary infiltrate	Urine discoloration
	Rash	Vertigo or dizziness

Interactions

- Alcohol can produce a disulfiram reaction with furazolidone.

- Citalopram, escitalopram, and sertraline enhance the toxicity of furazolidone.

- Levodopa can be more toxic when combined with furazolidone.

- MAO inhibitors, opiates, tricyclic antidepressants, and tyramine can produce hypertensive crisis with furazolidone.

Spectrum

Note: This drug is also effective against a variety of gram-negative bacterial species.

Blastocystis hominis	*Giardia intestinalis (lamblia)*	*Trichomonas*

Trade Names

Atapec	Enterobion	Fuzotyl
Attafur	Enterolidon	Giarlam
Caopecfar	Exofur	Lisquinol
Coccila	Furasian	Lomofen
Colestase	Furazolin	Magnostase
Coralzul	Furazolon	Med-Kafuzone
Dialgin	Furion	Neo-Kap
Dibapec	Furopectin	Nifuran
Compuesto	Furoxane	Novafur
Difuran	Furoxona	Optazol
Di-Su-Frone	Furoxone	Plasmocolit
Emantid	Fuxol	Salmocide

Seforman   Suspectim   Trilor
Seleton   Tratocoli   Yodozona
Solfurol   Tricofur

Halofantrine
Note: Fatal cardiac arrhythmias have been associated with use of this drug.

Mechanism of Action
9 phenanthrenemethanol.
Possibly complexes with ferriprotoporphyrin IX.
    Resulting substance toxic to cell membranes.

Typical Adult Dosage
500 mg PO Q6h $\times$ 3 doses; not to exceed 24 mg/kg/d

Typical Pediatric Dosage
Weight $<$ 40 kg: 8 mg/kg PO at 0, 6, and 12h
Weight $>$ 40 kg: 500 mg PO at 0, 6, and 12h

Potential Side Effects
Abdominal pain
Cardiac toxicity/
    conduction
    disturbance
Diarrhea
Hemolysis
Hepatic
    dysfunction/
    hepatitis
Myalgia or
    myopathy
Pregnancy—
    contra-
    indicated
Pruritis
Psychosis
Rash
Seizures
Torsade de
    points/
    prolonged QT
    interval

Interactions
The following drugs could increase the risk for arrhythmias with halofantrine:

Adenosine
Ajmaline
Amiodarone
Amisulpride
Amoxapine
Aprindine
Arsenic trioxide
Astemizole
Aurothioglucose
Azimilide
Bepridil
Bretylium
Chloral hydrate
Chlorpromazine
Cisapride
Colchicine
Dibenzepin
Droperidol
Enflurane
Erythromycin
Fluoxetine
Gatifloxacin
Hydroquinidine
Isoflurane
Lidoflazine
Mefloquine
Mesoridazine
Moxifloxacin
Nortriptyline
Octreotide
Perphenazine
Phenothiazine(s)
Prajmaline
Probucol
Prochlorperazine
Protriptyline
Quinidine
Sematilide
Sertindole
Sotalol
Sultopride
Tedisamil
Terfenadine
Thioridazine
Tricyclic
   antidepres-
   sant(s)
Trifluoperazine
Trimipramine
Vasopressin
Zolmitriptan

Spectrum
Plasmodium (all species, including resistant strains)

Trade Name
Halfan

Hydroxychloroquine

Mechanism of Action
A 4-aminoquinoline.
Competes for degradation of ferriprotoporphyrin IX by
   glutathione. The resulting substance possibly
   interferes with vacuole acidification.

Typical Adult Dosage
800 PO; then 400 mg at 6, 24, and 48h
Prophylaxis = 400 mg/w

Typical Pediatric Dosage

13 mg/kg (base) PO; then 6.5 mg/kg at 6, 24, and 48h
Prophylaxis = 6.5 mg/kg/w

Potential Side Effects

Allergy
Alopecia
Altered skin or
nail color
Amnesia
Ataxia
Cardiac toxicity/
conduction
disturbance
Confusion
Delusions
Depression
Diarrhea
G6PD-related
hemolysis

Hallucinations
Headache
Hearing loss
Hypoglycemia
Leukopenia/
neutropenia
Mania
Methemoglo-
binemia
Nausea/vomiting
Neuropathy
Photosensitivity
Porphyria—
exacerbation
Pruritis

Psoriasis—
exacerbation
reported
Rash
Retinopathy
Stevens-Johnson
syndrome
Thrombo-
cytopenia
Tinnitus
Visual
disturbance

Interactions

- Antacids, famotidine, kaolin preparations, ranitidine,
  and roxatidine reduce absorption of
  hydroxychloroquine.

- Aurothioglucose increases the risk for hematotoxicity
  from hydroxychloroquine.

- Cimetidine increases levels of hydroxychloroquine.

- Digoxin increases the risk for arrhythmias with
  hydroxychloroquine.

- Mefloquine and quinacrine enhance the potential for
  toxicity of hydroxychloroquine.

Spectrum

Plasmodium falciparum,
   chloroquine sensitive
Plasmodium malariae

Plasmodium ovale
Plasmodium vivax

Trade Names

Apo- Hydroxyquine	Haloxin Oxiklorin	Quineprox Toremonil
Dimard	Plaquenil	Yuma
Ercoquin	Plaquinol	
Geniquin	Quensyl	

Ivermectin

Mechanism of Action

Macrocyclic lactones (avermectins)
Derived from *Streptomyces avermitilis*
Paralysis of parasite
Affects GABA and GluCl channels
Inhibits development and release of microfilariae from
   parasite uterus

Typical Adult Dosage

200 mcg/kg PO $\times$ 1

Typical Pediatric Dosage

Safety and efficacy < 15 kg have not been established.

Potential Side Effects

Abdominal pain	Conjunctivitis	Myalgia or
Breast-feeding—	Constipation	myopathy
contraindi-	Fever	Optic neuritis or
cation	Headache	atrophy
Coagulopathy		

Pregnancy—
    contraindi-
    cated

Pruritis
Rash
Tremor

Vertigo or
    dizziness

Interactions
None reported

Spectrum

*Ascaris
    lumbricoides*
*Brugia malayi**
*Brugia timori**
Cutaneous larva
    migrans**
*Enterobius
    vermicularis*

Loa loa
*Mansonella
    ozzardi**
*Mansonella
    streptocerca*
*Onchocerca
    volvulus**
Scabies

Strongyloides
*Trichuris
    trichiura*
*Wuchereria
    bancrofti**

Trade Names
Mectizan
Revectina
Stromectol

Levamisole
Note: This drug is no longer available.

Mechanism of Action
Active levo-isomer of tetramisole
Acts through muscular paralysis of parasite

Typical Adult Dosage
120 to 150 mg PO $\times$ 1

Typical Pediatric Dosage
3 mg/kg PO $\times$ 1

Potential Side Effects

Abdominal pain	Fever	Tremor
Alopecia	Headache	Vertigo or
Arthralgia or	Leukopenia/	dizziness
arthritis	neutropenia	Visual
Ataxia	Nausea/vomiting	disturbance
Conjunctivitis	Proteinuria	
Dysgeusia	Seizures	

Interactions

- Alcohol can produce a disulfiram reaction with levamisole.

- Fluorouracil increases the risk for hepatotoxicity from levamisole.

- Phenytoin levels are increased by levamisole.

- Rifampin decreases levels of levamisole.

- Warfarin activity is increased by levamisole.

Spectrum

Ascaris lumbricoides	*Strongyloides*
Enterobius vermicularis	*Trichostrongylus*
Hookworm	*Trichuris trichiura*

Trade Names

Ascaridil	Dewormis	Solaskil
Ascaryl	Ergamisol	Vermisol
Decaris	Immunol	Vizole
Decas	Ketrax	
Detrax 40	Newkentax	

Lumefantrine/Artemether

Mechanism of Action
Synthetic racemic fluorene artemether
Dichlorobenzylidine schizonticide (action as for
   halofantrine artimesinin)

Typical Adult Dosage
Artemether 80 mg/lumefantrine 480 mg PO at 0, 8, 24,
36, 48, and 60h

Typical Pediatric Dosage
Weight < 15 kg: 1/4 adult dose
Weight 15 to 25 kg: 1/2 adult dose
Weight 25 to 35 kg: 3/4 adult dose
Weight > 35 kg: adult dose

Potential Side Effects

Abdominal pain	Insomnia	Rash
Anemia	Nausea/	Tremor
Diarrhea	vomiting	Vertigo or
Headache	Nystagmus	dizziness
Hemolysis	Pruritis	

Interactions

- Aurothioglucose increases the risk for hematotoxicity
  from lumefantrine/artemether.

- Droperidol and quinine increase the risk for
  arrhythmias with lumefantrine/artemether.

- Mefloquine decreases levels of
  lumefantrine/artemether.

Spectrum
Plasmodium (all species, including resistant strains)

Trade Names

Benflumelol	Coartem	Riamet
Benflumetol	Co-Artemether	

Mebendazole

Mechanism of Action
A benzimidazole
Binds to free beta tubulin and inhibits tubulin
   polymerization—resultant inhibition of glucose
   uptake

Typical Adult Dosage
100 mg PO $\times$ 1 for 1–3d

Typical Pediatric Dosage
Age $\geq$ 2 years: As for adult

Potential Side Effects

Abdominal pain	Headache	Nausea/vomiting
Allergy	Hepatic	Pregnancy—
Alopecia	dysfunction/	contraindi-
Anemia	hepatitis	cated
Constipation	Leukopenia/	Vertigo or
Diarrhea	neutropenia	dizziness

Interactions

- Carbamazapine and phenytoin increase
  metabolism/clearance of mebendazole.

- Cimetidine increases levels of mebendazole.

- Insulin dosage requirement might be altered by mebendazole.

Spectrum

*Angiostrongylus cantonensis**
Ascaris lumbricoides
Capillaria philippinensis
Dracunculus medinensis
Echinococcus granulosus
Echinococcus multilocularis
Enterobius vermicularis
Gnathostoma spinigerum
Hookworm
Loa loa
Mansonella perstans
Onchocerca volvulus
Strongyloides
Taenia saginata
Taenia solium
Toxocara
Trichinella spiralis
Trichomonas
Trichostrongylus
Trichuris trichiura

Trade Names

Amycil
Anelmin
Anhelmin
Anthex
Antiox
Ascariobel
Ascaritor
Ascarobex
Athelmin
Averpan
Bantenol
Belmirax
Benda
Bendosan
Bendrax
Bensolmin
Bepmokc
Bestelar
Bivalem
Carbatil
Certovermil
Cessaverm
Chemist's Own De Worm
Cipex
Combantrin-1
Conquer
Daben
Damaben
Diazolen
Divermil
Drivermide
D-Worm
Elmetin
Eraverm
Exaverm
Exbenzol
Exelmin
Exteny
Fanciadazol
Feller
Flenverme
Forverm
Fugacar
Gamax
Geophagol
Gran-Verm
Hedazol

Helmib
Helmiben
Helmidrax
Helminzole
Helmio-Ped
Helmizil
Ibdazol
Idibend
Kaizole
Kindelmin
Lomper
Lumbicid
Madicure
Marben
Masaworm-1
M-Bentabs
Meba
Meban
Mebandozer
Mebasol
Mebeciclol
Mebelmin
Meben
Mebendan
Mebenda-P
Mebendazotil
Mebendil
Mebenlax
Mebensole
Mebentiasis
Mebentine
Mebentral
Mebex
Meb-Overoid
Mebzol
Mediazole

Meforasol
Mindol
Mizolmex
Moben
Necamin
Nemapres
Neovermin
Novelmin
Noverme
Noxworm
Octelmin
Ovex
Oxitover
Oxizole
Panfugan
Pantelmin
Panvermin
Paracicar
Paranzol
Paraverm
Parelmin
Penalcol
Petazole
Pharaxis
Pluriverm
Pluvivermil
Poliben
Poltelmin
Pripsen
Prodazol
Profenzol
Profium
Prohelmin
Propsen
Quemox
Quintelmin

Revapol
Sirben
Soltric
Sqworm
Sufil
Sulfil
Surfont
Tetrahelmin
Thelmox
Toloxim
Vagaka
Vermepen
Vermicidin
Vermicol
Vermin-Dazol
Vermirax
Vermol
Vermonon
Vermoplex
Vermoral
Vermoran
Vermorex
Vermox
Vertex
Vertizole
Virmidil
Warca
Wormgo
Wormin
Wormstop
Zadomen
Zakor
Zoles
Zol-Triq
Zumin

Mefloquine
Note: Contraindicated in patients with a history of seizures or neuropsychiatric disorders.

Mechanism of Action
A methanoquinoline
Possibly, formation of toxic complex with
　ferriprotoporphyrin IX

Typical Adult Dosage
750 mg PO; additional 500 mg after 6h
Prophylaxis = 250 mg weekly, continue for 4w after
　exposure ends

Typical Pediatric Dosage
Therapy: 25 mg/kg PO as single dose
Prophylaxis:
Weight 15 to 20 kg: 1/4 tab
Weight 20 to 30 kg: 1/2 tab
Weight 30 to 45 kg: 3/4 tab

Potential Side Effects

Alopecia
Cholestasis or
　cholelithiasis
Conduction
　disturbance
Confusion
Depression
Diarrhea
Encephalitis/
　opathy
Hallucinations
Headache
Hepatic
　dysfunction
Hepatitis
Insomnia
Lymph-
　adenopathy
Nausea/vomiting
Pruritis
Psychosis
Rash
Seizures
Stevens-Johnson
　syndrome
Toxic epidermal
　necrolysis
Vertigo or
　dizziness
Visual
　disturbance

Interactions

- Ampicillin increases levels of mefloquine.

- Aurothioglucose increases the risk for hematotoxicity from mefloquine.

- Chloroquine, hydroxychloroquine, quinacrine and quinine enhance the toxicity of mefloquine.

- Lumefantrine/artemether levels are decreased by mefloquine.

- Rifampin decreases levels of mefloquine.

- Valproic acid can cause seizures with mefloquine.

The following drugs can increase the risk for arrhythmias with mefloquine:

Acecainide	Colchicine	Probucol
Adenosine	Dibenzepin	Prochlorperazine
Ajmaline	Droperidol	Propanolol
Amisulpride	Enflurane	Protriptyline
Amoxapine	Erythromycin	Quinidine
Aprindine	Fluoxetine	Sematilide
Arsenic trioxide	Gatifloxacin	Sertindole
Azimilide	Halofantrine	Sotalol
Beta-adrenergic	Hydroquinidine	Sultopride
blocker(s)	Isoflurane	Tedisamil
Bretylium	Lidoflazine	Trifluoperazine
Calcium channel	Mesoridazine	Vasopressin
blocker(s)	Moxifloxacin	Zolmitriptan
Chloral hydrate	Octreotide	
Chlorpromazine	Prajmaline	

Spectrum

Plasmodium (all species)

Trade Names

Apo-Mefloquine	Laricam	Mephaquin
Lariam	Mefliam	Mephaquine
Lariamar	Meflotas	Mequin

Melarsoprol

Note: Fatal side effects are reported in 4 to 12% of patients.

Mechanism of Action
A trivalent arsenical
Binds to trypanothione
Inhibits pyruvate kinase and possibly other enzymes

Typical Adult Dosage
2.5 mg/kg/d i.v. $\times$ 3; increase to 3.6 mg/kg/d $\times$ 3 after 7d

Typical Pediatric Dosage
0.36 mg/kg i.v.; increasing to 3.6 mg/kg/d i.v. $\times$ 10

Potential Side Effects

Allergy
Cardiac arrhythmia
Cardiac toxicity/ conduction disturbance
Cerebral edema
Confusion
Conjunctivitis
Diarrhea
Encephalitis or encephalopathy
Fever
G6PD-related hemolysis
Guillain-Barré syndrome
Headache
Hepatic dysfunction
Hyponatremia
Nausea/vomiting
Neuropathy
Proteinuria
Pruritis
Rash
Seizures
Somnolence
Tremor

Interactions
None reported

Spectrum
Trypanosoma brucei gambiense
Trypanosoma brucei rhodesiense

Trade Names
Arsobal
Mel B

Metrifonate
Note: Metrifonate has been largely replaced by praziquantel.

Mechanism of Action
An organophosphorus compound
Converted in vivo to an active metabolite, dichlorvos
Inhibits parasite cholinesterase

Typical Dosage
7.5 mg/kg PO every 2w × 3

Potential Side Effects

Abdominal pain	Pregnancy contraindicated
Diarrhea	Somnolence
Headache	Tremor
Nausea/vomiting	Vertigo or dizziness

Interaction
Neuromuscular blockers can be more toxic when combined with metrifonate.

Spectrum

Cysticercosis	*Schistosoma haematobium*

Trade Name
Bilarcil

Metronidazole

Mechanism of Action
A 5-nitroimidazole derivative
Activated in vivo by cellular pyruvate: ferredoxin
   oxidoreductase
Resultant compound interferes with electron transport
   in metabolic pathways

Typical Adult Dosage
500 to 750 mg PO t.i.d. or b.i.d.
500 mg i.v. q6h

Typical Pediatric Dosage
Newborn < 2000 g: 7.5 mg/kg i.v. q24h
Newborn > 2000 g: 7.5 mg/kg PO/i.v. q12h
Age 8–28d: 15 mg/kg PO/i.v. q12h
Age > 28d: 5 to 15 mg/kg PO/i.v. q8h

Potential Side Effects
Allergy
Anemia
Breast-feeding—
   contraindi-
   cation
Depression
Diarrhea
Dysgeusia
Gynecomastia
Hallucinations
Headache
Hepatic

dysfunction/
   hepatitis
Hyperpig-
   mentation
Leukopenia/
   neutropenia
Metallic
   phantogeusia
Nausea/vomiting
Neuropathy
Pancreatitis
Paresthesia

Porphyria—
   exacerbation
Pregnancy—
   contraindi-
   cated
Pruritis
Pseudomem-
   branous colitis
Pulmonary
   infiltrate
Rash
Seizures

Skin discoloration	Thrombo-cytopenia	Vertigo or dizziness
Somnolence	Urine discoloration	
Stomatitis		

Interactions

- Alcohol and sulfa-trimethoprim can produce a disulfiram reaction with metronidazole.

- Anisindione increases the risk for bleeding with metronidazole.

- Astemizole and terfenadine increase the risk for arrhythmias with metronidazole.

- Azathioprine increases the risk for hematotoxicity from metronidazole.

- Barbiturates and phenytoin increase metabolism/clearance of metronidazole.

- Carbamazapine levels are increased by metronidazole.

- Cimetidine increases levels of metronidazole.

- Cyclosporine and lithium might be more toxic when combined with metronidazole.

- Disulfiram exhibits enhanced CNS effects with metronidazole.

- Fluorouracil enhances the toxicity of metronidazole.

- Oral contraceptive activity is decreased by metronidazole.

- Tacrolimus can be more toxic when combined with metronidazole.

- Warfarin activity is increased by metronidazole.

• Zalcitabine (ddC) increases the risk for neurotoxicity from metronidazole.

Spectrum

Note: A wide variety of anaerobic bacteria are susceptible to metronidazole.

Balantidium coli
Dracunculus medinensis
*Entamoeba histolytica**
Entamoeba polecki

Giardia intestinalis
*(lamblia)**
*Trichomonas**

Trade Names

Abbonidazole	Aristogyl	Fagizol
Acromona	Asiazole	Fartricon
Acsacea	Asuzol	Flagenol
Acuzole	Bemetrazole	Flaginazol
Ambral	Berazol	Flagizole
Ameblin	Biogyl	Flagyl
Amevan	Biomona	Flasinyl
Amiyodazol	Biotazol	Flazol
Amotein	Camezol	Fossyol
Anabact	Clont	Fresenizol
Anaerobex	Cryozol	Frotin
Anaerobyl	Dasmetrol	Fungimax
Anaeromet	Dasolin	Fusanidazol
Anayodil	Debetrol	Gineflavir
Anerobia	Deflamon	Ginestatin
Antral	Dumozol	Ginovagin
Apo-	Dynametron	Gynoplix
Metronidazole	Elyzol	Hemestal
Arcazol	Endazole	Infectoclont
Arilin	Epaq	Juaflor
Ariline		

Klion
Klont
Labitrix
Lagyl
Lagylan
Lamblit
Meclon
Medamet
Medazol
Medazyl
Medizol
Med-Tricocide
Mefiron
Menisole
Mepagyl
Meredazol
Meronidal
Mesolex
Metagyl
Metarsal
Metizol
Metole
Metrazol
Metric
Metricom
Metrizol
Metro
Metrocide
Metrogel
Metrolag
Metrolex
Metrolyl
Metromeba
Metromidol

Metronib
Metronid
Metronide
Metronix
Metronour
Metront
Metrosa
Metroson
Metrostat
Metrotop
Metroxyn
Metrozin
Metrozine
Metrozol
Metryl
Mibazol
Milanidazole
MND
Monasin
Monizole
Nabact
Nalox
Narobic
Negazole
Neo-Metric
Niacel
Nida
Nidatron
Nidazol
Nidazolem
Nidralon
Nitromidager
Nitrozol
Nizole

Noritate
Nor-Metrogel
Norzol
Novazole
Novo-Nidazol
Oecozol
Ortrizol
Otrozole
Perilox
Periodontil
Pernyzol
Pharmaflex
Planizol
Profargil
Proflag
Promibasol
Protogyl
Protostat
Protozol
Prozolin
Ranigyl
Rathimed
Retofar
Rhodogil
Rivozol
Robaz
Rodermil
Rodogyl
Rosaced
Rosalox
Rosased
Rosiced
Rozagel
Rozex

Salmonil
Sarcoton
Satric
Sawagyl
Selegil
Servizol
Sharizole
Solumidazol
Supplin
Takimetol
Trichazole
Trichex
Tricho Cordes
Trichonazole
Trichozol
Tricowas B
Trikacide
Trikozol
Trisdazol
Trizele
Trofonil
Ulcolind Metro
Unigo
Unimezol
Urometron
Vagi Biotic
Vagilen
Vagimax
Vagimid
Vaginyl
Valpar
Vatrix-S
Venogyl
Vertisal
Zadstat
Zagyl
Zidoval
Zobacide
Zolerol
Zyomet

Miltefosine

Mechanism of Action
A phosphocholine analogue.
Antitumor agent which could affect lipid remodeling, membrane synthesis and cell signaling pathways.
Cell apoptosis induced by proteases could also be involved.

Typical Adult Dosage
50 to 150 mg PO daily $\times$ 4–6w
Or 100 to 150 mg PO daily $\times$ 28d

Typical Pediatric Dosage
Ages 2 to 12: 1.5 to 2.5 mg/kg PO daily $\times$ 28d

Potential Side Effects
Constipation
Diarrhea
Hepatic
   dysfunction
Leukocytosis
Nausea/vomiting

Pregnancy—
   contraindi-
   cated
Pruritis

Rash
Renal toxicity/
   dysfunction
Retinopathy

Thrombocytosis

Interactions
None reported

Spectrum
Leishmaniasis—*visceral*

Trade Names
Hexadecylphosphocholine
Impavido
Miltefosin
Miltefosina
Miltefosinum
Miltex

Niclosamide
Note: This drug is no longer manufactured.

Mechanism of Action
A nitrosalicylanilide
Interferes with respiration and glucose uptake
Blocks ATP production

Typical Adult Dosage
1 g PO $\times$ 2

Typical Pediatric Dosage
Weight 11 to 34 kg: 2 tabs (1 g)
Weight > 34 kg: 3 tabs (1.5 g)

Potential Side Effects
Alopecia
Nausea/vomiting

Pruritis
Rash

Interactions
None reported

Spectrum
Diphyllobothrium latum
Dipylidium caninum
Fasciolopsis buski

Hymenolepis diminuta
Hymenolepis nana

Taenia saginata
Taenia solium

Trade Names
Atenase
Kontal
Niclocide
Niclosan

Overoid
Telmitin
Tredemine
Unicide

Yomesan
Yomesane
Zenda

Nifurtimox

Mechanism of Action
A nitrofuran derivative
Generates hydrogen peroxide and active radicals
Produces breaks in DNA

Typical Adult Dosage
2 mg/kg PO q.i.d. $\times$ 120d

Typical Pediatric Dosage
Age 1–10y: 4 to 5 mg/kg PO q.i.d. $\times$ 90d
Age 11–16y: 3 to 4 mg/kg PO q.i.d. $\times$ 90d

Potential Side Effects

Abdominal pain
Arthralgia or
   arthritis
G6PD-hemolysis
Headache
Hepatic
   dysfunction
Insomnia

Myalgia/
   myopathy
Nausea/vomiting
Neuropathy
Oligospermia
Paresthesia
Psychosis
Rash

Seizures
Somnolence
Tremor
Urinary
   frequency

Interactions
None reported

Spectrum
Note: This drug is also effective against a variety of anaerobic bacterial species.

Trypanosoma cruzi

Trade Names
Bayer 2502
Lampit

Niridazole
Note: This drug has been largely replaced by newer agents.

Mechanism of Action
A nitrothiazole
Phosphorylase inhibition
Glycogen depletion

Typical Adult Dosage
25 mg/kg PO (max. 1.5g) daily × 10

Typical Pediatric Dosage
25 mg/kg PO daily × 10

Potential Side Effects

Abdominal pain
Allergy
Coagulopathy
Conduction
    disturbance
Confusion
Depression
Diarrhea
Dysgeusia

G6PD-related
    hemolysis
Headache
Insomnia
Nausea/vomiting
Pregnancy—
    contraindi-
    cated
Psychosis

Rash
Seizures
Urine
    discoloration
Vertigo or
    dizziness

Interactions
None reported

Spectrum
Note: This drug is also effective against a variety of anaerobic bacterial species.

Dracunculus medinensis
Entamoeba histolytica

Schistosoma haematobium
Schistosoma mansoni

Trade Name
Ambilhar

Nitazoxanide

Mechanism of Action
A nitrothiazole (structurally similar to aspirin)
Converted to active drug, tizoxanide, by esterases
Interferes with the pyruvate: ferredoxin oxidoreductase

Typical Adult Dosage
500 mg PO; could require repeat doses (t.i.d. or q.i.d.)

Typical Pediatric Dosage
Age 1–3y: 5 ml (100 mg) PO daily
Age 4–11y: 10 mg (200 mg) PO daily

Potential Side Effects
Abdominal pain
Headache
Pregnancy—contraindicated

Interactions
Aspirin sensitivity can be a contraindication to nitazoxanide.

Spectrum
Note: A variety of anaerobic bacterial species are also susceptible.

Ascaris lumbricoides	*Enterobius vermicularis*	*Hymenolepis nana*
Balantidium coli	*Fasciola hepatica*	*Isospora belli*
Blastocystis hominis	*Giardia intestinalis (lamblia)*	*Strongyloides*
Cryptosporidium*	Hookworm	*Taenia saginata*
Entamoeba histolytica		*Trichuris trichiura*

Trade Names
Alinia
Cryptaz

Daxon
Heliton

Nitrofurazone

Mechanism of Action
A nitrofuran derivative (mechanism unknown)

Typical Adult Dosage
0.5 g PO q.i.d. × 7d

Typical Pediatric Dosage
Not established

Potential Side Effects
Allergy
G6PD-related hemolysis
Neuropathy

Interactions
None reported

Spectrum
Trypanosoma brucei gambiense
Trypanosoma brucei rhodesiense

Trade Names

Colpacid	Furanvit	Nifucin
Furacin	Furasept	Nifurol
Furacine	Germex	Rafuzone

Ornidazole

Mechanism of Action
A 5-nitroimidazole derivative
Interferes with electron transport in metabolic pathways

Typical Adult Dosage
1.5 g PO daily for 3d

Typical Pediatric Dosage
25 to 40 mg/kg PO daily for 3d

Potential Side Effects

Abdominal pain	Nausea/vomiting	Pruritis
Diarrhea	Neuropathy	Somnolence
Headache	Neutropenia	Vertigo

Interactions

- Barbiturates interact with ornidazole (details not given).

- Cimetidine increases levels of ornidazole.

- Disulfiram exhibits enhanced CNS effects with ornidazole.

- Lithium can be more toxic when combined with ornidazole.

- Phenytoin levels are increased by ornidazole.

- Warfarin activity is increased by ornidazole.

Spectrum

Note: A variety of anaerobic bacteria are also susceptible to this drug.

Balantidium coli	*Entamoeba polecki*
Blastocystis hominis	*Giardia intestinalis*
Entamoeba histolytica	*Trichomonas*

Trade Names

Avrazor	Tiberal
Danubial	Tinerol
Oniz	

Oxamniquine

Mechanism of Action

A tetrahydroquinoline

Possibly anticholinergic
Displaces male from female adult worm
Interacts with parasite DNA

Typical Adult Dosage
15 mg/kg PO
30 mg/kg in Africa

Typical Pediatric Dosage
20 mg/kg PO > age 14y and below 30 kg
30 mg/kg in Africa

Potential Side Effects
Allergy
Diarrhea
Fever
Hallucinations
Headache
Hepatic
  dysfunction
Myalgia/
  myopathy
Nausea/
  vomiting
Psychosis
Rash
Seizures
Somnolence
Vertigo or
  dizziness

Interactions
None reported

Spectrum
Schistosoma mansoni

Trade Names
Mansil
Vansil

Pentamidine

Mechanism of Action
An aromatic diamidine derivative

Possibly interferes with polyamines and nucleic acid
metabolism

Typical Dosage
4 mg/kg i.v. daily × 14d

Potential Side Effects

Allergy	Hyperkalemia	Rhabdomyolysis
Anemia	Hypocalcemia	Rhinitis
Blepharitis	Hypogeusia	Stevens-Johnson
Cardiac toxicity	Hypoglycemia	syndrome
Coagulopathy	Hypomagne-	Thrombocy-
Conduction	semia	topenia
disturbance	Hyposmia	Torsade de
Confusion	Insomnia	points/
Conjunctivitis	Leukopenia/	Toxic
Diarrhea	neutropenia	epidermal
Dysgeusia	Metallic	necrolysis
Electrolyte	phantogeusia	Tremor
imbalance	Nausea/vomiting	Vasodilation
Esophagitis	Pancreatitis	
Hallucinations	Paresthesia	
Headache	Proteinuria	
Hepatic	Psychosis	
dysfunction/	Renal toxicity/	
hepatitis	dysfunction	

Interactions

- Aminoglycosides increase the risk for nephrotoxicity
  with pentamidine.

- Amphotericin B, capreomycin, cidofovir, cisplatin,
  methoxyflurane, polymyxins and vancomycin increase
  the risk for nephrotoxicity with pentamidine.

- Didanosine (DDI), zalcitabine (ddC) and zidovudine increase the risk for pancreatitis from pentamidine.

- Cimetidine interacts with pentamidine (details not given).

- Foscarnet could produce hypocalcemia with pentamidine.

The following drugs increase the risk for arrhythmias with pentamidine:

Acecainide	Droperidol	Probucol
Adenosine	Enflurane	Prochlorperazine
Ajmaline	Erythromycin	Protriptyline
Amisulpride	Fluoxetine	Sematilide
Amoxapine	Gatifloxacin	Sertindole
Aprindine	Grepafloxacin	Sotalol
Arsenic trioxide	Hydroquinidine	Sparfloxacin
Azimilide	Isoflurane	Sultopride
Bretylium	Lidoflazine	Tedisamil
Chloral hydrate	Mesoridazine	Thioridazine
Chlorpromazin	Moxifloxacin	Trifluoperazine
Colchicine	Octreotide	Vasopressin
Dibenzepin	Prajmaline	Zolmitriptan

Spectrum

Babesia (in combination)
Leishmaniasis—*cutaneous*
Leishmaniasis—*mucocutaneous*
Leishmaniasis—*visceral*
Trypanosoma brucei gambiense

Trade Names

Benambex	Lomidine	Pentacarinat
Fisoneb	Nebupent	Pentam 300

Pentamina   Penticarinat   Pneumopent

Pentavalent Antimonials

Mechanism of Action
Pentavalent antimonials
Stibogluconate and N-methylglucamine inhibit
   glycolysis (fructose-6-PO4 phosphorylation) and fatty
   acid oxidation

Typical Adult Dosage
20 mg/kg i.v. or i.m. daily × 14–28d

Typical Pediatric Dosage
As for adult
Or 542 mg Sb/sq m/d

Potential Side Effects
Abdominal pain	Hemolysis	Proteinuria
Arthralgia or arthritis	Hepatic dysfunction/ hepatitis	Pruritis
Cardiac toxicity/ conduction disturbance	Nausea/vomiting Pancreatitis	Rash Renal toxicity/ dysfunction

Interactions
Amphotericin B increases the risk for arrhythmias with
pentavalent antimonials.

Spectrum
Leishmaniasis (all forms)

Trade Names
Glucantim Glucaratime	Meglumine antimoniate	N-Methyl- glucamine

Pentostam   Stibogluconate   Tricostam
Protostib

Piperazine Citrate

Mechanism of Action
Muscular paralysis in parasite (GABA agonist at the extrasynaptic muscle receptor)

Typical Dosage
75 mg/kg (max 3.5g) PO daily $\times$ 2d

Potential Side Effects

Abdominal pain	Headache	Somnolence
Allergy	Nausea/vomiting	Tremor
Ataxia	Nystagmus	Vertigo or dizziness
Conduction disturbance	Pregnancy— contraindicated	Visual disturbance
Diarrhea		
G6PD-related hemolysis	Rash	
	Seizures	

Interactions

- Phenothiazines can cause seizures with piperazine citrate.

- Pyrantel activity is decreased by piperazine citrate.

Spectrum
Ascaris lumbricoides
Enterobius vermicularis

Trade Names

Adelmintex	Antcucs	Antepar
Aloxin	Antelmina	Anticucs

Ascalix
Ascarient
Ascarin
Carudol
Citrazine
Citropiperazina
Ectodyne
Entacyl
Epilix
Expellin
Girheulit H
Licor De Cacau
Lombrimade
Lumbriquil
Multifuge
Neox

Ortovermim
Oxiurazina
Pip-A-Ray
Piperazil
Pipertox
Pipervermin
Pipralen
Piprine
Pirvikain
  (pyrvinium)
Pripsen
Rotape
SB Tox
Solucamphre
Tasnon
Thioderazine B1

Trivermon
Ultraseptine
  Rogier
Uvilon
Vermex
Vermi
Vermichem
Vermidol
Vermifuge
Vermilen
Vermizine
Worm
Wormdix
Wormex

Praziquantel

Mechanism of Action
A pyrazinoisoquinoline derivative
Altered calcium flux through parasite tectum
Muscular paralysis and detachment of the worm

Typical Dosage
20 mg/kg PO b.i.d. to t.i.d. × 1d (use below age 4y not established)

Potential Side Effects

Abdominal pain
Allergy
Diarrhea
Headache

Hepatic
  dysfunction/
  hepatitis
Nausea/vomiting

Porphyria—
  exacerbation
Pruritis
Rash

Somnolence
Vertigo or
dizziness

Interactions

- Albendazole levels are increased by praziquantel.

- Carbamazapine and dexamethasone decrease levels of praziquantel.

- Chloroquine and cimetidine increase levels of praziquantel.

- Phenytoin levels are decreased by praziquantel.

Spectrum

*Clonorchis
  sinensis**
Cysticercosis**
*Diphyllobothrium
  latum**
*Dipylidium
  caninum**
*Fasciolopsis
  buski**
*Gastrodiscoides
  hominis*
*Heterophyes
  heterophyes**

*Hymenolepis
  diminuta**
*Hymenolepis
  nana**
*Metagonimus
  yokogawai**
*Metorchis
  conjunctus**
*Opisthorchis**
*Paragonimus**
*Schistosoma
  haematobium**

*Schistosoma
  japonicum**
*Schistosoma
  mansoni**
*Taenia saginata**
*Taenia solium**

Trade Names

Biltricide
Cesol
Cesticid

Cestox
Cisticid
Cysticide

Distocide
Ehliten
Kalcide

Opticide   Prazite   Teniken
Pontel

Primaquine
Note: This drug poses a major risk for severe hemolysis in G6PD-deficient individuals.

Mechanism of Action
An 8-aminoquinoline
Mimics ubiquinone (disrupts with mitochondria and golgi apparatus)
Stops pyrimidine synthesis

Typical Adult Dosage
Therapy: 15 mg (base) PO daily × 14d
Prophylaxis: 30 mg daily, continue for 1w after exposure ends

Typical Pediatric Dosage
Prophylaxis: 0.3 mg/kg (base) daily × 14d

Potential Side Effects

Abdominal pain
Anemia
Cardiac toxicity/ conduction disturbance
G6PD-related hemolysis
Headache
Leukocytosis
Leukopenia/ neutropenia
Methemo- globinemia
Nausea/ vomiting
Pregnancy— contraindi- cated
Pruritis
Visual disturbance

Interactions

- Antacids reduce absorption of primaquine.

- Aurothioglucose increases the risk for hematotoxicity from primaquine.

- Cimetidine increases levels of primaquine.

- Digoxin increases the risk for arrhythmias with primaquine.

- Quinacrine enhances the toxicity of primaquine.

Spectrum
Plasmodium (all species—hepatic phase)

Trade Names
Palum	Primachin
PMQ-INGA	Primacin

Proguanil

Mechanism of Action
A biguanide
Metabolized in-vivo to active agent, cycloguanil
Inhibition of dihydrofolate reductase

Typical Adult Dosage
Prophylaxis: 200 mg PO daily

Typical Pediatric Dosage
Prophylaxis:
Age < 1 year: 25 mg/d PO
Age 1–5 years: 50 mg/d PO
Age 6–10 years: 100 mg/d PO

Potential Side Effects
Abdominal pain	Anemia—	Diarrhea
Alopecia	aplastic	

Hepatic dysfunction	Renal toxicity/ dysfunction	Stomatitis
Nausea/vomiting		

Interactions

- Aurothioglucose increases the risk for hematotoxicity from proguanil.

- Warfarin activity is increased by proguanil.

Spectrum
Plasmodium (all species)

Trade Names
Lapdap (combined with dapsone)
Paludrine

Pyrantel Pamoate

Mechanism of Action
A depolarizing neuromuscular blocking agent
Nicotinic activation results in spastic paralysis of the target worm

Typical Adult Dosage
10 mg/kg (max 1 g) PO × 1

Typical Pediatric Dosage
Age ≥ 2 years: 11 mg/kg PO once (maximum 1g)

Potential Side Effects

Abdominal pain	Hepatic dysfunction/ hepatitis	Insomnia
Diarrhea		Nausea/ vomiting
Headache		

Rash
Vertigo or
dizziness

Interactions

- Piperazine activity is decreased by pyrantel pamoate.

- Theophylline levels are increased by pyrantel pamoate.

Spectrum

Ascaris lumbricoides   Hookworm
Enterobius vermicularis   *Trichostrongylus*

Trade Names

Anthel	Helmintox	Pinworm
Antiminth	Lombriareu	Medicine
Ascarical	Nemocid	Pin-X
Cobantril	One Step	Reese's Pinworm
Combantrin	Pin-Rid	Trilombrin
Early Bird	Pinworm	Vertel
Helmex		

Pyrimethamine

Mechanism of Action
A diaminopyrimidine
Interferes with dihydrofolate reductase

Typical Adult Dosage
25 mg PO daily (with sulfonamide for toxoplasmosis) × 21d

Typical Pediatric Dosage
2 mg/kg/d PO × 2, then 1 mg/kg/d × 21d (with sulfonamide for toxoplasmosis)

Potential Side Effects

Allergy	Insomnia	Seizures
Cardiac arrhythmia	Leukopenia/ neutropenia	Stevens-Johnson syndrome
Carnitine deficiency	Nausea/vomiting	Thrombocyto- penia
Erythema multiforme	Porphyria— exacerbation	Toxic epidermal necrolysis
Hematuria	Pregnancy— contraindi- cated	
Hyperpigmen- tation	Rash	

Interactions

- Artemisinin increases levels of pyrimethamine.

- Aurothioglucose, dapsone, methotrexate, sulfa-trimethoprim, and sulfomamides increase the risk for hematotoxicity from pyrimethamine.

- Benzodiazepines increase the risk for hepatotoxicity from pyrimethamine.

- Zidovudine reduces the activity of pyrimethamine.

- Zinc salts reduce the absorption of pyrimethamine.

Spectrum

Giardia intestinalis (lamblia)	*Plasmodium falciparum,* chloroquine sensitive	*Plasmodium vivax*
Isospora belli		*Toxoplasma*
Plasmodium falciparum, chloroquine resistant	*Plasmodium malariae*	
	Plasmodium ovale	

Trade Names

Daraprim

Erbaprelina

Malocide

Pirimecidan

Pyrimethamine/Sulfadoxine

Mechanism of Action

Diaminopyrimidine/para-aminobenzoate analog

Interferes with dihydrofolate reductase

Typical Adult Dosage

Therapy: 3 tablets PO as single dose

Prophylaxis: 1 tablet weekly

Typical Pediatric Dosage

Dosage for single dose stand by therapy:

Age < 1 year: 1/4 tablet

Age 1–3 years: 1/2 tablet

Age 4–8 years: 1 tablet

Age 9–14 years: 2 tablets

Potential Side Effects

Allergy

Amblyopia

Breast-feeding—
   contraindi-
   cation

Cardiac
   arrhythmia

Carnitine
   deficiency

Erythema
   multiforme

G6PD-related
   hemolysis

Glossitis

Hematuria

Hepatic
   dysfunction/
   hepatitis

Iritis

Kernicterus

Leukopenia/
   neutropenia

Nausea/vomiting

Photosensitivity

Porphyria—
   exacerbation

Pregnancy—
   contraindi-
   cated

Pulmonary
   infiltrate

Rash

Seizures

| Stevens-Johnson syndrome | Toxic epidermal necrolysis | Visual disturbance |
| Thrombocyto-penia | | |

Interactions

- Aurothioglucose, dapsone, methotrexate, sulfa-trimethoprim, and sulfonamides increase the risk for hematotoxicity from pyrimethamine/sulfadoxine.

- Benzodiazepines increase the risk for hepatotoxicity from pyrimethamine/sulfadoxine.

- Chloroquine and hydroxychloroquine can be more toxic when combined with pyrimethamine/sulfadoxine.

- Cyclosporine levels are decreased by pyrimethamine/sulfadoxine.

- Theophylline levels are increased by pyrimethamine/sulfadoxine.

- Zidovudine reduces the activity of pyrimethamine/sulfadoxine.

- Zinc salts reduce the absorption of pyrimethamine/sulfadoxine.

Spectrum

Isospora belli
Plasmodium falciparum, chloroquine-resistant
Plasmodium falciparum, chloroquine-sensitive
Plasmodium malariae
Plasmodium ovale
Plasmodium vivax

Trade Names

Cryodoxin
Falcidin
Fansidar
Gvdoxin

Laridox
Malostat
Maxoline
Metakelfin

Methipox
Orodar
Periodine
Anti-Malarico

Pyrvinium
Note: Pyrvinium has been largely replaced by newer drugs.

Mechanism of Action
A cyanine dye
Inhibits carbohydrate metabolism

Typical Dosage
5 mg/kg PO as single dose—maximum 350 mg

Potential Side Effects

Abdominal pain
Allergy
Diarrhea
Discoloration of
  stools

Erythema
  multiforme
Nausea/vomiting
Photosensitivity
Rash

Stevens-Johnson
  syndrome

Interactions
None reported

Spectrum
Enterobius vermicularis

Trade Names

Antioxiur
Molevac
Pamoxan
Polyquil

Povan
Povanyl
Pyrcon
Pyr-Pam

Pyrvin
Vanquin

Quinacrine

Note: Quinacrine has been largely replaced by chloroquine and other antimalarials.

Mechanism of Action
4-aminoacridine
Possibly intercalates onto parasite DNA

Typical Adult Dosage
100 mg PO t.i.d. × 7d

Typical Pediatric Dosage
2 mg/kg PO t.i.d. × 7d

Potential Side Effects

Alopecia
Altered skin or
    nail color
Anemia
Anemia—
    aplastic
G6PD-related
    hemolysis
Headache
Hepatic
    dysfunction
Nausea/
    vomiting
Psoriasis—
    exacerbation
Psychosis
Pulmonary
    infiltrate
Rash
Seizures
Skin
    discoloration
Urine
    discoloration
Vertigo or
    dizziness
Visual
    disturbance

Interactions

- Alcohol can produce a disulfiram reaction with quinacrine.

- Aurothioglucose increases the risk for hematotoxicity from quinacrine.

- Mefloquine and primaquine enhance the toxicity of quinacrine.

- Rifampin interacts with quinacrine (details not given).

Spectrum

Blastocystis hominis
Diphyllobothrium latum
Giardia intestinalis (lamblia)
Hymenolepis nana
Plasmodium falciparum
    (chloroquine sensitive)

Plasmodium malariae
Plasmodium ovale
Plasmodium vivax
Taenia saginata
Taenia solium

Trade Names

Atabil
Atabrine
Mepacrine

Quinine

Mechanism of Action

4-methanoquinoline
A cinchona alkaloid
Possibly, formation of toxic complex with
    ferriprotoporphyrin IX

Typical Adult Dosage

650 mg PO t.i.d. × 3–7d (in combination with tetracycline, sulfone, etc. for therapy)

Typical Pediatric Dosage

8 mg/kg PO t.i.d. × 3–7d (in combination with sulfone, tetracycline, etc. for therapy)

Potential Side Effects

Abdominal pain   Allergy   Alopecia

Altered skin or nail color
Amblyopia
Ataxia
Cardiac toxicity/conduction disturbance
Coagulopathy
Diarrhea
Diplopia
Erythema multiforme
Fever
G6PD-related hemolysis
Headache
Hearing loss
Hemolysis
Hepatic dysfunction/hepatitis
Hypoglycemia
Interstitial nephritis
Leukopenia/neutropenia
Myasthenia gravis—exacerbation
Nausea/vomiting
Nystagmus
Photophobia
Photosensitivity
Pregnancy—contraindicated
Pruritis
Psychosis
Rash
Retinopathy
Scotomata
Seizures
Stevens-Johnson syndrome
Thrombocytopenia
Tinnitus
Torsade de points/prolonged QT interval
Toxic epidermal necrolysis
Vertigo or dizziness
Visual disturbance

Interactions

- Acetazolamide, cimetidine, and rifampin increase metabolism/clearance of quinine.

- Aminoglycosides can be more toxic when combined with quinine.

- Anisindione increases the risk for bleeding with quinine.

- Antacids reduce absorption of quinine.

- Aurothioglucose increases the risk for hematotoxicity from quinine.

- Cyclosporine and heparin activity are decreased by quinine.

- Diltiazem interacts with quinine (details not given).

- Encainide, flecainide, lorcainide, and metformin levels are increased by quinine.

- Famotidine and roxatidine reduce the absorption of quinine.

- Neuromuscular blockers increase the risk for apnea with quinine.

- Ritonavir increases levels of quinine.

- Warfarin activity is increased by quinine.

The following drugs increase the risk for cardiac arrhythmias with quinine:

Acecainide	Digoxin	Probucol
Adenosine	Droperidol	Prochlor-
Ajmaline	Enflurane	perazine
Amisulpride	Gatifloxacin	Protriptyline
Amoxapine	Hydroquinidine	Sematilide
Aprindine	Isoflurane	Sertindole
Arsenic trioxide	Lidoflazine	Sotalol
Astemizole	Lumefantrine/	Sultopride
Azimilide	artemether	Tedisamil
Bretylium	Mefloquine	Trifluoperazine
Chloral hydrate	Mesoridazine	Vasopressin
Chlorpromazine	Moxifloxacin	Zolmitriptan
Colchicine	Octreotide	
Dibenzepin	Prajmaline	

Trade Names

Adaquin	Aflukin	BiChinine

Biquin

Biquinate

Bisulquin

Chinine

Circonyl N

Coco-Quinine

Genin

Impalud

Kinin

Kininh

Legatrin

Myoquin

Novo-Quinine

Paluquina

Q200

Q300

Qm-260

Quin-Amino

Quinaminoph

Quinamm

Quinasul

Quinate

Quinbisu

Quinbisul

Quindan

Quine

Quinidan

Quinimax

Quinite

Quinoctal

Quinsan

Quinsul

Quiphile

Salquin

Spectrum
Babesia (in combination)*
Plasmodium (all species)

Secnidazole

Mechanism of Action
A 5-nitroimidazole derivative
Activated in-vivo by cellular pyruvate: ferredoxin
    oxidoreductase.
Interferes with electron transport in metabolic pathways

Typical Adult Dosage
2 g PO as single dose; 1.5 g daily for 5d in hepatic amebiasis

Typical Pediatric Dosage
30 mg/kg PO as single dose. Repeat for 5 days for amebiasis.

Potential Side Effects

| Allergy | Anemia | Ataxia |

Depression
Diarrhea
Dysgeusia
Gynecomastia
Hallucinations
Headache
Hepatic
  dysfunction
Hyperpigmen-
  tation
Leukocytosis
Leukopenia/
  neutropenia
Nausea/vomiting
Neuropathy
Pancreatitis
Paresthesia
Porphyria—
  exacerbation
Pregnancy—
  contraindi-
  cated
Pruritis
Pulmonary
  infiltrate
Rash
Renal toxicity/
  dysfunction
Seizures
Skin
  discoloration
Somnolence
Stomatitis
Thrombocyto-
  penia
Urine
  discoloration
Vertigo or
  dizziness

Interactions

- Alcohol and sulfa-trimethoprim can produce a disulfiram reaction with secnidazole.

- Astemizole and terfenadine increase the risk for arrhythmias with secnidazole.

- Azathioprine increases the risk for hematotoxicity from secnidazole.

- Barbiturates and phenytoin increase metabolism/clearance of secnidazole.

- Carbamazapine levels are increased by secnidazole.

- Cimetidine increases levels of secnidazole.

- Cyclosporine, lithium, and tacrolimus can be more toxic when combined with secnidazole.

- Disulfiram exhibits enhanced CNS effects with secnidazole.

- Fluorouracil enhances the toxicity of secnidazole.

- Oral contraceptive activity is decreased by secnidazole.

- Warfarin activity is increased by secnidazole.

- Zalcitabine (ddC) increases the risk for neurotoxicity from secnidazole.

Trade Name
Flagentyl

Spectrum
Note: This drug is also active against a variety of bacterial species.

Dientamoeba fragilis	*Trichomonas*
Entamoeba histolytica	
Giardia intestinalis (lamblia)	

Suramin
Note: Severe reactions at initiation of therapy have been reported—a small test dose recommended.

Mechanism of Action
Inhibits glycerol phosphate oxidase and digestive and membrane functions in the parasite

Typical Adult Dosage
1 g i.v. days 1, 3, 7, 14, and 21 (after test dose 100 mg)

Typical Pediatric Dosage
20 mg/kg i.v. days 1, 3, 7, 14, and 21 (after test dose 100 mg)

Potential Side Effects
Abdominal pain	Allergy	Blepharitis

Conjunctivitis
Fever
Hemolysis
Hepatic
    dysfunction/
    hepatitis
Keratopathy
Leukopenia/
    neutropenia
Myalgia or
    myopathy

Nausea/vomiting
Neuropathy
Optic neuritis or
    atrophy
Paresthesia
Photophobia
Pregnancy—
    contraindi-
    cated
Proteinuria
Pruritis

Rash
Renal toxicity/
    dysfunction
Thrombocyto-
    penia
Visual
    disturbance

Interactions
Foscarnet increases the risk for nephrotoxicity with suramin.

Spectrum
Onchocerca volvulus
Trypanosoma brucei gambiense
Trypanosoma brucei rhodesiense

Trade Names
Antrypol
Bayer 205
Germanin
Moranyl Fourneau 309
Naphuride

Tetrachloroethylene
Note: This drug has been largely replaced by several newer drugs.

Mechanism of Action
A chlorinated hydrocarbon (mechanism unknown)

Typical Dosage
0.1 ml/kg (max 5.0 ml) PO × 1

Potential Side Effects

Abdominal pain	Nausea/	Rash
Headache	vomiting	Somnolence

Interactions

- Alcohol enhances the toxicity of tetrachloroethylene.
- Laxatives enhance the toxicity of tetrachloroethylene.

Trade Name
NEMA

Spectrum

Fasciolopsis buski	*Heterophyes*	*Metagonimus*
Gastrodiscoides	*heterophyes*	*yokogawai*
hominis	Hookworm	

Thiabendazole

Mechanism of Action
A benzimidazole
Binds to free beta tubulin and inhibits tubulin
   polymerization
Resultant inhibition of glucose uptake

Typical Dosage
25 mg/kg PO b.i.d. × 2

Potential Side Effects

Headache	Leukopenia/	Nausea/vomiting
Hepatic	neutropenia	Photosensitivity
dysfunction/	Myalgia or	
hepatitis	myopathy	

Pregnancy—
    contraindi-
    cated
Pruritis
Psychosis
Rash

Seizures
Somnolence
Tinnitus
Toxic epidermal
    necrolysis

Vertigo or
    dizziness
Visual
    disturbance

Interactions
Theophylline levels are increased by thiabendazole.

Spectrum
*Angiostrongylus
    cantonensis*
*Angiostrongylus
    costaricensis**
Anisakis
*Ascaris
    lumbricoides*
*Capillaria
    philippinensis*

Cutaneous larva
    migrans
*Dracunculus
    medinensis*
*Enterobius
    vermicularis*
Hookworm
Strongyloides

*Syngamus
    laryngeus*
Toxocara
*Trichinella
    spiralis*
Trichostrongylus

Trade Names
Foldan
Folderm
Micoplex
Mintezol
Thiaben

Thiabena
Tiabiose
Triasox
Tutiverm

Tinidazole

Mechanism of Action
A 5-nitroimidazole derivative
Activated in vivo by cellular pyruvate: ferredoxin
    oxidoreductase
Interferes with electron transport in metabolic path-
    ways

Typical Adult Dosage
2 g PO as single dose

Typical Pediatric Dosage
50 mg/kg PO as single dose

Potential Side Effects

Allergy	Leukopenia/	Stomatitis
Anemia	neutropenia	Urine
Breast-feeding—	Nausea/vomiting	discoloration
contraindi-	Neuropathy	Vertigo or
cation	Pancreatitis	dizziness
Candidiasis	Pregnancy—	
Constipation	contraindi-	
Diarrhea	cated	
Gynecomastia	Pruritis	
Headache	Rash	
Hepatic	Seizures	
dysfunction/	Serum sickness	
hepatitis	Somnolence	

Interactions

- Alcohol can produce a disulfiram reaction with tinidazole.

- Barbiturates reduce the activity of tinidazole.

- Cimetidine reduces absorption of tinidazole.

- Disulfiram exhibits enhanced CNS effects with tinidazole.

- Phenytoin levels are decreased by tinidazole.

- Warfarin activity is increased by tinidazole.

Trade Names

Abdogyl	Fasigyne	Tiniba
Amplium	Pletil	Tricolam
Dyzol	Protocide	Tricolane
Fa-Cyl	Simplotan	Trimonase
Fasigin	Sorquetan	Trinizol
Fasigyn	Timidex	

Spectrum

Note: This drug is also effective against *Clostridium difficile* and *Helicobacter pylori*.

Blastocystis hominis
Entamoeba histolytica
Giardia intestinalis

Triclabendazole

Mechanism of Action

A benzimidazole.
Mechanism can be related to microtubule formation and protein synthesis.

Typical Dosage

Fascioliasis: 10 mg/kg PO as single postprandial dose
Paragonimiasis: give second dose after 12 hours

Potential Side Effects

Abdominal pain
Headache
Vertigo or dizziness

Interactions

None reported

Spectrum
Fasciola hepatica*
Paragonimus

Trade Name
Fasinex

Parasite Name Index